Clinical Imaging Applications in Obstetrics and Gynecology

Clinical Imaging Applications in Obstetrics and Gynecology

Editors

Florian Recker
Brigitte Strizek
Ulrich Gembruch

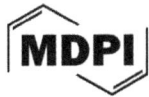

Basel • Beijing • Wuhan • Barcelona • Belgrade • Novi Sad • Cluj • Manchester

Editors

Florian Recker
University Hospital Bonn
Bonn
Germany

Brigitte Strizek
University Hospital Bonn
Bonn
Germany

Ulrich Gembruch
University Hospital Bonn
Bonn
Germany

Editorial Office
MDPI
St. Alban-Anlage 66
4052 Basel, Switzerland

This is a reprint of articles from the Special Issue published online in the open access journal *Journal of Clinical Medicine* (ISSN 2077-0383) (available at: https://www.mdpi.com/journal/jcm/special_issues/Imaging_Obstetrics_Gynecology).

For citation purposes, cite each article independently as indicated on the article page online and as indicated below:

Lastname, A.A.; Lastname, B.B. Article Title. *Journal Name* **Year**, *Volume Number*, Page Range.

ISBN 978-3-7258-0517-4 (Hbk)
ISBN 978-3-7258-0518-1 (PDF)
doi.org/10.3390/books978-3-7258-0518-1

© 2024 by the authors. Articles in this book are Open Access and distributed under the Creative Commons Attribution (CC BY) license. The book as a whole is distributed by MDPI under the terms and conditions of the Creative Commons Attribution-NonCommercial-NoDerivs (CC BY-NC-ND) license.

Contents

About the Editors .... **vii**

Florian Recker, Ulrich Gembruch and Brigitte Strizek
Clinical Ultrasound Applications in Obstetrics and Gynecology in the Year 2024
Reprinted from: *J. Clin. Med.* **2024**, *13*, 1244, doi:10.3390/jcm13051244 .... **1**

**Hector Borboa-Olivares, Johnatan Torres-Torres, Arturo Flores-Pliego,
Aurora Espejel-Nuñez, Ignacio Camacho-Arroyo, Mario Guzman-Huerta, et al.**
AI-Enhanced Analysis Reveals Impact of Maternal Diabetes on Subcutaneous Fat Mass in Fetuses without Growth Alterations
Reprinted from: *J. Clin. Med.* **2023**, *12*, 6485, doi:10.3390/jcm12206485 .... **7**

**Anne Dathan-Stumpf, Massimiliano Lia, Christof Meigen, Karoline Bornmann,
Mireille Martin, Manuela Aßmann, et al.**
Novel Three-Dimensional Body Scan Anthropometry versus MR-Pelvimetry for Vaginal Breech Delivery Assessment
Reprinted from: *J. Clin. Med.* **2023**, *12*, 6181, doi:10.3390/jcm12196181 .... **20**

**Adeline Walter, Elina Calite, Annegret Geipel, Brigitte Strizek, Florian Recker,
Ulrike Herberg, et al.**
Spectrum and Outcome of Prenatally Diagnosed Fetal Primary Cardiomyopathies—A Twenty-Year Overview
Reprinted from: *J. Clin. Med.* **2023**, *12*, 4366, doi:10.3390/jcm12134366 .... **33**

**Constanza A. Pontones, Adriana Titzmann, Hanna Huebner, Nina Danzberger,
Matthias Ruebner, Lothar Häberle, et al.**
Feasibility and Acceptance of Self-Guided Mobile Ultrasound among Pregnant Women in Routine Prenatal Care
Reprinted from: *J. Clin. Med.* **2023**, *12*, 4224, doi:10.3390/jcm12134224 .... **45**

**Luigi Manzo, Giuliana Orlandi, Olimpia Gabrielli, Paolo Toscano, Enrica Di Lella,
Antonia Lettieri, et al.**
Fetal Cerebellar Area: Ultrasound Reference Ranges at 13–39 Weeks of Gestation
Reprinted from: *J. Clin. Med.* **2023**, *12*, 4080, doi:10.3390/jcm12124080 .... **59**

**Alina-Madalina Luca, Raluca Haba, Luiza-Maria Cobzeanu, Dragos Nemescu,
Anamaria Harabor, Raluca Mogos, et al.**
Predicting Preterm Birth with Strain Ratio Analysis of the Internal Cervical Os: A Prospective Study
Reprinted from: *J. Clin. Med.* **2023**, *12*, 3885, doi:10.3390/jcm12123885 .... **70**

**Ana L. Moreno-Espinosa, Ameth Hawkins-Villarreal, David Coronado-Gutierrez,
Xavier P. Burgos-Artizzu, Raigam J. Martínez-Portilla, Tatiana Peña-Ramirez, et al.**
Prediction of Neonatal Respiratory Morbidity Assessed by Quantitative Ultrasound Lung Texture Analysis in Twin Pregnancies
Reprinted from: *J. Clin. Med.* **2022**, *11*, 4895, doi:10.3390/jcm11164895 .... **85**

**Elena Jost, Philipp Kosian, Jorge Jimenez Cruz, Shadi Albarqouni,
Ulrich Gembruch, Brigitte Strizek and Florian Recker**
Evolving the Era of 5D Ultrasound? A Systematic Literature Review on the Applications for Artificial Intelligence Ultrasound Imaging in Obstetrics and Gynecology
Reprinted from: *J. Clin. Med.* **2023**, *12*, 6833, doi:10.3390/jcm12216833 .... **96**

Dieter M. Matlac, Tolga Tonguc, Nikola Mutschler, Florian Recker, Olga Ramig, Holger M. Strunk, et al.
Study Protocol of a Prospective, Monocentric, Single-Arm Study Investigating the Safety and Efficacy of Local Ablation of Symptomatic Uterine Fibroids with US-Guided High-Intensity Focused Ultrasound (HIFU)
Reprinted from: *J. Clin. Med.* 2023, 12, 5926, doi:10.3390/jcm12185926 127

Ruben Plöger, Mateja Condic, Damian J. Ralser, Hannah M. Plöger, Eva K. Egger, Lucia A. Otten and Alexander Mustea
Intraoperative Utilization of Indocyanine Green (ICG) Dye for the Assessment of Ovarian Perfusion—Case Report and Review of the Literature
Reprinted from: *J. Clin. Med.* 2023, 12, 5923, doi:10.3390/jcm12185923 136

Giuliana Orlandi, Paolo Toscano, Olimpia Gabrielli, Enrica Di Lella, Antonia Lettieri, Luigi Manzo, et al.
Prenatal Diagnosis of an Intrathoracic Left Kidney Associated with Congenital Diaphragmatic Hernia: Case Report and Systematic Review
Reprinted from: *J. Clin. Med.* 2023, 12, 3608, doi:10.3390/jcm12113608 145

Moira Barbieri, Giulia Zamagni, Ilaria Fantasia, Lorenzo Monasta, Leila Lo Bello, Mariachiara Quadrifoglio, et al.
Umbilical Vein Blood Flow in Uncomplicated Pregnancies: Systematic Review of Available Reference Charts and Comparison with a New Cohort
Reprinted from: *J. Clin. Med.* 2023, 12, 3132, doi:10.3390/jcm12093132 157

Elisa Pappalardo, Ferdinando Antonio Gulino, Carla Ettore, Francesco Cannone and Giuseppe Ettore
Body Stalk Anomaly Complicated by Ectopia Cordis: First-Trimester Diagnosis of Two Cases Using 2- and 3-Dimensional Sonography
Reprinted from: *J. Clin. Med.* 2023, 12, 1896, doi:10.3390/jcm12051896 173

About the Editors

Florian Recker

Florian Recker is an associate professor for Obstetrics and Gynecology and the Head of the Centre for Medical Education in Obstetrics and the Centre for Ultrasound Research and Innovations in Obstetrical Science (CURIOS) in the Department of Obstetrics and Prenatal Medicine of the University Hospital Bonn, Germany. His research focuses in particular on new and innovative technologies and concepts in ultrasound education and training as well as the latest technologies, such as artificial intelligence and 3D printing technology. A particular focus of his is on the application of point-of-care ultrasound and its multidisciplinary areas of application in training.

Brigitte Strizek

Brigitte Strizek, a distinguished professor in the field of Obstetrics and Prenatal Medicine, is currently the Head of the Department of Obstetrics and Prenatal Medicine at the University Hospital of Bonn. Her academic and research pursuits are deeply rooted in prenatal medicine, with a particular emphasis on advancing prenatal ultrasound diagnostics and fetal therapies. Her expertise and insights have not only been disseminated through numerous scholarly articles but also encapsulated in several co-authored books that focus on prenatal and obstetrical ultrasound and fetal interventions.

Ulrich Gembruch

Ulrich Gembruch is a professor emeritus of Obstetrics and Gynecology and was the Director of the Department of Obstetrics and Prenatal Medicine at the University Hospital of Bonn from 2002 to 2022. U. Gembruch has been, throughout his career, an outstanding researcher and teacher and has made substantial contributions to the medical literature in areas of prenatal diagnosis of congenital heart defects, rare congenital malformation syndromes, multiple gestation, first trimester diagnosis of fetal anomalies, diagnosis and monitoring of fetal growth restriction, and fetal therapy. He is the editor of several textbooks on obstetrics and prenatal medicine, including, together with Simcha Yagel and Norman Silverman, the textbook Fetal cardiology, now in its 3rd edition.

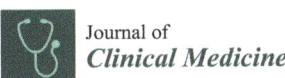

Editorial

Clinical Ultrasound Applications in Obstetrics and Gynecology in the Year 2024

Florian Recker *, Ulrich Gembruch and Brigitte Strizek

Department of Obstetrics and Prenatal Medicine, University Hospital Bonn, Venusberg Campus 1, 53127 Bonn, Germany; ulrich.gembruch@ukbonn.de (U.G.); brigitte.strizek@ukbonn.de (B.S.)
* Correspondence: florian.recker@ukbonn.de

Citation: Recker, F.; Gembruch, U.; Strizek, B. Clinical Ultrasound Applications in Obstetrics and Gynecology in the Year 2024. *J. Clin. Med.* **2024**, *13*, 1244. https://doi.org/10.3390/jcm13051244

Received: 1 February 2024
Revised: 16 February 2024
Accepted: 20 February 2024
Published: 22 February 2024

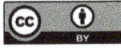

Copyright: © 2024 by the authors. Licensee MDPI, Basel, Switzerland. This article is an open access article distributed under the terms and conditions of the Creative Commons Attribution (CC BY) license (https:// creativecommons.org/licenses/by/ 4.0/).

Ultrasound imaging stands as a fundamental technology in the realms of obstetrics and gynecology, utilizing high-frequency sound waves to create detailed images of the internal structures of the body [1]. This non-invasive, safe, and cost-effective imaging modality has revolutionized the fields of prenatal and gynecological care [2]. Its ability to provide real-time visualization has transformed diagnostic processes, allowing for immediate assessment and monitoring. The evolution of ultrasound technology, particularly with the advent of Doppler, three-dimensional (3D), and four-dimensional (4D) imaging, has expanded its scope of applications, thereby enhancing both diagnostic accuracy and the quality of patient care [3].

Ultrasound imaging operates on the principle of echolocation. High-frequency sound waves, when transmitted into the body by a transducer, are reflected back by internal tissues and organs. These reflected sound waves, or echoes, are then captured by the transducer and translated into visual images by a computer. The varying densities and compositions of bodily tissues result in different echo patterns, enabling the visualization of structures within the body, such as organs, blood vessels, and, in the case of obstetrics, the developing fetus [4].

In obstetrics, ultrasound is a vital tool throughout all stages of pregnancy. During the first trimester, it is indispensable for confirming intrauterine pregnancy, assessing the viability of the fetus, estimating gestational age, and performing nuchal translucency screening to evaluate the risk of chromosomal abnormalities such as Down syndrome. The second trimester brings the critical anatomy scan, where a detailed examination of the fetal anatomy is conducted to identify any structural anomalies. This scan also assesses the placental location and the volume of amniotic fluid, both of which are crucial for fetal well-being [5].

The third trimester focuses on fetal growth and well-being. Ultrasound during this phase is used to monitor the growth of the fetus, particularly in pregnancies deemed high-risk, such as those with gestational diabetes or hypertension. A biophysical profile, combining ultrasound imaging with fetal heart rate monitoring, is often performed to assess the health of the fetus.

Doppler ultrasound, a specialized form, is employed to evaluate the blood flow in fetal and placental vessels. This is particularly important in cases where there is a concern for conditions such as fetal growth restriction or placental insufficiency.

The introduction of 3D and 4D ultrasound technologies has further revolutionized obstetric imaging. These advanced forms of ultrasound provide detailed, three-dimensional images of the fetus, offering an unprecedented view of fetal anatomy that aids in the diagnosis of certain abnormalities. Additionally, 4D ultrasound, which shows real-time fetal movements, has added a new dimension to prenatal care, enhancing the bonding experience for expectant parents and providing a unique opportunity for early interaction with the fetus [6].

In the field of gynecology, ultrasound serves as a key diagnostic tool for a variety of conditions. It is routinely used to evaluate the uterus, ovaries, and fallopian tubes, helping in the diagnosis and management of conditions such as uterine fibroids, ovarian cysts, and endometriosis. Ultrasound is pivotal in fertility assessments, where it aids in monitoring follicular development and guiding procedures like egg retrieval in assisted reproductive technologies.

This modality is also fundamental in the evaluation of pelvic pain, a common symptom in gynecological practice. It helps in the diagnosis of conditions such as ectopic pregnancy, pelvic inflammatory disease, and ovarian torsion. In the realm of gynecologic oncology, ultrasound serves as an initial assessment tool for cancers of the reproductive organs, although its findings are often supplemented with more comprehensive imaging techniques for accurate staging and management.

While ultrasound is a versatile and invaluable tool in obstetrics and gynecology, it is not without its limitations. The quality and accuracy of ultrasound imaging can be affected by factors such as operator skill, patient body habitus, and the presence of intervening structures like gas or bone. The technology also has limitations in terms of deep tissue penetration and may not always provide comprehensive information on certain pathologies, necessitating the use of complementary imaging modalities for a thorough evaluation [7].

The future of ultrasound imaging in obstetrics and gynecology is marked by continuous innovation and advancement. Emerging technologies and techniques, such as elastography and the integration of artificial intelligence (AI) for enhanced image analysis, are expected to overcome some of the current limitations and expand the capabilities of ultrasound imaging [8]. These advancements promise to further refine diagnostic accuracy and improve patient outcomes in these vital fields of medicine.

In gynecology, adnexal masses are frequently cited as a primary reason for undergoing ultrasonography (US) in the field of gynecology, primarily driven by the critical need for the early detection of ovarian cancer. Distinguishing between benign and malignant tumors is not only crucial for accurate diagnosis but also significantly impacts the direction of subsequent diagnostic procedures and therapeutic planning. In clinical practice, the examination of adnexal masses typically involves transvaginal US, which combines grayscale 2D images with color Doppler imaging to evaluate vascularization. However, the accurate identification and classification of adnexal masses presents substantial challenges, even for seasoned examiners. In response to these challenges, the International Ovarian Tumor Analysis (IOTA) group has devised US-based guidelines to aid in the classification of adnexal tumors.

In recent years, the field has seen a notable shift towards the automated analysis of US images of adnexal masses. This approach has been recognized for its potential to support diagnostic decision making by assisting both inexperienced and experienced examiners. From the 11 studies examined, research conducted between 2009 and 2023 highlighted the initial use of AI in sonographic assessment by the research group led by Amor et al., employing pattern recognition analysis for classifying adnexal masses within a new reporting system [9]. The majority of these studies analyzed 2D images, with a subset also incorporating color Doppler imaging to enhance diagnostic accuracy.

A significant focus of current research is the automated differentiation between benign and malignant tumors, with six studies dedicated to this endeavor. The application of AI in this context aims to improve diagnostic accuracy, reduce examination times, and facilitate early detection, which is particularly crucial in managing breast cancer. Breast US has been emphasized for its advantages, especially in women with dense breast tissue and in underserved areas, where it serves as a critical diagnostic and screening tool.

Despite the promising results, including AI's ability to outperform average trained radiologists in some instances, challenges remain. These include the limitations imposed by small sample sizes for algorithm training, data homogeneity, absence of external validation, and the necessity for algorithms to consider clinical contexts. Moreover, studies have indicated potential issues with AI interpretation, such as the misinterpretation of metastases or secondary ovarian cancer due to their rare representation in datasets and differences in clinical presentation.

Beyond adnexal masses, AI's role in evaluating the endometrium, pelvic floor, and other gynecological conditions like endometriosis, premature ovarian failure, uterine fibroids, follicle tracking, and ectopic pregnancies has been explored. Each area presents unique challenges but also demonstrates the potential for AI to enhance diagnostic accuracy, efficiency, and patient care. For instance, the application of AI in assessing endometrial thickness and texture, and in the management of pelvic floor dysfunction, shows promise in improving patient outcomes through more precise and quicker diagnostics.

Ultrasound imaging remains an indispensable tool in the field of obstetrics and gynecology, continually evolving to offer safe, cost-effective, and detailed visualization of the female reproductive system and developing fetus. Its extensive applications, ranging from routine prenatal screenings to complex gynecological evaluations, underscore its integral role in enhancing patient care and clinical outcomes [10]. As technology advances, ultrasound imaging is poised to overcome current challenges and further extend its capabilities, solidifying its position as a cornerstone in the realm of women's health care.

In this Special Issue, selected subjects on new imaging applications and insights are presented.

In this context, Borboa-Olivares et al. present a study where they evaluated subcutaneous fat tissue in the fetuses of women with well-controlled diabetes using 3D ultrasound, and AI classifiers were investigated, finding larger fat areas in fetuses from diabetic mothers compared to a healthy control group. The study's comprehensive classifier model, including variables like subcutaneous fat measure and maternal BMI, effectively predicted the impact of maternal diabetes on fetal subcutaneous fat, independent of fetal growth.

Danathan-Stumpf et al. show in a prospective study the effectiveness of a novel three-dimensional (3D) body scanner with MR pelvimetry for assessing pelvic dimensions in planning vaginal breech deliveries. Among 73 singleton pregnancies intended for vaginal breech birth, the study found that the 3D body scanner, particularly the ratio of waist girth to maternal height, was at least as effective as MRI in predicting successful vaginal delivery. However, further large-scale studies are needed to confirm these findings.

Walter et al. conducted a retrospective study over 20 years at a tertiary center, examining the course and outcome of 21 cases of fetuses diagnosed with primary cardiomyopathy (CM). They found a 40% overall survival rate, with genetic etiology confirmed in 50% of cases and prenatal isolated right ventricular involvement as a significant parameter for survival. The study suggests that while the prenatal detection of CM is feasible, it requires a classification method for improved consultation and management, noting a poor outcome in many cases but emphasizing that increased examiner awareness could influence optimal multispecialized care.

In this context, Pontones et al. conducted a study to assess the feasibility and acceptance of self-guided mobile ultrasound by pregnant women in routine prenatal care. The study included 46 women who used mobile ultrasound systems to examine fetal heartbeat, profile, and amniotic fluid, finding that while two-thirds could imagine performing the examination at home, most preferred professional support. The success rates for locating target structures varied, and the study concludes that while there is acceptance for self-examination, further research is needed to determine its role in prenatal care and its impact on fetomaternal outcomes.

Manzo and colleagues established two-dimensional ultrasonographic (2D-US) reference ranges for the normal fetal cerebellar area from 13 to 39 weeks of gestation. Analyzing 252 normal singleton pregnancies, they found a significant positive correlation between cerebellar area and gestational age, providing several 2D-US nomograms for the cerebellar area. The study suggests that understanding the typical dimensions of the fetal cerebellar area could aid in identifying cerebellar abnormalities and enhance the detection of posterior fossa anomalies in future prenatal assessments.

Luca et al. evaluate in a prospective study the effectiveness of strain ratio (SR) analysis at the internal cervical US in predicting spontaneous preterm birth (PTB). Involving 114 high-risk pregnant patients, the study found that SR, particularly when combined with other parameters, showed high accuracy in predicting PTB before 37 weeks of gestation, with even higher predictive accuracy for extremely preterm births before 28 weeks. The study concludes that SR is a promising tool for predicting PTB and warrants further evaluation in diverse patient cohorts.

Likewise, Moreno-Espinosa et al. evaluate the effectiveness of quantitative ultrasound lung texture analysis using quantusFLM® version 3.0 (quantusFLM, Barcelona, Spain) for predicting neonatal respiratory morbidity (NRM) in twin pregnancies. Involving 166 cases between 27.0 and 38.6 weeks of gestation, the study found that quantusFLM® predicted NRM with a sensitivity of 42.9%, specificity of 95.9%, and an accuracy of 89.2%. The study demonstrates the potential of this non-invasive method for predicting NRM in twin pregnancies, highlighting its high specificity, negative predictive value, and overall good performance.

Orlandi and colleagues report on a case of prenatal-diagnosed intrathoracic left kidney (ITK) associated with congenital diaphragmatic hernia (CDH), complemented by a systematic review of similar cases. Their findings, based on eleven documented cases, indicate that CDH is a rare cause of ITK, typically diagnosed around 29 weeks of gestation. The study highlights that prenatal diagnosis and counseling are crucial for planning effective prenatal and postnatal management, leading to favorable outcomes after surgical repair of the herniated kidney and associated CDH.

In comparison, Barbieri et al. conducted a systematic review of umbilical vein blood flow volume (UV-Q) reference ranges in uncomplicated pregnancies and compared these findings with data from a local cohort. Their research, which followed the PRISMA guidelines and included 15 datasets, revealed substantial heterogeneity among the reported UV-Q central values. However, they found that when using consistent sampling methodologies and formulae, UV-Q assessment is accurate and reproducible. This suggests potential clinical applications for UV-Q measurement in obstetric practice.

In this context, Pappalardo et al. describe their experience in the prenatal diagnosis of body stalk anomaly complicated by ectopia cordis, a severe defect where the heart is located outside the thorax, as part of first-trimester sonographic screening. They report two cases, diagnosed at 9 and 13 weeks of gestation, respectively, using high-quality two- and three-dimensional ultrasonographic images with the Realistic Vue and Crystal Vue techniques. Despite normal fetal karyotype and CGH-array results, both pregnancies were terminated due to the poor prognosis of this anomaly. This study highlights the importance of early diagnosis, achievable between 10 and 14 weeks of gestation, using advanced sonographic techniques.

Matlac et al. show a prospective, monocentric, single-arm study to investigate the safety and efficacy of using US-guided High-Intensity Focused Ultrasound (HIFU) for treating symptomatic uterine fibroids. As the only center in German-speaking countries utilizing this technology, their study aims to evaluate not only the clinical outcomes of HIFU, such as symptom relief and fibroid size reduction, but also its effects on laboratory parameters and the structural integrity of uterine tissue. This research addresses the gap in data regarding the impact of HIFU on these specific aspects.

Plöger et al. report on the successful intraoperative use of indocyanine green (ICG) dye for assessing ovarian perfusion in a 17-year-old patient with ovarian torsion who underwent ovary-preserving surgery. Their case, supported by a systematic literature review, indicates that ICG angiography is a feasible and safe technique in the surgical treatment of ovarian torsion, with potential implications for reducing the need for oophorectomy, although further research is needed to confirm these findings.

The overview by Jost et al. provides a systematic literature review on the applications of artificial intelligence (AI) in obstetrics and gynecology (OB/GYN) ultrasound imaging. AI-assisted ultrasound applications in OB/GYN encompass fetal biometry, echocardiography, neurosonography, as well as the identification of adnexal and breast masses, and the assessment of the endometrium and pelvic floor. While AI shows promise in automating plane acquisition, measurements, and pathology detection, this review emphasizes the need for further research in emerging and experimental fields within OB/GYN ultrasound imaging to harness the full potential of AI technology.

In this Special Issue, various aspects of prenatal and obstetric care have been explored, leveraging advanced technologies and innovative approaches. This comprehensive examination has been made possible through the judicious utilization of cutting-edge technologies and the application of pioneering methodologies. The collective body of work presented in these studies exemplifies the relentless pursuit of enhanced knowledge and improved practices in the field of maternal–fetal healthcare. In summary, this compilation of studies represents a testament to the relentless pursuit of excellence in maternal–fetal healthcare. Through the judicious amalgamation of cutting-edge technologies and innovative methodologies, these endeavors collectively contribute to the continuous enhancement of prenatal and obstetric care, paving the way for improved maternal and fetal outcomes.

Conflicts of Interest: The authors declare no conflict of interest.

List of Contributions

1. Borboa-Olivares, H.; Torres-Torres, J.; Flores-Pliego, A.; Espejel-Nuñez, A.; Camacho-Arroyo, I.; Guzman-Huerta, M.; Perichart-Perera, O.; Piña-Ramirez, O.; Estrada-Gutierrez, G. AI-Enhanced Analysis Reveals Impact of Maternal Diabetes on Subcutaneous Fat Mass in Fetuses without Growth Alterations. *J. Clin. Med.* **2023**, *12*, 6485. https://doi.org/10.3390/jcm12206485

2. Dathan-Stumpf, A.; Lia, M.; Meigen, C.; Bornmann, K.; Martin, M.; Aßmann, M.; Kiess, W.; Stepan, H. Novel Three-Dimensional Body Scan Anthropometry versus MR-Pelvimetry for Vaginal Breech Delivery Assessment. *J. Clin. Med.* **2023**, *12*, 6181. https://doi.org/10.3390/jcm12196181

3. Walter, A.; Calite, E.; Geipel, A.; Strizek, B.; Recker, F.; Herberg, U.; Berg, C.; Gembruch, U. Spectrum and Outcome of Prenatally Diagnosed Fetal Primary Cardiomyopathies—A Twenty-Year Overview. *J. Clin. Med.* **2023**, *12*, 4366. https://doi.org/10.3390/jcm12134366

4. Pontones, C.A.; Titzmann, A.; Huebner, H.; Danzberger, N.; Ruebner, M.; Häberle, L.; Eskofier, B.M.; Nissen, M.; Kehl, S.; Faschingbauer, F.; et al. Feasibility and Acceptance of Self-Guided Mobile Ultrasound among Pregnant Women in Routine Prenatal Care. *J. Clin. Med.* **2023**, *12*, 4224. https://doi.org/10.3390/jcm12134224

5. Manzo, L.; Orlandi, G.; Gabrielli, O.; Toscano, P.; Di Lella, E.; Lettieri, A.; Mazzarelli, L.L.; Sica, G.; Di Meglio, L.; Di Meglio, L.; et al. Fetal Cerebellar Area: Ultrasound Reference Ranges at 13–39 Weeks of Gestation. *J. Clin. Med.* **2023**, *12*, 4080. https://doi.org/10.3390/jcm12124080

6. Luca, A.-M.; Haba, R.; Cobzeanu, L.-M.; Nemescu, D.; Harabor, A.; Mogos, R.; Adam, A.-M.; Harabor, V.; Nechita, A.; Adam, G.; et al. Predicting Preterm Birth with Strain Ratio Analysis of the Internal Cervical Os: A Prospective Study. *J. Clin. Med.* **2023**, *12*, 3885. https://doi.org/10.3390/jcm12123885

7. Moreno-Espinosa, A.L.; Hawkins-Villarreal, A.; Coronado-Gutierrez, D.; Burgos-Artizzu, X.P.; Martínez-Portilla, R.J.; Peña-Ramirez, T.; Gallo, D.M.; Hansson, S.R.; Gratacòs, E.; Palacio, M. Prediction of Neonatal Respiratory Morbidity Assessed by Quantitative Ultrasound Lung Texture Analysis in Twin Pregnancies. *J. Clin. Med.* **2022**, *11*, 4895. https://doi.org/10.3390/jcm11164895

8. Orlandi, G.; Toscano, P.; Gabrielli, O.; Di Lella, E.; Lettieri, A.; Manzo, L.; Mazzarelli, L.L.; Sica, C.; Di Meglio, L.; Di Meglio, L.; et al. Prenatal Diagnosis of an Intrathoracic Left Kidney Associated with Congenital Diaphragmatic Hernia: Case Report and Systematic Review. *J. Clin. Med.* **2023**, *12*, 3608. https://doi.org/10.3390/jcm12113608

9. Barbieri, M.; Zamagni, G.; Fantasia, I.; Monasta, L.; Lo Bello, L.; Quadrifoglio, M.; Ricci, G.; Maso, G.; Piccoli, M.; Di Martino, D.D.; et al. Umbilical Vein Blood Flow in Uncomplicated Pregnancies: Systematic Review of Available Reference Charts and

Comparison with a New Cohort. *J. Clin. Med.* **2023**, *12*, 3132. https://doi.org/10.3390/jcm12093132

10. Pappalardo, E.; Gulino, F.A.; Ettore, C.; Cannone, F.; Ettore, G. Body Stalk Anomaly Complicated by Ectopia Cordis: First-Trimester Diagnosis of Two Cases Using 2- and 3-Dimensional Sonography. *J. Clin. Med.* **2023**, *12*, 1896. https://doi.org/10.3390/jcm12051896

11. Matlac, D.M.; Tonguc, T.; Mutschler, N.; Recker, F.; Ramig, O.; Strunk, H.M.; Dell, T.; Pieper, C.C.; Coenen, M.; Fuhrmann, C.; et al. Study Protocol of a Prospective, Monocentric, Single-Arm Study Investigating the Safety and Efficacy of Local Ablation of Symptomatic Uterine Fibroids with US-Guided High-Intensity Focused Ultrasound (HIFU). *J. Clin. Med.* **2023**, *12*, 5926. https://doi.org/10.3390/jcm12185926

12. Plöger, R.; Condic, M.; Ralser, D.J.; Plöger, H.M.; Egger, E.K.; Otten, L.A.; Mustea, A. Intraoperative Utilization of Indocyanine Green (ICG) Dye for the Assessment of Ovarian Perfusion—Case Report and Review of the Literature. *J. Clin. Med.* **2023**, *12*, 5923. https://doi.org/10.3390/jcm12185923

13. Jost, E.; Kosian, P.; Jimenez Cruz, J.; Albarqouni, S.; Gembruch, U.; Strizek, B.; Recker, F. Evolving the Era of 5D Ultrasound? A Systematic Literature Review on the Applications for Artificial Intelligence Ultrasound Imaging in Obstetrics and Gynecology. *J. Clin. Med.* **2023**, *12*, 6833. https://doi.org/10.3390/jcm12216833

References

1. Benson, C.B.; Doubilet, P.M. The History of Imaging in Obstetrics. *Radiology* **2014**, *273*, S92–S110. [CrossRef] [PubMed]
2. Harrison, B.P.; Crystal, C.S. Imaging modalities in obstetrics and gynecology. *Emerg. Med. Clin. N. Am.* **2003**, *21*, 711–735. [CrossRef] [PubMed]
3. Merz, E.; Pashaj, S. Advantages of 3D Ultrasound in the Assessment of Fetal Abnormalities. *J. Perinat. Med.* **2017**, *45*, 643–650. [CrossRef] [PubMed]
4. Abramowicz, J.S. Obstetric ultrasound: Where are we and where are we going? *Ultrasonography* **2021**, *40*, 57–74. [CrossRef] [PubMed]
5. Salomon, L.J.; Alfirevic, Z.; Da Silva Costa, F.; Deter, R.L.; Figueras, F.; Ghi, T.A.; Glanc, P.; Khalil, A.; Lee, W.; Napolitano, R.; et al. ISUOG Practice Guidelines: Ultrasound assessment of fetal biometry and growth. *Ultrasound Obstet. Gynecol.* **2019**, *53*, 715–723. [CrossRef]
6. Kurjak, A. 3D/4D Sonography. *J. Perinat. Med.* **2017**, *45*, 639–641. [CrossRef] [PubMed]
7. Abinader, R.; Warsof, S.L. Benefits and Pitfalls of Ultrasound in Obstetrics and Gynecology. *Obstet. Gynecol. Clin. N. Am.* **2019**, *46*, 367–378. [CrossRef] [PubMed]
8. Jost, E.; Kosian, P.; Jimenez Cruz, J.; Albarqouni, S.; Gembruch, U.; Strizek, B.; Recker, F. Evolving the Era of 5D Ultrasound? A Systematic Literature Review on the Applications for Artificial Intelligence Ultrasound Imaging in Obstetrics and Gynecology. *J. Clin. Med.* **2023**, *12*, 6833. [CrossRef] [PubMed]
9. Amor, F.; Vaccaro, H.; Alcázar, J.L.; León, M.; Craig, J.M.; Martinez, J. Gynecologic imaging reporting and data system: A new proposal for classifying adnexal masses on the basis of sonographic findings. *J. Ultrasound Med.* **2009**, *28*, 285–291. [CrossRef] [PubMed]
10. Leung, K.Y. Applications of Advanced Ultrasound Technology in Obstetrics. *Diagnostics* **2021**, *11*, 1217. [CrossRef] [PubMed]

Disclaimer/Publisher's Note: The statements, opinions and data contained in all publications are solely those of the individual author(s) and contributor(s) and not of MDPI and/or the editor(s). MDPI and/or the editor(s) disclaim responsibility for any injury to people or property resulting from any ideas, methods, instructions or products referred to in the content.

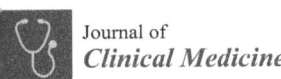

Article

AI-Enhanced Analysis Reveals Impact of Maternal Diabetes on Subcutaneous Fat Mass in Fetuses without Growth Alterations

Hector Borboa-Olivares [1,*], Johnatan Torres-Torres [2], Arturo Flores-Pliego [3], Aurora Espejel-Nuñez [3], Ignacio Camacho-Arroyo [4], Mario Guzman-Huerta [5], Otilia Perichart-Perera [6], Omar Piña-Ramirez [7] and Guadalupe Estrada-Gutierrez [8,*]

1. Community Interventions Research Branch, Instituto Nacional de Perinatología, Mexico City 11000, Mexico
2. Clinical Research Division, Instituto Nacional de Perinatología, Mexico City 11000, Mexico; torresmmf@gmail.com
3. Department of Immunobiochemistry, Instituto Nacional de Perinatología, Mexico City 11000, Mexico; arturo.flores@inper.gob.mx (A.F.-P.); aurora.espejel@inper.gob.mx (A.E.-N.)
4. Unidad de Investigación en Reproducción Humana, Instituto Nacional de Perinatologia-Facultad de Química, Universidad Nacional Autónoma de México, Mexico City 11000, Mexico; camachoarroyoi@quimica.unam.com
5. Department of Translational Medicine, Instituto Nacional de Perinatología, Mexico City 11000, Mexico; mguzmanhuerta@yahoo.com.mx
6. Nutrition and Bioprogramming Department, Instituto Nacional de Perinatología, Mexico City 11000, Mexico; oti_perichart@yahoo.com
7. Bioinformatics and Statistical Analysis Department, Instituto Nacional de Perinatología, Mexico City 11000, Mexico; omar.pina@inper.gob.mx
8. Research Division, Instituto Nacional de Perinatología, Mexico City 11000, Mexico
* Correspondence: hector.borboa@inper.gob.mx (H.B.-O.); guadalupe.estrada@inper.gob.mx (G.E.-G.); Tel.: +52-5555209900 (ext. 120) (H.B.-O.); +52-5555209900 (ext. 160) (G.E.-G.)

Abstract: Pregnant women with diabetes often present impaired fetal growth, which is less common if maternal diabetes is well-controlled. However, developing strategies to estimate fetal body composition beyond fetal growth that could better predict metabolic complications later in life is essential. This study aimed to evaluate subcutaneous fat tissue (femur and humerus) in fetuses with normal growth among pregnant women with well-controlled diabetes using a reproducible 3D-ultrasound tool and offline TUI (Tomographic Ultrasound Imaging) analysis. Additionally, three artificial intelligence classifier models were trained and validated to assess the clinical utility of the fetal subcutaneous fat measurement. A significantly larger subcutaneous fat area was found in three-femur and two-humerus selected segments of fetuses from women with diabetes compared to the healthy pregnant control group. The full classifier model that includes subcutaneous fat measure, gestational age, fetal weight, fetal abdominal circumference, maternal body mass index, and fetal weight percentile as variables, showed the best performance, with a detection rate of 70%, considering a false positive rate of 10%, and a positive predictive value of 82%. These findings provide valuable insights into the impact of maternal diabetes on fetal subcutaneous fat tissue as a variable independent of fetal growth.

Keywords: diabetes and pregnancy; ultrasound evaluation; fetal subcutaneous fat mass

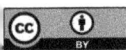

1. Introduction

Abnormal fetal growth is linked to higher rates of perinatal morbidity and mortality and an increased risk of metabolic diseases later in life, including diabetes, hypertension, obesity, metabolic syndrome, and dyslipidemia [1,2]. In pregnant women, pre-existing diabetes and inadequate metabolic control can negatively impact embryogenesis during early gestation and significantly influence growth and body composition later in pregnancy [3]. Poor glucose control in pregnancies complicated by diabetes, whether insulin-dependent or gestational, often results in identifiable characteristics such as selective macrosomia (excessive fetal growth) and organomegaly (enlargement of organs) [4]. Furthermore, diabetic pregnant women with complications such as preeclampsia or pre-existing vascular disease may experience reduced uterine flow and morphological changes in the placenta, which affect nutrient exchange, leading to intrauterine growth restriction [5].

Maternal hyperglycemia induces fetal hyperglycemia, stimulating pancreatic activity resulting in hypertrophy, hyperplasia, and increased insulin secretion. Insulin is the primary anabolic hormone for fetal growth and development, contributing to macrosomia and organomegaly [1,3,6,7]. Current evidence suggests that maintaining reasonable glycemic control in pregnant women with diabetes can disrupt the cycle of hyperglycemia and hyperinsulinemia, thus preventing complications associated with abnormal fetal growth [8,9]. However, it remains uncertain whether poor metabolic control in the latter half of pregnancy exclusively impairs fetal growth [10].

Changes in fetal body composition have implications for both the life period within the uterus and after birth, leading to alterations in metabolism and inflammation, increasing the fetus's vulnerability to higher morbidity and long-term consequences [11,12]. As a result, evaluating fetal body composition provides numerous advantages over conventional methods used to assess fetal growth. Previous studies have investigated fat levels in fetuses of diabetic mothers, revealing elevated subcutaneous or abdominal fat areas [13–15]. However, these techniques for evaluating fat are impractical for routine clinical use due to their limited reproducibility attributed to operator bias involved in manually selecting the ultrasound plane for measurement [16–19]. Consequently, ongoing research aims to develop innovative tools capable of detecting changes in fetal body composition, enabling early and comprehensive assessments of growth disorders, and ultimately enhancing clinical management and perinatal outcomes.

Artificial intelligence (AI) has shown some benefits in clinical research. These tools in obstetrics have been used to incorporate data and images in machine learning models to predict preterm birth, birth weight, preeclampsia, mortality, hypertensive disorders, and postpartum depression and placental abnormalities, offering a reduction in inter- and intraoperator variability, time reduction in procedures, and improving overall diagnostic performance [20–22].

The present study evaluated subcutaneous fat tissue in fetuses with normal growth among pregnant women with well-controlled maternal diabetes using a more reproducible 3D-ultrasound tool and offline TUI (Tomographic Ultrasound Imaging) analysis [23]. Additionally, three artificial intelligence (AI) classifier models were trained and validated to assess the impact of maternal diabetes on subcutaneous fat mass in fetuses, identifying the offspring of a diabetic mother.

2. Materials and Methods

2.1. Ethics Statement

This study was conducted as part of the ongoing OBESO (Biochemical and Epigenetic Origins of Overweight and Obesity) perinatal cohort at the Instituto Nacional de Perinatologia (INPer) in Mexico City, which aims to investigate the association between obesity, maternal metabolic profile, and their predictive roles in fetal body composition, obesity, and neurodevelopment during infancy. The project was approved by the Ethics and Research Internal Review Board (2016-1-568/2017-2-79). Enrolled women were provided with detailed information regarding the risks and benefits of the study, and their participation was voluntary. Informed consent was obtained from all recruited participants.

2.2. Study Population

Sixty singleton pregnant women were conveniently selected during their third-trimester ultrasound appointments from January to December 2019. Thirty of these women had well-controlled diabetes, including sixteen with pregestational (type 2) diabetes without pre-existing vascular disease and fourteen with gestational diabetes. The other thirty women were selected as healthy controls, matched by gestational age. The control group underwent an oral glucose tolerance test between 24 and– 28 weeks of gestation to rule out diabetes. Patients used as controls were paired for gestational age, fetal gender, BMI classification (underweight, normal weight, overweight), and weight gain at the time of the study (adequate, insufficient, or excessive) [24]. The diabetic participants maintained good glycemic control throughout pregnancy based on the guidelines set by the American Diabetes Association, which included fasting capillary glycemia $\leq$ 95 mg/dL and one-hour postprandial capillary glycemia $\leq$ 140 mg/dL in at least 80% of measurements, with glycosylated hemoglobin HbA1c levels below 6.0% [25]. Women were enrolled after 31 weeks of gestation, as determined by the last menstrual period and confirmed by the first-trimester ultrasound. Participants with chronic or pregnancy-induced high blood pressure, type 1 diabetes, diabetes with vasculopathy, and intrauterine fetal growth alterations were excluded from the study. All enrolled women received routine prenatal care at INPer, and relevant clinical data were extracted from their medical records. Women with diabetes received medical nutrition therapy provided by a dietitian, and in some cases, pharmacological treatment with metformin was necessary to achieve adequate metabolic control. The Department of Endocrinology at INPer adjusted the metformin dosage to maintain optimal glycemic standards. Maternal anthropometric measurements, including pre-gestational weight, height, and body mass index, were obtained from the medical records. All patients included were followed up to pregnancy ended to collect perinatal outcomes. No sample size calculation was performed beforehand, but the statistical power was calculated for all variables with significant differences to verify that it was greater than 80%.

2.3. Fetometry

Fetometry was performed using a Voluson E8 (GE Healthcare, Chicago, IL, USA) 3D ultrasound with a volumetric transducer (4–8 MHz). Measurements such as biparietal diameter, head circumference, abdominal circumference, and femoral length were taken to estimate fetal weight using the Hadlock 2 formula. Weight percentiles were calculated based on gestational age, according to the Hadlock reference values, preloaded in the ultrasound machine; all fetuses included were weighed between the 10th and 90th percentile. The ultrasound examination involved acquiring a 3D volume scan with a 30° sweep angle and an acquisition time of 10 s. To ensure accuracy, the transducer was placed as close as possible to the extremity without applying pressure and with minimal fetal and maternal movement. The arm and thigh closest to the mother's abdominal wall were selected for measurement.

2.4. Assessment of Fat Mass Area

Volumetry was performed on the arm and thigh (humerus/femur) anterior to the maternal abdominal wall, placing the transducer as close as possible to the limb without exerting pressure in the absence of fetal and maternal movement. The volumetry transducer was selected (4–8 MHz), and the initial settings were the same as used in the 2D evaluation; only contrast and zoom were increased in order to see the complete structure in 70 to 80% of the screen, the focus was placed in the area of interest and the gains to optimize the image. A volume acquisition angle of 80° was selected, and the limb was centered correctly. The quality of the images depended on the exposure speed; a rotational scan was selected in a sagittal Z plane with an acquisition time of 10 s [26].

In the offline evaluation, the ViewPoint program, GE Healthcare, was used; select the "explore submenu", and then the acquired file was chosen. The sagittal plane of the bone was displayed as the main screen, and the proximal epiphysis lateralized to the left. A Sepia filter was applied in the image to delineate the lean and fat mass contours. In the TUI (Tomographic Ultrasound Imaging) tool, three tomographic slices were programmed, and the diaphysis was centered to have the center, 1 to the right and 1 to the left [26].

The fat mass area was determined by subtracting the central area representing lean mass, consisting of bone and muscle, from the total area obtained in the image. At least two measurements were taken for each tomographic plane, and the average of these observations was used for analysis. Three planes of the humerus/femur were utilized: the union of the proximal third with the middle, the middle of the bone, and the union of the distal third with the middle third (Figure 1). The acquisition of images and the subsequent offline analysis were performed by three ultrasound experts specialized in maternal–fetal medicine, who followed a standardized technique. Prior to the study, the technique was standardized among these three operators. The inter- and intra-observer variability was calculated using the intraclass correlation coefficient, yielding a value greater than 0.90 for all three selected planes.

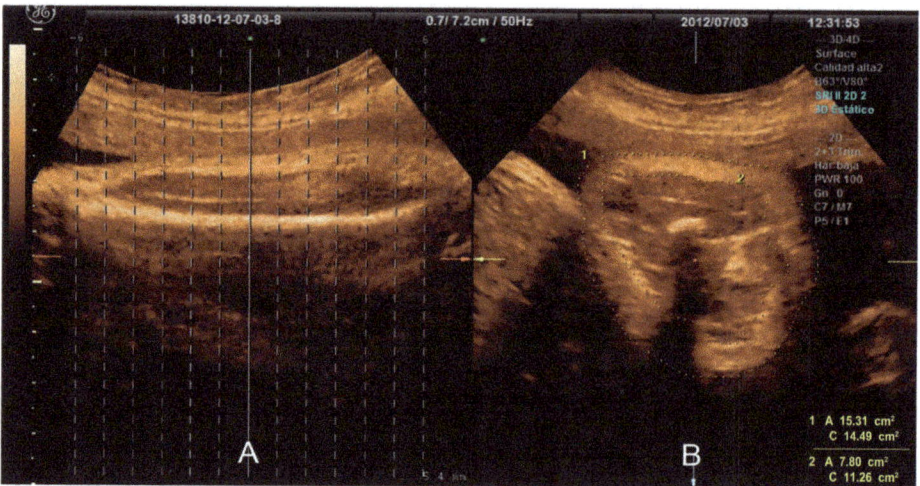

Figure 1. Offline Tomographic Ultrasound Imaging analysis. (**A**) Sagittal plane of the fetal femur. (**B**) Axial plane selected, fat area obtained by subtracting the lean tissue area (muscle and bone) from the total area (covering the total area).

2.5. Statistical Analysis

Statistical analysis was performed using IBM® SPSS® Statistics, version 20, and descriptive statistics were employed to characterize the general population. The paired t-test and Wilcoxon rank test were used to assess differences based on data normality and the requirement for non-parametric tests, respectively. Statistical significance was considered for $p < 0.05$.

2.6. Classifier Models

Data analysis comprised two stages: (A) Feature Selection, during which relevant variables were identified using a 70-30% bootstrapping technique, and (B) Classifiers Training and Validation, which involved training and evaluating three Linear Discriminant Analysis with Shrinkage models via a cross-validation process. Each model accounted for a different group of features. For the classification task, control and diabetes case data were labeled with 0 and 1, respectively.

(A)   Feature Selection

The Least Absolute Shrinkage Selector Operator (LASSO) is a regularized version of linear regression that assigns zero weight to non-relevant features and, therefore, serves as a feature selector.

An optimal LASSO model was trained using 70% of the class-stratified data in each bootstrapping iteration. The remaining 30% was discarded as this stage focused on determining the variables that contributed the most relevant information (Figure 2a). Optimal LASSO models were obtained using Python's sci-kit-learn library. This process was repeated across ten blocks, each comprising five bootstrapping iterations (Figure 2b).

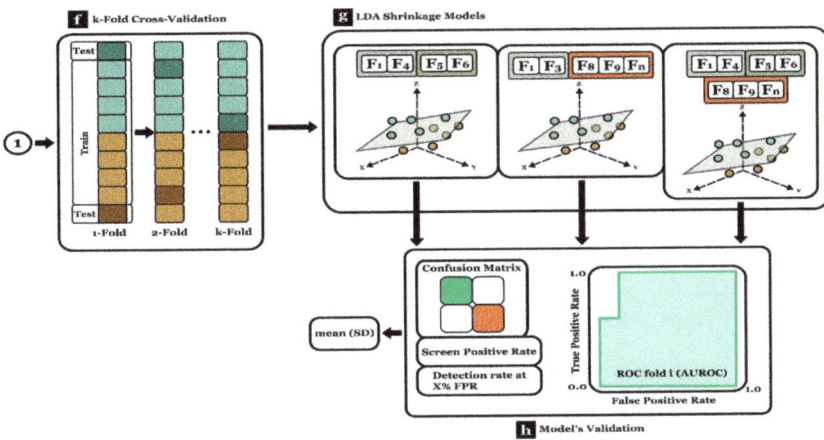

Figure 2. Classifier model development process, variable selection, training, and validation.

Features were selected based on variables that did not register any non-zero-weight counts of LASSO (Figure 2c). These were grouped according to variable nature: biometric, free fat-mass, and fat-mass. The average weight of the features is displayed in bar plots (Figure 2e).

(B) Classifier Training and Validation

The classifier utilized was the Linear Discriminant Analysis, which employed a shrinkage approach with Ledoit–Wolf parameter optimization. Three models were trained, and each included a different combination of feature groups: biometric + free fat mass, biometric + fat mass, and biometric + free fat mass + fat mass (Figure 2g). Classification performances were assessed using a class-stratified 10-fold cross-validation technique (Figure 2f). Finally, the mean and standard deviation of the Area under the ROC (AUROC), Detection Rate adjusted with False Positive Rate percentage, and Screen Positive Rate are reported (Figure 2h).

Three artificial intelligence classifier models were trained and validated to assess the clinical utility of fetal subcutaneous fat measurement. Model 1, referred to as "full", included the following variables: subcutaneous fat measured by ultrasound, gestational age, fetal weight (ultrasound), fetal abdominal circumference, maternal BMI, and fetal weight percentile (ultrasound). Model 2, named "ft fat", exclusively incorporated measurements of subcutaneous fat in the fetal arm and thigh. Model 3, termed "ft no fat", was similar to model 1 but excluded the subcutaneous fat measure. For each of the proposed models, the detection rate (DR) was calculated considering a false positive rate (FPR) = 5, 10, 15, 20%, Area Under the Curve (AUC), and Positive Predictive Value (PPV).

To ensure the interpretability of the classifier models and verify that differences were attributed to the set of features used rather than the classifier itself, Regularized Linear Discriminant Analysis (Shrinkage-LDA) was employed. Model training and validation were conducted using Python 3.8 software with the scikit-learn machine learning library. The data were divided using an 8-way cross-validation strategy, with 70% used for training and 30% for validation. The strategy aimed to maintain a similar number of items per class in both training and validation sets (Figure 2).

3. Results

3.1. Characteristics of the Study Population

Baseline characteristics were similar between the study groups (Table 1). However, mothers with diabetes showed higher pre-gestational weight and pre-gestational BMI than mothers in the control group ($p = 0.034$ and 0.046, respectively). No significant difference was found between the study groups in biparietal diameter, head circumference, abdominal circumference, femoral length, ratio between male and female fetuses, as well as gestational age at birth. All newborns were evaluated by neonatologists from the institute staff, weight was measured, and somatometry was performed; all had a diagnosis of "normal weight for gestational age," according to local reference values.

Table 1. Clinical characteristics of the population.

	Control $n = 30$	Diabetes $n = 30$	p Value
Maternal age (Years, mean ± SD)	30.76 ± 6.4	32.9 ± 7.13	0.247
Gestational age (Weeks, mean ± SD)	34.63 ± 1.7	34.61 ± 1.71	0.609
Pre-gestational maternal weight (kg, ± SD)	69.69 ± 9.7	77.87 ± 15.38	0.034 *
Pre-gestational BMI (kg/m^2, mean ± SD)	28.33 ± 3.99	31.00 ± 5.20	0.046 *
Parity (Median, minimum, and maximum range)	2 (1–5)	2 (1–6)	0.432
Fetal weight by ultrasound (Grams, mean ± SD)	2447 ± 397	2533 ± 459	0.198
Biparietal diameter (cm)	8.60	8.65	0.322
Cephalic circumference (cm)	30.97	31.26	0.134
Abdominal circumference (cm)	30.57	30.96	0.091
Femoral length (cm)	7.21	6.57	0.074
Newborn weight (Grams, mean ± SD)	3257 ± 298	3389 ± 389	0.233
Gestational age at birth (Weeks, median)	39.1 (37.3–40.1)	38.5 (36.6–39.4)	0.191
Male/female proportion	15/15	15/15	0.478

SD: standard deviation; BMI: body mass index. Student's t-test. * $p < 0.05$.

In the group of pregnant diabetic patients, all received counseling from a clinical nutritionist and were assigned a nutritional plan according to their weight, physical activity, and weeks of gestation. Twenty patients (66%) received treatment with metformin (adjusting the dose to achieve the goals of glycemic control), and five (16%) received subcutaneous insulin treatment (adjusting the dose to achieve the goals of glycemic control).

3.2. Association between Maternal Diabetes and Fetal Subcutaneous Fat Tissue

The mean fat area (in square centimeters, cm^2) obtained from six measurements (three from the humerus and three from the femur) was compared between the study groups. A significantly larger fat area was observed in the three selected femur segments of fetuses from women with diabetes than in the control group. These segments included the junction of the proximal third and middle third ($p = 0.024$), the middle third ($p = 0.026$), and the junction of the distal third and middle third ($p = 0.005$) (Table 2 and Figure 3). In the humerus, an increase in fat area was detected at the junction of the proximal third and middle third ($p = 0.045$), as well as at the junction of the distal third and middle third ($p = 0.023$) in fetuses from pregnant women with diabetes, in comparison to healthy controls (Table 2 and Figure 3). When women with pregestational diabetes and gestational diabetes were analyzed separately, no differences were found in the segments evaluated in the fetal arm or thigh (Table 3).

Table 2. Fat area in three axial planes of the femur and humerus among the study groups.

	Control (cm^2, Mean ± SD) n = 30	Diabetes (cm^2, Mean ± SD) n = 30	p Value
FEMUR			
Proximal third-middle union	8.9 ± 2.0	10.1 ± 2.0	0.024 *
Middle	7.8 ± 1.7	9.0 ± 2.0	0.026 *
Distal third-middle	7.3 ± 1.7	8.8 ± 1.8	0.005 **
HUMERUS			
Proximal third-middle union	5.4 ± 1.6	6.1 ± 1.4	0.045 *
Middle	5.1 ± 1.4	5.8 ± 1.8	0.069
Distal third-middle	4.7 ± 1.2	5.3 ± 1.2	0.023 *

SD: standard deviation; Paired student's *t*-test. * $p < 0.05$, ** $p < 0.01$.

Table 3. Fat area in three axial planes of the femur and humerus among women with pregestational and gestational diabetes.

	Pregestational Diabetes (cm^2, Mean ± SD) n = 16	Gestational Diabetes (cm^2, Mean ± SD) n = 14	p Value
FEMUR			
Proximal third-middle union	9.9 ± 1.6	10.2 ± 1.8	0.34
Middle	8.7 ± 2.1	9.3 ± 2.4	0.42
Distal third-middle	7.9 ± 1.9	8.6 ± 2.1	0.06
HUMERUS			
Proximal third-middle union	5.9 ± 1.8	6.4 ± 1.8	0.35
Middle	5.6 ± 1.2	5.4 ± 1.9	0.69
Distal third-middle	5.1 ± 1.5	5.6 ± 1.4	0.23

SD: standard deviation; Paired student's *t*-test.

3.3. Classifier Models between Fetal Subcutaneous Fat Tissue and Ultrasonographic Tools

Analysis using classifier models to identify whether a patient belonged to the "gestational diabetes" group showed that model 1, which included all the "full model" variables, had a detection rate of 70% considering a false positive rate of 10%, with a positive predictive value of 82%, and an area under the curve of 0.88. Model 2, "ft fat," had a DR of 38%, considering a false positive rate of 10%, with a PPV of 67% and an AUC of 0.71. Model 3, "ft non-fat," had a DR of 45%, considering an FPR of 10%, with a PPV of 68% and an AUC of 0.68. The performance of the different models calculated with false positive rates of 5, 10, 15, and 20% are shown in Table 4.

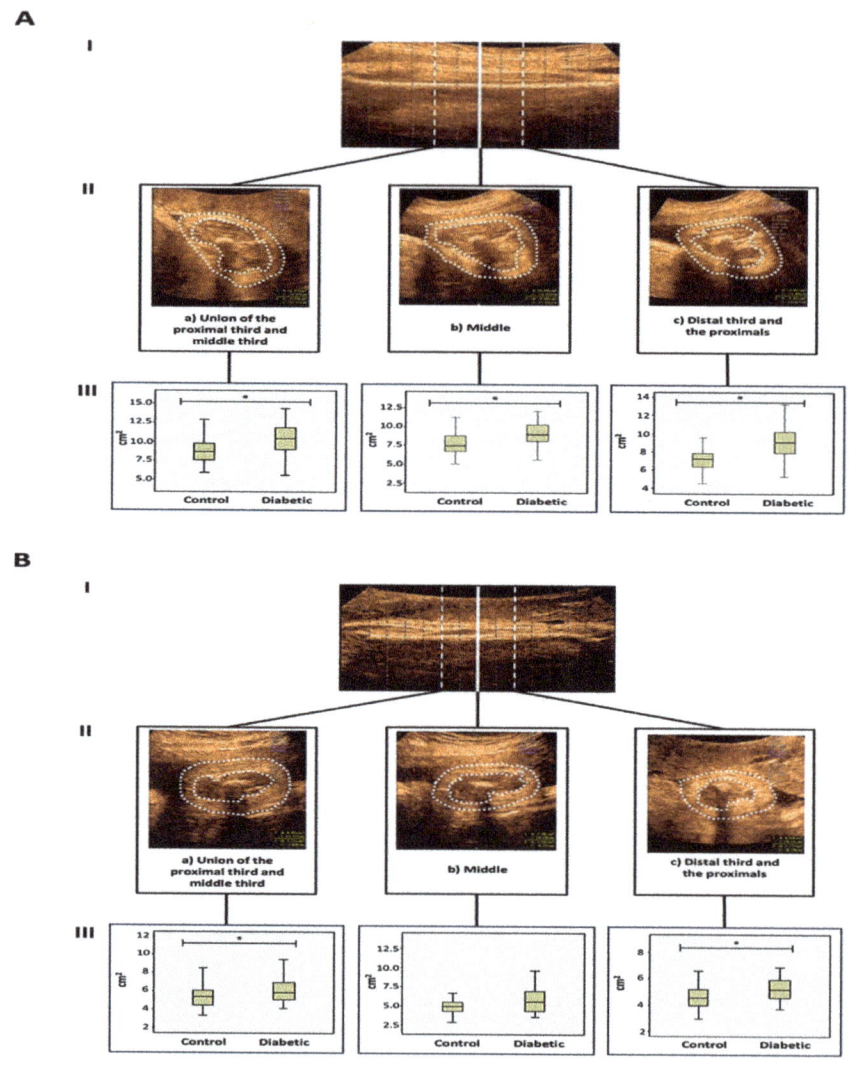

Figure 3. Differences in the fat area around the fetal femur and humerus were analyzed with 3D-View Tomographic Ultrasound Imaging. (A) femur; (I) Sagittal plane of the femur in the offline analysis. (II) Axial plane: Areas corresponding to subcutaneous fatty tissue in offline analysis. (III) Boxplots showing comparison between fetuses from diabetic pregnant women vs. healthy pregnant women. (B) humerus; (I) Sagittal plane of the femur in the offline analysis. (II) Axial plane: Areas corresponding to subcutaneous fatty tissue in offline analysis. (III) Boxplots showing comparison between fetuses from diabetic pregnant women vs. healthy pregnant women * $p < 0.05$.

Table 4. Performance of the three proposed models: "full model", "ft-fat", and "ft-no fat".

Model	DR at FPR				AUC	PPV
	0.05	0.10	0.15	0.2		
Full model	0.704 (0.214)	0.704 (0.214)	0.738 (0.204)	0.778 (0.182)	0.881 (0.100)	0.823 (0.188)
Ft-fat	0.385 (0.292)	0.385 (0.292)	0.468 (0.279)	0.573 (0.255)	0.719 (0.143)	0.676 (0.190)
Ft no-fat	0.458 (0.269)	0.458 (0.269)	0.501 (0.284)	0.591 (0.269)	0.746 (0.156)	0.682 (0.205)

DR: detection rate; FPR: false positive rate; AUC: area under curve; PPV: positive predictive value. Full model: subcutaneous fat measured by ultrasound, gestational age, fetal weight (ultrasound), fetal abdominal circumference, maternal BMI, and fetal weight percentile (ultrasound); Ft-fat: exclusively incorporated measurements of subcutaneous fat in the fetal arm and thigh; Ft no-fat: excluded the subcutaneous fat measure.

4. Discussion

4.1. Main Findings

The most striking finding was the significantly larger fat area observed in specific segments of fetuses from mothers with diabetes, regardless of adequate glycemic control compared to the control group. This suggests that maternal diabetes should directly impact the accumulation of subcutaneous fat in certain fetal segments.

4.2. Comparison with Existing Literature

This finding is consistent with a prior investigation conducted by Larciprete et al., who utilized ultrasound examinations to illustrate an increase in fetal subcutaneous fat in pregnancies affected by gestational diabetes [27]. However, our study diverges from that research since we exclusively enrolled women with well-controlled diabetes and fetuses of normal weight. In a related study, De Santis et al. in 2010 also documented variations in subcutaneous fat levels among fetuses born to diabetic mothers, highlighting the utility of fat assessment as a third-trimester gestational tool, irrespective of the specific maternal diabetes treatment employed [16]. Building upon their observations, our study concentrated on fetal fat measurements exclusively in the third trimester without stratification by treatment modality.

It is reasonable to assume that the rise in fetal adipose tissue is concomitant with the increase in fetal weight, which is clinically indicative of maternal diabetes decompensation [13]. Therefore, the most noteworthy discovery in our study is the absence of disparities in estimated fetal weight or birth weight between the groups but the increased fat area in the extremities of fetuses born to well-controlled diabetic mothers. Given the insulin sensitivity of adipose tissue, our findings imply that alterations in fetal adipose tissue may function as a more sensitive indicator of the ramifications of maternal metabolic changes, even before significant shifts in fetal weight become apparent [28].

Hence, we can infer that if this cohort of pregnant women with well-controlled diabetes had undergone routine ultrasound assessments without the inclusion of fetal fat measurements, their fetuses would likely have been categorized as having normal weight and presumed to be in good health. This approach, however, would underestimate the metabolic risk associated with changes in body composition. In 2017, Venkataraman et al. provided additional evidence of the "thin but fat" phenotype within the Asian population. They characterized fetuses with a disproportional increase in adipose tissue, even when lean body mass was smaller or comparable, occurring before the biochemical diagnosis of gestational diabetes mellitus. They introduced fetal anterior abdominal wall thickness as an early indicator of this condition [29]. Nevertheless, it is worth noting that this measurement can be influenced by fetal position, orientation, attitude, and the volume of amniotic fluid, potentially reducing its reproducibility. In our study, we assessed the limbs because this approach is not influenced by the variables mentioned earlier. Additionally, the adoption of TUI analysis allows for precise selection of measurement planes, thereby diminishing dependence on inter-observer variability [29,30].

In recent years, there have been notable advancements in ultrasonography, leading to improved resolution. This enhancement enables more precise tissue characterization and accurate quantification of fetal fat accumulation. Additionally, a novel metric called fetal fractional limb volume has emerged, designed to measure the volume of fetal soft tissues, encompassing both fat mass and lean mass [31,32]. It has become evident that substantial physiological diversity and heterogeneity exist in fetal growth velocity patterns, particularly during the third trimester of pregnancy. Furthermore, the growth trajectory of fetal soft tissue volume, primarily comprising fat mass, experiences acceleration in the early stages of the third trimester. Based on these insights, it is suggested that serial assessments of fetal fat mass and fractional limb volume in the third trimester, spaced at intervals of 2–4 weeks, could offer valuable clinical insights. Such assessments have the potential to differentiate between constitutionally small/large fetuses and malnourished/overnourished fetuses, thus facilitating a deeper understanding of the "thrifty" or "drifty" phenotype, both of which are predisposed to the development of metabolic syndrome [33]. By detecting significant variations in fetal fat accumulation, researchers may gain fresh perspectives into the underlying causes of altered fetal body composition observed in conditions such as fetal growth restriction or fetal macrosomia. Further studies must be conducted to evaluate clinical interventions to address altered fetal growth and body composition, with the ultimate goal of primary prevention of future metabolic dysfunction [32,34].

In the forthcoming years, these novel approaches have the potential to reveal that alterations in fetal body composition are equally, if not more, crucial than birth weight alone in identifying newborns with an elevated risk of developing metabolic syndrome, diabetes, heart disease, obesity, and high blood pressure later in life. To rigorously assess this hypothesis, ongoing studies are underway to investigate the influence of changes in fetal body composition on metabolic and neurodevelopmental outcomes in a follow-up cohort at the age of 8 [35,36]. Furthermore, we advocate for the inclusion of comprehensive evaluations at birth and follow-up assessments for fetuses exhibiting growth alterations, such as intrauterine growth restriction and macrosomia. This approach is vital as these fetuses may exhibit similar modifications as previously documented in studies focused on body composition at birth [37,38].

The research also explored the potential of using AI-enhanced classifier models to distinguish between patients with gestational diabetes and those without it. The "full model" achieved a detection rate of 70% at a false positive rate of 10%, indicating a promising ability to identify patients with gestational diabetes.

AI methods in medical care could facilitate individual pregnancy management and improve public health, especially in low- and middle-income countries. Classifier models are one of the methods of analysis that uses AI. Using statistical analysis methods different from those we are conventionally accustomed to seeing in the medical literature is becoming more common to demonstrate the association between variables. Particularly in obstetrics, these analysis methods have been used to evaluate the risk of preeclampsia [39]. We found no history of their use in comorbidities such as diabetes in pregnancy.

4.3. Strengths and Limitations

A weakness of our study is the limited number of included patients; however, we assessed the statistical power of the observed differences, all of which exceeded 0.80. Additionally, our study is limited by the exclusion of certain variables that may influence birth weight, such as maternal weight, supplementation, and the use of medications to manage underlying diseases. Nevertheless, existing evidence suggests that various treatments for diabetes do not appear to impact fetal fat measurements.

On the other hand, a strength of our study lies in the comprehensive clinical management provided to all women by the Department of Endocrinology at INPer. Rigorous glycemic control was confirmed through regular measurements of pre- and postprandial capillary and venous blood glucose levels, along with periodic quantification of glycosylated hemoglobin. The employed TUI technique offers the advantage of eliminating operator dependence or bias, as axial cuts are predetermined in the software, accounting for bone edges. The software consistently maintains the same distance between axial planes in all 3D volumes, ensuring consistency across measurements. This contrasts with previous studies that relied on ultrasound-based subcutaneous fat tissue measurement, where operators subjectively selected the measurement plane.

To our knowledge, no other work has utilized classifier models to assess fetal fat measurement as a clinical contributor to diabetes. Thus, this represents the primary strength of our research.

4.4. Clinical Interpretation

Fetal weight and the quantity of amniotic fluid are the primary clinical indicators of poorly controlled diabetes during pregnancy. It is worth noting that fetal body composition is also affected in pregnant women with well-controlled diabetes. Consequently, assessing fetal fat content can be a valuable tool, offering advantages over assessing fetal weight alone. This allows clinicians to detect early changes in body composition even before fetal weight is impacted. Detecting such changes during the fetal period provides an opportunity to design and implement early interventions that can positively impact the metabolic control of pregnant women with diabetes, thereby improving perinatal outcomes.

However, establishing reference values for fetal fat is still pending to determine what would be considered normal. Additionally, our findings raise questions about whether the variables currently used in the ultrasonographic evaluation of fetuses from diabetic mothers are adequate or if it is necessary to implement new and more sensitive tools to classify fetuses more accurately at an increased risk of developing metabolic issues later in life [40,41].

The development of a classifier model represents an innovative approach to examining the clinical relevance of subcutaneous fat measurement in fetuses through the utilization of artificial intelligence. In this study, we conducted training and validation of three models. By inputting various variables into the analysis, these models can determine whether the mother–fetus dyad belongs to the diabetic or control group. The analyses of the classifier models indicate that the inclusion of subcutaneous fetal fat measurement via ultrasound leads to a more precise prediction of whether the dyad belongs to the diabetic group. Specifically, this inclusion enhances the detection capability by 10%, raising it from 0.688 to 0.781. These findings support our initial hypothesis that maternal diabetes significantly affects fetal fat.

5. Conclusions

This study provides valuable insights into the impact of maternal diabetes on fetal subcutaneous fat tissue. Our findings demonstrate an increase in fat accumulation in fetuses of mothers with well-controlled diabetes. Furthermore, the application of AI-enhanced classifier models allows us to identify the offspring of a diabetic mother. These findings contribute to our comprehension of maternal diabetes and its potential consequences on fetal development, even when the patient is under good glycemic control.

Author Contributions: Conceptualization: H.B.-O., M.G.-H. and G.E.-G. Methodology: H.B.-O., J.T.-T. and G.E.-G. Formal analysis: H.B.-O., J.T.-T. and O.P.-R. Investigation: H.B.-O., A.F.-P. and I.C.-A. Resources: H.B.-O., A.F.-P., A.E.-N., O.P.-P. and I.C.-A. Data curation: H.B.-O., O.P.-P. and A.F.-P. Writing—original draft preparation: H.B.-O., J.T.-T. and G.E.-G. Writing—review and editing: H.B.-O., J.T.-T., G.E.-G., I.C.-A., O.P.-P., A.F.-P. and A.E.-N. Project administration: H.B.-O. and G.E.-G. Funding acquisition: H.B.-O. All authors have read and agreed to the published version of the manuscript.

Funding: This research was funded by the Instituto Nacional de Perinatologia in Mexico City, grant number (2016-1-568/2017-2-79).

Institutional Review Board Statement: The research protocol received approval from the Ethics and Research Internal Review Board (2016-1-568/2017-2-79).

Informed Consent Statement: Informed consent was obtained from all subjects involved in the study.

Data Availability Statement: The data presented in this study are available on request from the corresponding author. The data are not publicly available due to privacy or ethical issues.

Conflicts of Interest: The authors declare no conflict of interest.

References

1. Padmanabhan, V.; Cardoso, R.C.; Puttabyatappa, M. Developmental Programming, a Pathway to Disease. *Endocrinology* **2016**, *157*, 1328–1340. [CrossRef] [PubMed]
2. Estrada-Gutiérrez, G.; Zambrano, E.; Polo-Oteyza, E.; Cardona-Pérez, A.; Vadillo-Ortega, F. Intervention during the first 1000 days in Mexico. *Nutr. Rev.* **2020**, *78*, 80–90. [CrossRef]
3. Ornoy, A.; Reece, E.A.; Pavlinkova, G.; Kappen, C.; Miller, R.K. Effect of maternal diabetes on the embryo, fetus, and children: Congenital anomalies, genetic and epigenetic changes and developmental outcomes. *Birth Defects Res. Part C Embryo Today* **2015**, *105*, 53–72. [CrossRef]
4. Kc, K.; Shakya, S.; Zhang, H. Gestational diabetes mellitus and macrosomia: A literature review. *Ann. Nutr. Metab.* **2015**, *66* (Suppl. 2), 14–20. [CrossRef] [PubMed]
5. Jensen, L.A.; Chik, C.L.; Ryan, E.A. Review of gestational diabetes mellitus effects on vascular structure and function. *Diabetes Vasc. Dis. Res.* **2016**, *13*, 170–182. [CrossRef] [PubMed]
6. Casey, B. Gestational Diabetes—On Broadening the Diagnosis. *N. Engl. J. Med.* **2021**, *384*, 965–966. [CrossRef]
7. HAPO Study Cooperative Research Group. Hyperglycemia and Adverse Pregnancy Outcome (HAPO) Study: Associations with neonatal anthropometrics. *Diabetes* **2009**, *58*, 453–459. [CrossRef]
8. Szmuilowicz, E.D.; Josefson, J.L.; Metzger, B.E. Gestational Diabetes Mellitus. *Endocrinol. Metab. Clin. N. Am.* **2019**, *48*, 479–493. [CrossRef]
9. Alexopoulos, A.S.; Blair, R.; Peters, A.L. Management of Preexisting Diabetes in Pregnancy: A Review. *JAMA* **2019**, *321*, 1811–1819. [CrossRef]
10. Balsells, M.; García-Patterson, A.; Gich, I.; Corcoy, R. Ultrasound-guided compared to conventional treatment in gestational diabetes leads to improved birthweight but more insulin treatment: Systematic review and meta-analysis. *Acta Obstet. Gynecol. Scand.* **2014**, *93*, 144–151. [CrossRef]
11. Staud, F.; Karahoda, R. Trophoblast: The central unit of fetal growth, protection and programming. *Int. J. Biochem. Cell Biol.* **2018**, *105*, 35–40. [CrossRef]
12. Godfrey, K.M.; Costello, P.M.; Lillycrop, K.A. Development, Epigenetics and Metabolic Programming. *Nestle Nutr. Inst. Workshop Ser.* **2016**, *85*, 71–80. [CrossRef] [PubMed]
13. Desoye, G.; Herrera, E. Adipose tissue development and lipid metabolism in the human fetus: The 2020 perspective focusing on maternal diabetes and obesity. *Prog. Lipid Res.* **2021**, *81*, 101082. [CrossRef] [PubMed]
14. Catalano, P.M.; Thomas, A.; Huston-Presley, L.; Amini, S.B. Increased fetal adiposity: A very sensitive marker of abnormal in utero development. *Am. J. Obstet. Gynecol.* **2003**, *189*, 1698–1704. [CrossRef] [PubMed]
15. Stanirowski, P.J.; Majewska, A.; Lipa, M.; Bomba-Opoń, D.; Wielgoś, M. Ultrasound evaluation of the fetal fat tissue, heart, liver and umbilical cord measurements in pregnancies complicated by gestational and type 1 diabetes mellitus: Potential application in the fetal birth-weight estimation and prediction of the fetal macrosomia. *Diabetol. Metab. Syndr.* **2021**, *13*, 22. [CrossRef] [PubMed]
16. de Santis, M.S.; Taricco, E.; Radaelli, T.; Spada, E.; Rigano, S.; Ferrazzi, E.; Milani, S.; Cetin, I. Growth of fetal lean mass and fetal fat mass in gestational diabetes. *Ultrasound Obstet. Gynecol.* **2010**, *36*, 328–337. [CrossRef]
17. Lingwood, B.E.; Henry, A.M.; d'Emden, M.C.; Fullerton, A.M.; Mortimer, R.H.; Colditz, P.B.; KA, L.C.; Callaway, L.K. Determinants of body fat in infants of women with gestational diabetes mellitus differ with fetal sex. *Diabetes Care* **2011**, *34*, 2581–2585. [CrossRef]
18. Elessawy, M.; Harders, C.; Kleinwechter, H.; Demandt, N.; Sheasha, G.A.; Maass, N.; Pecks, U.; Eckmann-Scholz, C. Measurement and evaluation of fetal fat layer in the prediction of fetal macrosomia in pregnancies complicated by gestational diabetes. *Arch. Gynecol. Obstet.* **2017**, *296*, 445–453. [CrossRef]
19. Orsso, C.E.; Silva, M.I.B.; Gonzalez, M.C.; Rubin, D.A.; Heymsfield, S.B.; Prado, C.M.; Haqq, A.M. Assessment of body composition in pediatric overweight and obesity: A systematic review of the reliability and validity of common techniques. *Obes. Rev.* **2020**, *21*, e13041. [CrossRef]
20. Sarno, L.; Neola, D.; Carbone, L.; Saccone, G.; Carlea, A.; Miceli, M.; Iorio, G.G.; Mappa, I.; Rizzo, G.; Girolamo, R.D.; et al. Use of artificial intelligence in obstetrics: Not quite ready for prime time. *Am. J. Obstet Gynecol. MFM* **2023**, *5*, 100792. [CrossRef]
21. Borboa-Olivares, H.; Rodríguez-Sibaja, M.J.; Espejel-Nuñez, A.; Flores-Pliego, A.; Mendoza-Ortega, J.; Camacho-Arroyo, I.; González-Camarena, R.; Echeverría-Arjonilla, J.C.; Estrada-Gutierrez, G. A Novel Predictive Machine Learning Model Integrating Cytokines in Cervical-Vaginal Mucus Increases the Prediction Rate for Preterm Birth. *Int. J. Mol. Sci.* **2023**, *24*, 13851. [CrossRef]
22. Ramakrishnan, R.; Rao, S.; He, J.R. Perinatal health predictors using artificial intelligence: A review. *Womens Health* **2021**, *17*, 17455065211046132. [CrossRef] [PubMed]
23. Markov, D. Tomographic ultrasound imaging (TUI)—Technique and methodological study. *Akush. Ginekol.* **2008**, *47*, 9–15.

24. National Academies of Sciences Engineering and Medicine. The National Academies Collection: Reports funded by National Institutes of Health. In *Weight Gain during Pregnancy: Reexamining the Guidelines*; Rasmussen, K.M., Yaktine, A.L., Eds.; National Academies Press: Washington, DC, USA, 2009.
25. American Diabetes Association. 14. Management of Diabetes in Pregnancy: Standards of Medical Care in Diabetes-2020. *Diabetes Care* **2020**, *43*, S183–S192. [CrossRef] [PubMed]
26. Lee, W. Soft tissue assessment for fetal growth restriction. *Minerva Obstet. Gynecol.* **2021**, *73*, 442–452. [CrossRef]
27. Larciprete, G.; Valensise, H.; Vasapollo, B.; Novelli, G.P.; Parretti, E.; Altomare, F.; Di Pierro, G.; Menghini, S.; Barbati, G.; Mello, G.; et al. Fetal subcutaneous tissue thickness (SCTT) in healthy and gestational diabetic pregnancies. *Ultrasound Obstet. Gynecol.* **2003**, *22*, 591–597. [CrossRef]
28. Toro-Ramos, T.; Paley, C.; Pi-Sunyer, F.X.; Gallagher, D. Body composition during fetal development and infancy through the age of 5 years. *Eur. J. Clin. Nutr.* **2015**, *69*, 1279–1289. [CrossRef] [PubMed]
29. Venkataraman, H.; Ram, U.; Craik, S.; Arungunasekaran, A.; Seshadri, S.; Saravanan, P. Increased fetal adiposity prior to diagnosis of gestational diabetes in South Asians: More evidence for the 'thin-fat' baby. *Diabetologia* **2017**, *60*, 399–405. [CrossRef]
30. Herath, M.P.; Beckett, J.M.; Hills, A.P.; Byrne, N.M.; Ahuja, K.D.K. Gestational Diabetes Mellitus and Infant Adiposity at Birth: A Systematic Review and Meta-Analysis of Therapeutic Interventions. *J. Clin. Med.* **2021**, *10*, 835. [CrossRef]
31. Sacks, D.A. Fetal macrosomia and gestational diabetes: What's the problem? *Obstet. Gynecol.* **1993**, *81*, 775–781.
32. Ikenoue, S.; Kasuga, Y.; Endo, T.; Tanaka, M.; Ochiai, D. Newer Insights Into Fetal Growth and Body Composition. *Front. Endocrinol.* **2021**, *12*, 708767. [CrossRef] [PubMed]
33. Sato, N.; Miyasaka, N. Heterogeneity in fetal growth velocity. *Sci. Rep.* **2019**, *9*, 11304. [CrossRef] [PubMed]
34. Ikenoue, S.; Akiba, Y.; Endo, T.; Kasuga, Y.; Yakubo, K.; Ishii, R.; Tanaka, M.; Ochiai, D. Defining the Normal Growth Curve of Fetal Fractional Limb Volume in a Japanese Population. *J. Clin. Med.* **2021**, *10*, 485. [CrossRef] [PubMed]
35. Uthaya, S.; Bell, J.; Modi, N. Adipose tissue magnetic resonance imaging in the newborn. *Horm. Res.* **2004**, *62* (Suppl. 3), 143–148. [CrossRef] [PubMed]
36. De Lucia Rolfe, E.; Modi, N.; Uthaya, S.; Hughes, I.A.; Dunger, D.B.; Acerini, C.; Stolk, R.P.; Ong, K.K. Ultrasound estimates of visceral and subcutaneous-abdominal adipose tissues in infancy. *J. Obes.* **2013**, *2013*, 951954. [CrossRef]
37. Lobelo, F. Fetal programming and risk of metabolic syndrome: Prevention efforts for high-risk populations. *Pediatrics* **2005**, *116*, 519. [CrossRef]
38. Lee, W.; Balasubramaniam, M.; Deter, R.L.; Hassan, S.S.; Gotsch, F.; Kusanovic, J.P.; Gonçalves, L.F.; Romero, R. Fractional limb volume—a soft tissue parameter of fetal body composition: Validation, technical considerations and normal ranges during pregnancy. *Ultrasound Obstet. Gynecol.* **2009**, *33*, 427–440. [CrossRef] [PubMed]
39. Garcés, M.F.; Sanchez, E.; Cardona, L.F.; Simanca, E.L.; González, I.; Leal, L.G.; Mora, J.A.; Bedoya, A.; Alzate, J.P.; Sánchez, Á.Y.; et al. Maternal Serum Meteorin Levels and the Risk of Preeclampsia. *PLoS ONE* **2015**, *10*, e0131013. [CrossRef] [PubMed]
40. Monteiro, L.J.; Norman, J.E.; Rice, G.E.; Illanes, S.E. Fetal programming and gestational diabetes mellitus. *Placenta* **2016**, *48* (Suppl. 1), S54–S60. [CrossRef]
41. Rinaudo, P.; Wang, E. Fetal programming and metabolic syndrome. *Annu. Rev. Physiol.* **2012**, *74*, 107–130. [CrossRef]

Disclaimer/Publisher's Note: The statements, opinions and data contained in all publications are solely those of the individual author(s) and contributor(s) and not of MDPI and/or the editor(s). MDPI and/or the editor(s) disclaim responsibility for any injury to people or property resulting from any ideas, methods, instructions or products referred to in the content.

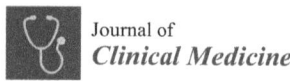

Article

Novel Three-Dimensional Body Scan Anthropometry versus MR-Pelvimetry for Vaginal Breech Delivery Assessment

Anne Dathan-Stumpf [1,*,†], Massimiliano Lia [1,†], Christof Meigen [2], Karoline Bornmann [1], Mireille Martin [3], Manuela Aßmann [2], Wieland Kiess [2,4] and Holger Stepan [1]

1. Department of Obstetrics, University Hospital Leipzig, 04103 Leipzig, Germany; massimiliano.lia@medizin.uni-leipzig.de (M.L.); karoline.bornmann@medizin.uni-leipzig.de (K.B.); holger.stepan@medizin.uni-leipzig.de (H.S.)
2. LIFE Leipzig Research Center for Civilization Diseases, University of Leipzig, 04103 Leipzig, Germany; christof.meigen@medizin.uni-leipzig.de (C.M.); manuela.assmann@medizin.uni-leipzig.de (M.A.); wieland.kiess@medizin.uni-leipzig.de (W.K.)
3. Department of Diagnostic and Interventional Radiology, University Hospital Leipzig, 04103 Leipzig, Germany; mireille.martin@medizin.uni-leipzig.de
4. Department of Pediatrics, University Hospital Leipzig, 04103 Leipzig, Germany
* Correspondence: anne.dathan-stumpf@medizin.uni-leipzig.de
† These authors contributed equally to this work.

Abstract: In this prospective, monocentric study, we investigated the potency of a novel three-dimensional (3D) body scanner for external pelvic assessment in birth planning for intended vaginal breech delivery. Between April 2021 and June 2022, 73 singleton pregnancies with intended vaginal birth from breech presentation (>36.0 weeks of gestation) were measured using a pelvimeter by Martin, a three-dimensional body scanner, and MR-pelvimetry. Measures were related to vaginal birth and intrapartum cesarean section. A total of 26 outer pelvic dimensions and 7 inner pelvic measurements were determined. The rate of successful vaginal breech delivery was 56.9%. The AUC (area under the curve) of the obstetric conjugate (OC) measured by MRI for predicting the primary outcome was 0.62 (OR 0.63; $p = 0.22$), adjusted for neonatal birth weight 0.66 (OR 0.60; $p = 0.19$). Of the 22 measured 3D body scanner values, the ratio of waist girth to maternal height showed the best prediction (AUC = 0.71; OR 1.27; $p = 0.015$). The best predictive pelvimeter value was the distantia spinarum with an AUC of 0.65 (OR = 0.80). The 3D body scanner technique is at least equal to predict successful vaginal breech delivery compared to MRI diagnostics. Further large-scale, prospective studies are needed to verify these results.

Keywords: breech delivery; birth planning; MR-pelvimetry; three-dimensional pelvimetry; body scan; obstetric conjugate

Citation: Dathan-Stumpf, A.; Lia, M.; Meigen, C.; Bornmann, K.; Martin, M.; Aßmann, M.; Kiess, W.; Stepan, H. Novel Three-Dimensional Body Scan Anthropometry versus MR-Pelvimetry for Vaginal Breech Delivery Assessment. *J. Clin. Med.* **2023**, *12*, 6181. https://doi.org/10.3390/jcm12196181

Academic Editors: Ulrich Gembruch, Florian Recker and Brigitte Strizek

Received: 23 August 2023
Revised: 21 September 2023
Accepted: 23 September 2023
Published: 25 September 2023

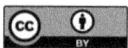

Copyright: © 2023 by the authors. Licensee MDPI, Basel, Switzerland. This article is an open access article distributed under the terms and conditions of the Creative Commons Attribution (CC BY) license (https://creativecommons.org/licenses/by/4.0/).

1. Introduction

The prevalence of fetal breech presentation around term is reported at 2–4% [1,2]. Since the Term Breech Trial, which showed significantly higher perinatal morbidity and mortality after vaginal birth [3], the planned cesarean section has been practiced internationally as the preferred mode of delivery [4], even though numerous studies have disproved the results of the Term Breech Trial [5–7] and the study itself was withdrawn due to methodological errors.

In Germany, a number of perinatal centers practice vaginal delivery from breech presentation. Although birth planning currently includes MR-pelvimetry in primiparous women with measurement of the obstetric conjugate (target > 12.0 cm) to detect a feto-pelvic disproportion, the role of MR-pelvimetry is unclear. Compared to women with a successful vaginal delivery, those with a cesarean section more frequently showed a lower value of the obstetric conjugate (OC) [8–11] and interspinous distance (ISD) [12]. Although some studies have shown that a higher OC is a predictive value for a successful vaginal birth from breech presentation, the predictive value of this parameter is conflicting.

Before MRI pelvimetry was established to determine the inner pelvic distances, efforts were made to determine a possible feto-pelvic disproportion by measuring the outer pelvis. As a tool for pelvic measurement, the pelvimeter was used. The external conjugate minus 9 cm was used as an approximation for the Obstetric conjugate [13]. Although there are hardly studies on measuring the outer pelvis using the pelvimeter in literature, the determination of a single outer pelvic value seems to hardly allow any conclusions about a feto-pelvic disproportion [14].

Recently, the anthropometric measurement of the outer pelvis was investigated using three-dimensional (3D) camera technology to detect such a disproportion [15,16]. Especially in developing countries with poor infrastructural conditions and long distances to the next maternity hospital, it could be shown that this inexpensive, fast, and portable technology offers new possibilities in measuring pelvic anatomy and predicting a feto-pelvic imbalance. Compared to conventional manual anthropometry, measurement errors and inherent fluctuations can be significantly reduced and new parameters established [16].

Since 2011, as part of the LIFE-Child study [17,18], pregnant women have been measured three-dimensionally using eye-safe laser technology in a double-triangulation process [19]. This method offers the possibility to determine numerous defined body circumferences, distances, and ratios automatically and non-invasively within a few seconds.

So far, there are no studies on the 3D body scan in pregnant women or the correlation between three-dimensional external pelvic measurements and MR-pelvimetry. The aim of the study was to investigate whether outer measurements of the pelvis, using the pelvimeter and 3D body scanner, are related to MRI measures. Secondly, we wanted to answer the question of whether 3D body scan measurements are superior to MR-pelvimetry and can be used to predict a successful vaginal breech delivery.

2. Materials and Methods

2.1. Study Population and Design

We conducted a prospective single-center study in a purely Caucasian, Central European cohort. Between April 2021 and June 2022, mainly primiparous women with a singleton pregnancy and persistent breech presentation at >36.0 weeks of gestation were recruited for the study during their birth planning visit at the University Hospital Leipzig. Patients with a medical indication for a planned cesarean section (severe fetal malformations, gestational age ≤ 36.0 weeks of pregnancy, estimated birth weight below 2500 g or above 4000 g) were also excluded.

After recruitment, the three examination methods of inner (MR-pelvimetry) and outer pelvic measuring (pelvimeter, 3D body scan) were carried out with a maximum interval of 5 days.

In addition to the anthropometric examinations of the pelvis, the following data were recorded: Maternal age, BMI at the time of the MR-pelvimetry, gestational age at the time of the MRI examination, parity, delivery mode, need for maneuvers in a vaginal delivery, reason for cesarean, gestational age at delivery, pH-value, APGAR score after 1/5/10 min, and neonatal birth weight and sex. Information on maternal height and weight before pregnancy was taken from the maternity booklet.

Studies on humans are carried out in accordance with the Declaration of Helsinki (1975). The study was approved by the Ethical Committee of the University of Leipzig (reference number: 086/21-ek; IRB00001750, date of approval: 16 March 2021). Additionally, appropriate written informed consent was obtained from all patients included in this study.

2.2. Pelvimeter

A pelvimeter by Martin was used for manual outer pelvimetry. The following measurements were recorded: *Distantia spinarum* (distance between the two spinae iliacae anteriores superiores), *Distantia cristarum* (farthest distance between the two cristae iliacae), *Distantia trochanterica* (distance between the two greater trochanters), and *External Conjugate* (distance from the upper edge of the symphysis to the processus spinosus of the 5th lumbar vertebra, corresponds to the top point of the Michaelic rhombus). To minimize interpersonal measurement errors, the measurement of the pelvis with the pelvimeter was exclusively carried out by two midwives.

2.3. Magnetic Resonance Imaging (MR) Pelvimetry

At the University Hospital Leipzig, MR-pelvimetry is part of the standard clinical procedure in planning delivery from breech presentation. The primary target parameter is the Obstetric conjugate (OC, sagittal distance between the dorsal edge of the promontorium and the dorsal surface of the symphysis, target > 12.0 cm). Secondary target measures were pelvic width (PW, sagittal distance between the dorsal surface of the pubic symphysis and the middle of the 3rd sacral vertebrae), sacral pelvic outlet diameter (SOD, sagittal distance between the inferior border of the pubic symphysis and sacroiliac joint), coccygeal-pelvic outlet (CPO, sagittal distance from the coccyx tip to the inferior border of the pubic symphysis), interspinous distance (ISD, distance between the sciatic spines), and intertuberous distance (ITD, distance between the two sciatic tubes) [12].

The MRI examination takes place between the 36th and 38th weeks of gestation (wog) using a 1.5-T-MRI system (Symphonie, Siemens Healthcare, Erlangen, Germany) in the supine position. A T2-weighted single-shot turbo spin-echo sequence (HASTE) is used for the sagittal section, and a T1-weighted spin-echo sequence (SE) is used for the axial section. The slice thickness in both sequences is 5 mm. Special patient preparation and administration of contrast media are not necessary.

The evaluation of the MR-pelvimetry was carried out by two senior physicians from the Department of Diagnostic and Interventional Radiology, University Hospital Leipzig.

2.4. Three-Dimensional (3D) Body Scan

The 3D body scan anthropometry was performed with the Vitus Smart 3D scanner from Vitronic [19]. Using eye-safe laser technology, three-dimensional images are designed within a few seconds in a double-triangulation process. The images are generated in AnthroScan 2.9.9 software, which, like the scanner itself, conforms to the international standard ISO 20685 [20]. The images can also be edited in the software. Measurement planes can be corrected and supplemented as required.

With a resolution of 1 mm, an average of 350,000 points are recorded per scan. A total of 22 potentially relevant body scanner values were analyzed. The exact designation and schematic representation of the automatically generated body scanner measurement values are shown in Table S1. In addition, it is possible to define certain points even more precisely using marking points. For a better evaluation of the measurement planes and comparability of the body scanner measurements with the pelvimeter, the following bone structures were marked with validated "marking points" from the Institute for Applied Training Sciences Leipzig (IAT): Both spinae iliacae anteriores superiores, the highest points of the cristae iliacae, trochanteres majores, the midpoint of the upper edge of the symphysis, and the 5th lumbar vertebra (upper point of Michaelic rhombus). The marking points (diameter of approximately 1 × 1 cm) were glued to the skin over the corresponding bone structures. The marking of the bone structures and measurement in the body scanner were primarily carried out by two employees in order to keep interpersonal bias to a minimum. The values of the external conjugate, distantia spinarum, distantia intercristarum, distantia trochanterica, and the distance crista to trochanter major on the right side were generated as additional variables and subsequently measured with the help of the marking points. There is a deviation in case numbers of the body scanner data, since three automatically generated datasets were missing values, while the additional measurements generated via the marking points could be measured.

The measurement in the body scanner was carried out while standing in an upright position with a foot closure approximately 5–10 cm open. The arms were spread out to the sides of the body (Figure 1). For the measurement, the pregnant woman only wore light-colored, tight-fitting underwear.

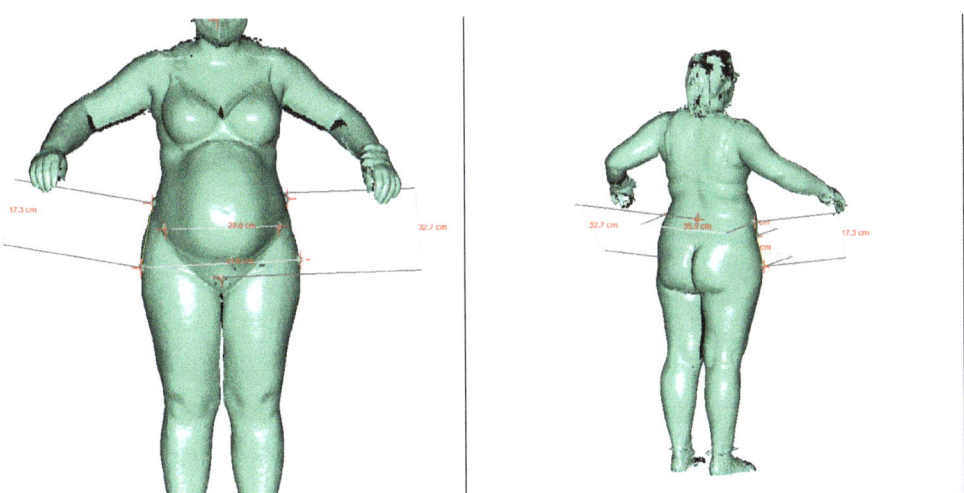

Figure 1. Example images of a measurement in the 3D body scanner from the front and side rear view.

The measurement in the body scanner was carried out while standing in an upright position with a slightly open footrest. The arms were spread out to the sides of the body. The red crosses are located in the center of the additionally glued marking points above the bony structures. Thus, the additional measurement values of the external conjugate, distantia spinarum, distantia intercristarum, distantia trochanterica, and the distance crista to trochanter major (right) could be determined.

2.5. Statistical Analysis

The main dependent variable and primary outcome was intrapartum cesarean section. The independent variables were selected based on the results of previous literature [8,9,12] and included all measures performed by the body scanner, as it was the main aim of the study to explore its clinical value. Different logistic regression models were built for the prediction of intrapartum cesarean section in our cohort. A descriptive analysis of the independent variables was performed and is presented in Tables 1 and 2. Continuous variables are presented as medians with interquartile ranges and categorical variables are presented as frequencies (%). The Mann–Whitney U test was used to compare continuous variables and the chi-square test for categorical variables. Univariable analysis was used to identify independent variables with an association with the primary outcome and were considered for inclusion in the multivariable logistic models. Since the number of the whole cohort and the events (intrapartum cesarean section) were limited, a maximum of two variables were included in these logistic models. Due to multiple model tests, adjusted *p*-values according to the false discovery rate by Benjamini–Hochberg were additionally indicated. Odds ratios (ORs) were obtained from the logistic regression analysis. The diagnostic accuracy of each model was assessed through sensitivity, specificity, receiver-operating characteristics (ROC) curves, and the area under the ROC curve (AUC) with a 95% CI. Paired ROC curves were compared by the DeLong method, and the reference was the ROC of the OC [21].

Table 1. Characteristics of the overall study cohort (N = 73), including the 10 pregnant women where the fetus turned spontaneously into a vertex position after the 36th week of gestation.

Character		N	%
Parity	0	68	93.2
	1	4	5.5
	2	1	1.4
Presentation	vertex	10	13.7
	breech	63	86.3
Delivery mode	vaginal	37	50.7
	planned (primary) cesarean	12	16.4
	Intrapartum (secondary) cesarean	24	32.9
Reason for cesarean	obstetric conjugate < 12.0 cm	12	34.3
	fetal estimated weight < 2500 g or >4000 g	1	2.9
	pathological CTG	3	8.6
	birth arrest	8	22.9
	difficult birth position	3	8.6
	maternal wish	5	14.3
	others	3	8.6

Shown are different study characteristics for the total cohort. Five women had a cesarean section in the previous pregnancy and therefore underwent birth planning with an MRI pelvimetry. Two of ten women with fetus in vertex presentation received an intrapartum cesarean section. In one case, the reason for intrapartum cesarean section (vertex presentation) could not be determined as birth took place in another hospital. N, number.

The statistical software package R (Version 4.1.0) [22] and the IBM Statistical Package for Social Sciences (IBM SPSS V.27) were used for data analysis and creation of graphics.

3. Results

3.1. Study Population

A total of 78 patients with a singleton pregnancy in breech presentation were recruited during the study period. Five of the included patients subsequently withdrew their consent or decided to undergo a planned cesarean section. After excluding 10 pregnant women where the fetus turned spontaneously into a vertex position after the 36th week of gestation and 12 planned cesareans (partly giving birth in external hospitals), a total of 51 patients were finally included in the analysis (Figure 2). The percentage of successful vaginal births from the breech presentation was 56.9%. Table 1 summarizes the examination characteristics of the total cohort.

The recruitment rate during the study period was almost 86% (78/91). After excluding deliveries from vertex positions and planned cesareans, a total of 51 patients were included in the analysis.

A total of five women had cesarean sections in previous pregnancies (one woman had two previous cesarean sections). Since these women have never given birth vaginally, they are treated as nulliparous according to hospital standards and undergo normal birth planning with MRI pelvimetry.

All women with an OC < 12.0 cm decided on planned cesarean section. The leading reason for an intrapartum cesarean section was birth arrest (22.9%). One patient who appeared suitable for vaginal delivery at the time of birth planning showed a macrosomic fetus estimated over 4000 g during labor, therefore a cesarean section was indicated.

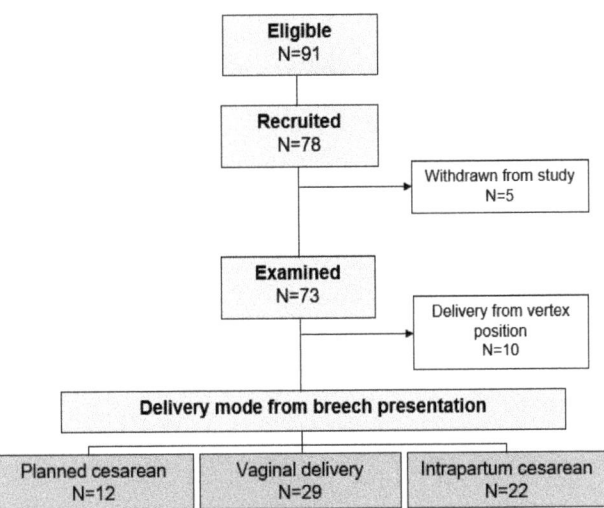

Figure 2. Presentation of the study cohort.

The mean gestational age at delivery was 39.4 wog. All children were born at term (>37.0 wog). On average, the measurements of the outer and inner pelvis were carried out in the 36.5 wog. With regard to the time of the outer and internal pelvic measurement, time of delivery, and neonatal birth weight, the two groups of successful vaginal breech delivery (N = 29) and intrapartum cesarean section (N = 22) were completely comparable. Also, the rate of epidural anesthesia did not differ significantly between the two delivery modes (vaginal delivery 62.1% (18/29), intrapartum cesarean section 59.1% (13/22), p = 0.83). The rate of obstetric maneuvers was 44.8% (13/29). As described before [23], neonates after intrapartum cesarean section showed significantly better pH values, but no differences could be found with regard to the 5 min APGAR scores (Table 2).

Table 2. Results of the outer and inner pelvic measurement.

Variables		Vaginal Delivery from Breech					Intrapartum (Secondary) Cesarean					p-Value	adj. p-Value
		N	Mean	SD	Median	95% CI	N	Mean	SD	Median	95% CI		
	gestational age at pelvimetry [weeks]	29	36.6	0.8	37.1	36.5; 37.1	22	36.6	0.5	37.0	36.5; 37.0	0.85	0.88
	BMI [kg/m²] before pregnancy	25	21.9	2.9	21.4	20.8; 23.0	22	23.1	3.4	22.2	21.6; 24.6	0.14	0.58
	BMI [kg/m²] at diagnostics	25	26.7	3.3	25.8	25.4; 28.1	22	28.7	3.9	28.6	27.1; 30.4	0.03	0.41
	BMI gain [kg/m²]	25	4.6	1.2	4.6	4.1; 5.1	22	5.7	1.7	5.8	4.9; 6.4	<0.001	0.04
MR pelvimetry	obstetrical conjugate [cm]	29	13.1	0.7	12.9	12.86; 13.36	22	12.8	0.9	12.8	12.45; 13.25	0.15	0.57
	pelvic width [cm]	29	13.8	0.9	13.9	13.49; 14.20	22	13.5	0.9	13.3	13.12; 13.92	0.28	0.55
	pelvic constriction [cm]	29	11.7	1.1	11.7	11.28; 12.13	22	12.0	0.8	12.1	11.65; 12.33	0.36	0.59
	sacral pelvic outlet diameter [cm]	29	13.6	0.7	13.7	13.36; 13.87	22	13.4	0.9	13.4	12.99; 13.79	0.31	0.56
	coccygeal-pelvic outlet [cm]	29	8.6	1.1	8.6	8.15; 8.96	22	8.7	0.9	8.7	8.32; 9.10	0.99	0.99
	interspinous distance [cm]	29	11.2	0.7	11.3	10.91; 11.47	22	10.9	1.0	11.0	10.46; 11.31	0.13	0.58
	intertuberous distance [cm]	29	14.3	1.1	14.2	13.93; 14.74	22	13.9	1.4	14.2	13.23; 14.51	0.36	0.57
Pelvimeter	external conjugate [cm]	29	23.9	2.2	24.0	23.01; 24.71	21	23.6	2.3	24.0	22.52; 24.61	0.76	0.92
	distantia spinarum [cm]	29	24.3	1.8	25.0	23.67; 25.02	21	23.7	1.6	24.0	22.98; 24.43	0.07	0.61
	distantia intercristarum [cm]	29	27.8	1.6	28.0	27.15; 28.37	21	28.0	2.5	27.5	26.83; 29.10	0.86	0.63
	distantia trochanterica [cm]	29	33.2	2.3	33.0	32.28; 34.06	20	33.1	2.6	32.1	31.85; 34.30	0.58	0.79

Table 2. Cont.

Variables		Vaginal Delivery from Breech					Intrapartum (Secondary) Cesarean				p-Value	adj. p-Value
		N	Mean	SD	Median	95% CI	N	Mean	SD	Median	95% CI		
3D bodyscan	waist to high hip back (5070) [cm]	25	7.7	1.5	7.6	1.06; 8.32	22	7.1	1.5	7.4	6.47; 7.83	0.25	0.55
	distance waistband to high hip back (5075) [cm]	25	4.1	2.7	4.0	2.95; 5.15	22	4.2	1.9	4.2	3.33; 4.97	0.89	0.94
	waist to buttock (5080) [cm]	25	21.7	1.6	21.7	21.02; 22.31	22	21.2	1.7	21.1	20.50; 21.97	0.34	0.58
	distance waistband to buttock (5085) [cm]	25	17.3	2.9	17.3	16.12; 18.48	22	17.2	2.0	17.2	16.31; 18.10	0.86	0.93
	scrotch length, rear (6012) [cm]	25	42.9	2.8	42.6	41.74; 44.01	22	43.1	2.6	42.7	41.98; 44.25	0.82	0.96
	scotch length at waistband (6015) [cm]	25	69.9	10.4	70.4	65.65; 74.24	22	72.7	10.1	74.9	68.27; 77.21	0.27	0.56
	waist girth (6510) [cm]	25	98.8	7.1	97.6	95.90; 101.73	22	102.5	6.8	103.7	99.49; 105.51	0.06	0.61
	middle hip (6512) [cm]	25	110.8	9.0	107.9	107.12; 114.56	22	113.8	8.7	114.7	109.99; 117.71	0.19	0.57
	waist band (6520) [cm]	25	103.6	7.2	102.2	100.66; 106.59	22	106.0	7.0	106.4	102.86; 109.11	0.23	0.53
	waist to buttock high right (7011) [cm]	25	21.4	1.6	20.9	20.71; 22.10	22	20.6	1.6	20.8	19.93; 21.34	0.19	0.65
	waistband to buttock hight right (7016) [cm]	25	15.0	3.5	16.0	13.54; 16.43	22	15.2	2.8	15.4	13.93; 16.42	0.90	0.92
	waist to hip right (7021) [cm]	25	36.1	2.0	36.0	35.26; 36.90	22	35.5	1.9	35.3	34.63; 36.31	0.31	0.57
	high hip girth (7510) [cm]	25	109.4	7.8	107.3	106.16; 112.60	22	112.2	8.2	112.7	108.61; 115.87	0.21	0.51
	buttock girth (7520) [cm]	25	109.4	9.5	107.2	105.51; 113.38	22	110.9	9.5	112.0	106.68; 115.13	0.52	0.73
	hip girth (7525) [cm]	25	110.5	9.8	108.5	106.42; 114.50	22	112.1	9.4	112.7	107.90; 116.28	0.48	0.70
	belly circumference (7540) [cm]	25	107.8	7.3	105.9	104.79; 110.82	22	110.6	7.8	111.0	107.10; 114.00	0.20	0.56
	maximum belly circumference (7545) [cm]	25	108.7	7.6	106.4	105.61; 111.88	22	111.6	8.0	111.9	108.10; 115.17	0.19	0.60
	external conjugate [cm]	26	29.3	2.5	28.7	28.25; 30.27	22	30.0	2.1	29.9	29.08; 30.98	0.09	0.59
	distantia spinarum [cm]	26	27.5	2.4	27.7	26.53; 28.44	22	27.3	2.1	27.0	26.42; 28.26	0.74	0.92
	distantia intercristarum [cm]	26	33.7	2.7	33.5	32.60; 34.75	22	34.6	2.8	34.8	33.32; 35.82	0.12	0.63
	distantia trochanterica [cm]	26	39.0	3.3	38.6	23.70; 30.35	22	38.9	3.7	38.4	27.25; 40.49	0.72	0.92
	distance crista to trochanter (right) [cm]	26	19.9	3.2	19.4	18.56; 21.16	22	18.7	3.7	17.7	17.08; 20.33	0.09	0.55
delivery	gestational age at delivery [weeks]	29	39.4	0.9	39.5	39.1; 39.6	22	39.5	1.2	40.0	39.1; 40.1	0.67	0.88
	birth weight [g]	28	3323.8	385.1	3270.0	3177.3; 3470.3	22	3397.5	262.6	3375.0	3281.1; 3513.9	0.21	0.54
	pH value	28	7.19	0.07	7.19	7.16; 7.22	22	7.25	0.10	7.27	7.21; 7.30	**0.005**	0.09
	APGAR score 5 min	28	9.2	0.7	9.0	8.9; 9.5	22	9.3	1.1	10.0	8.8; 9.8	0.41	0.62

Shown are the three different methods of inner and outer pelvis measuring, divided by delivery mode. Due to the small number of cases, the medians are given in addition to the mean values. Differences between the two different delivery modes were calculated using the Mann–Whitney U-test. A p-value < 0.05 was considered as significant and are shown in bold. Due to multiple model tests, the false discovery rate-adjusted p-values according to Benjamini–Hochberg are also given. The numbers in brackets behind the body scanner values correspond to the description from the measurement value catalog (Supplementary Materials). 5′ APGAR-value, Appearance-Pulse-Grimace-Activity-Respiration value 5 min after delivery; 95% CI, 95%-confidence interval; adj. p-value, adjusted p-value according Benjamini-Hochberg; BMI, Body-Mass-Index; max, maximum; min, minimum; N, number; SD, standard deviation.

3.2. Outer and Inner Measurement of the Pelvis and BMI Gain

Table S2 summarizes all of the inner and outer pelvic measurements for the total cohort, including the pregnancies with planned cesarean and vertex presentation. Table 2 shows the same table for the 51 included subjects, subdivided according to the delivery mode in 'successful vaginal delivery from a breech presentation' versus 'intrapartum cesarean section'. No significant difference between the two delivery modes could be shown for any of the measured values in the MR-pelvimetry, the external measurement with the pelvimeter, or the 3D body scan anthropometry (Table 2). A trend could be shown for the 3D anthropometry of the waist girth ($p = 0.059$): Women with successful vaginal delivery had a mean girth of 98.8 cm (median 97.6 cm) compared to women with an intrapartum cesarean section of 102.5 cm (median 103.7 cm). Notably, when waist circumference was related to the woman's height, this ratio was found to be significantly different between the two subgroups (0.58 ± 0.03 versus 0.61 ± 0.04, $p = 0.014$).

The two methods for measuring the outer pelvis using the pelvimeter and 3D body scanner showed, despite the additional marking points in the body scanner, large differences. Nevertheless, both methods showed significant dependencies for the external conjugate ($p = 0.002$), distantia spinarum ($p < 0.001$), and distantia trochanterica ($p < 0.001$) in the linear regression analysis, and the adjustment for the maternal BMI at the time of the measurement showed no influence.

The two subgroups of delivery mode differed significantly in terms of BMI gain during pregnancy. While the mean BMI gain in the group of vaginal births was 4.6 kg/m^2, the women with an intrapartum cesarean gained an average of 5.6 kg/m^2 ($p < 0.001$, adj. $p = 0.04$).

Figure 3 shows the relationship between BMI gain during pregnancy (kg/m^2) and the probability of a cesarean section. The graphic clearly shows a rapid increase in the probability of a cesarean section if the BMI gain is 5 kg/m^2.

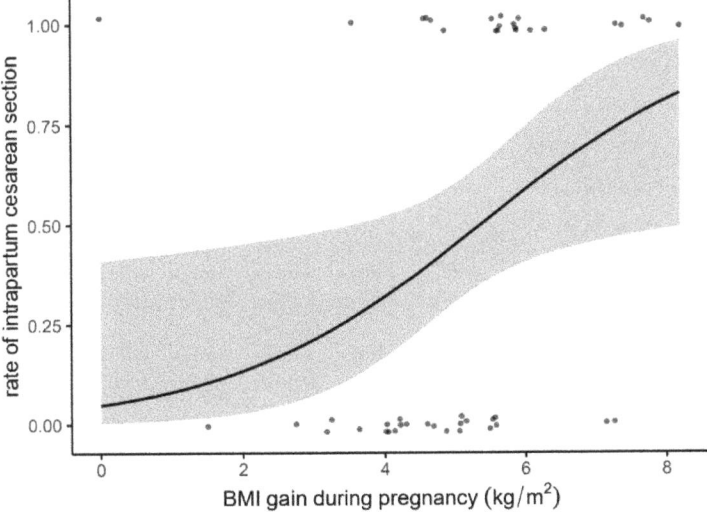

Figure 3. Presentation of the relation between BMI gain during pregnancy (kg/m^2) and probability for an intrapartum cesarean section by a regression line (black).

The gray area shows the 95% confidence interval. The points below the regression curve indicate successful vaginal births from a breech presentation, the points above the curve indicate women with an intrapartum cesarean section. Small random variation has been added to the dots in order to avoid overplotting and improve visualization. Women with a successful vaginal delivery from breech presentation showed a significantly lower BMI gain during pregnancy compared to women with intrapartum cesarean (mean 4.6 kg/m^2 versus 5.7 kg/m^2, $p < 0.001$).

3.3. Predictive Value of the Different Models

In the prediction of an intrapartum cesarean section, the obstetric conjugate showed an AUC of 0.62 (OR of 0.62, $p = 0.22$). Adjusted for neonatal birth weight the AUC was 0.66 (Table 3). Of the classic pelvic dimensions determined by the pelvimeter, the distantia spinarum showed the best prediction for the primary endpoint (AUC = 0.65, OR 0.80). The historical measure of the external conjugate minus 9 cm [13] showed the worst prediction of all represented models in Table 3 (AUC = 0.53, OR = 0.94). Significance was not found for any of these regression analyses (Table 3). In total, of the 22 analyzed body scanner measurements, the ratio of waist girth to maternal height showed the best discrimination with an AUC of 0.71 (OR 1.27, p = 0.015). However, the overall best prediction for the primary endpoint was achieved with the model of BMI gain during pregnancy (AUC = 0.79). With rising BMI gain, there was a significant increase in the odds of a cesarean section by a factor of 1.27 (p = 0.026).

Table 3. Logistic regression model for predicting a secondary cesarean section.

Independent Variable	Regr. Coefficient	95% CI		p-Value	OR	AUC	DeLong 1	DeLong 2
obstetric conjugate (MRI) [cm]	−0.47	0.29	1.33	0.22	0.63	0.62	Ref.	0.33
adj. obstetric conjugate * [cm]	−0.52	0.28	1.28	0.19	0.60	0.66		
interspinous distance (MRI) [cm]	−0.45	0.32	1.28	0.20	0.64	0.63		
external conjugate—9 cm [cm]	−0.06	0.73	1.22	0.64	0.94	0.53	0.33	Ref.
waist girth (body scan) [cm]	0.08	0.99	1.18	0.08	1.08	0.66	0.92	0.032
waist girth/body height (body scan)	0.24	1.05	1.55	0.015	1.27	0.71	0.35	0.013
adj. external conjugate # (body scan) [cm]	0.23	0.94	1.67	0.12	1.26	0.67		
distantia spinarum (pelvimeter) [cm]	−0.22	0.57	1.12	0.20	0.80	0.65	0.80	0.15
BMI gain during pregnancy [kg/m^2]	0.55	1.07	2.83	0.026	1.74	0.79	0.13	0.007

* Adjusted for neonatal birth weight; # adjusted for maternal hight. Shown are the predictive models for the primary endpoint of an intrapartum cesarean section. Identified independent variables of the three inner and outer pelvic measurements with a p-value of <0.15 in the univariate regression analysis were chosen for the multivariate logistic regression analysis. In total, the best predictive model was achieved using the BMI gain. A p-value < 0.05 was considered as significant. In prediction of the primary endpoint, all models were equivalent to the OC (DeLong 1). 95% CI, 95%-confidence interval; AUC, area under the curve; OR, Odds ratio; Ref., reference; Regr. Coefficient, Regression coefficient ß.

The models of the best predictive values of the three different examination methods of the inner and outer pelvis as well as the historical measure of the external conjugate minus 9 cm and the obstetric conjugate as a reference are shown as ROC curves in Figure 4.

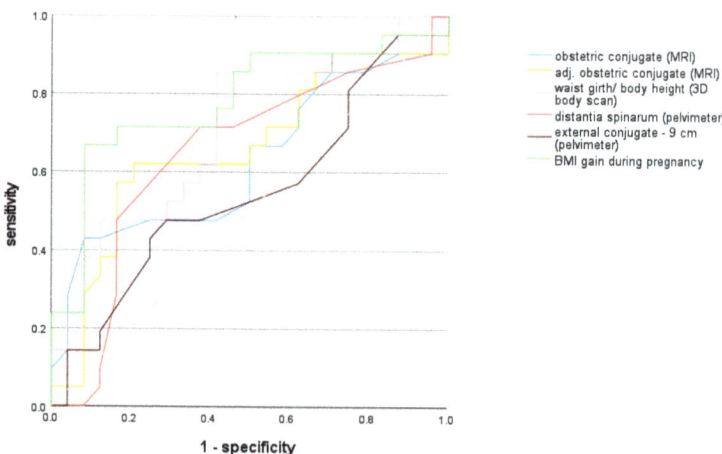

Figure 4. Presentation of the ROC curves with prediction of an intrapartum (secondary) cesarean section.

Shown are the best predictive values of the three different examination methods of the inner and outer pelvis as well as the historical measure of the external conjugate minus 9 cm. The diagonal reference line is shown in grey.

However, in paired comparisons of the ROC curves according to the DeLong method, each with the clinically relevant reference measure of the obstetric conjugate, no significant differences were found (Table 3).

The prediction models of waist girth ($p = 0.032$) and waist girth to height ($p = 0.013$) showed a significantly better prediction of the primary endpoint compared to the historical measure, while no difference was found between the historical measure and the OC (DeLong 2, Table 3).

4. Discussion

This is the first study in pregnant women using both an innovative 3D body scan and MRI to take pelvic measures in women planning vaginal breech delivery. We were able to show that an inexpensive, non-invasive, and fast measurement of the outer pelvis can achieve an at least equivalent prediction of a successful vaginal breech delivery as the standard reference measure of the obstetric conjugate.

Intended vaginal breech delivery requires birth planning and a selection of suitable women. At the University Hospital Leipzig, like others, the nationally and internationally recommended requirements for a vaginal breech birth apply [24,25]. In addition, MR-pelvimetry is performed to determine the obstetric conjugate, as various studies have shown a successful vaginal birth with an OC of ≥ 12.0 cm [8–10]. Nevertheless, the benefit of MR-pelvimetry in the prediction of a successful vaginal delivery is unclear, especially since previous publications do not name any specific prediction values.

Klemt et al. found a significant difference in OC between vaginal breech delivery and intrapartum cesarean section with an aOR of 1.56 per additional cm for a successful vaginal birth [9]. This corresponds to an adjusted OR of 0.64 for the intrapartum cesarean section (1/1.56), which is similar to our findings (OR = 0.63). This is also confirmed by comparing the mean values for the OC between the two delivery modes [9]. Also, Hoffmann et al. were able to show the same mean values for the obstetric conjugates for the two modes of delivery. Their study also found no significance for the OC between vaginal birth and cesarean section in the regression analysis, which also confirms the results of our study [12]. Hoffmann et al. named the ISD, measured in the MR-pelvimetry, with an AUC of 0.67 as a significant predictor of a successful vaginal birth from breech presentation. In our study, the AUC of the ISD was 0.63, although no significance could be demonstrated.

To our knowledge, there is no study that investigates the prediction of successful vaginal breech birth using anthropometric 3D body scan measurements. According to a systematic review, the 3D scanner allows automated, quick, and easy measurements of different body tissues. According to the authors, the measurements appear to be reproducible, reliable, accurate, and correlate with other measurement techniques [26]. The idea of a pelvic assessment without MRI might be an attractive alternative if MRI is not available. Moreover, an anthropometric 3D body scan measurement is able to challenge traditional outer pelvic measures. Interestingly, despite the marking of the bone structures via marking points, there were significant length differences between the same outer pelvic dimensions, measured by the pelvimeter and the body scanner. This results from the fact that the pelvimeter is specifically placed on the bony structures and, thus, changes the skin level. The 3D body scanner only scans the skin surface. Therefore, the measurement of subcutaneous fat tissue was considered during study preparation in order to adjust the results later accordingly. However, due to the different intra-individual and inter-individual distribution of subcutaneous fat, the measurement was removed from the study protocol [27]. Nevertheless, it can be assumed that a comparison of conventional anthropometry (e.g., measurement of waist girth) and body scanner anthropometry would result in reliable, comparable values [26] even in pregnant women.

In summary, the results show the limited prediction of the OC measured in the MRI. We were able to show that equivalent prediction can be achieved by time-saving, cost-effective anthropometric measurements like the waist girth. In our opinion, the strength of MR-pelvimetry is not in predicting birth success from breech presentation. Rather, research suggests that determining the ITD using MRI can predict the duration of the active second stage of labor as well as the rate of obstetrical maneuvers [28].

A limitation of this study is certainly the small number of cases. This results partly from the unusually high rate of spontaneous versions into vertex position (13.7%). In the literature, the incidence for a spontaneous version from the 37th week of gestation is given as 6–9%, and in primiparous women, it is as high as 2.3% [29,30].

Further large-scale, prospective studies should be carried out to confirm the effect of the BMI gain during pregnancy as well as the influence of waist girth on the success of vaginal breech delivery.

5. Conclusions

The usefulness and benefit of measuring the OC with MR-pelvimetry in predicting the success of a vaginal breech delivery is controversial. In our study, we show evidence that anthropometric outer measures can also be obtained by the 3D body scan technique, which may be at least equivalent in predicting an intrapartum cesarean section to measurements of internal pelvic dimensions. Future studies have to show which methods of pelvic assessment are best to forecast successful vaginal breech delivery.

6. Contribution

What are the novel findings of this work?

For the first time, we were able to show that the relation of waist girth to maternal height, measured anthropometrically in an innovative 3D body scanner, is at least equivalent to the prediction to the current standard measure of the obstetric conjugate measured by MR-pelvimetry.

What are the clinical implications of this work?

Anthropometric 3D body scan measurement is able to challenge traditional outer pelvic measures and might be an attractive alternative in birth planning in vaginally intended breech deliveries if MRI is not available.

Supplementary Materials: The following supporting information can be downloaded at: https://www.mdpi.com/article/10.3390/jcm12196181/s1, Table S1: Catalog of the body scanner values used in the study; Table S2: Characteristics of the overall study population (N = 73), including delivery from vertex position as well as primary cesarean section.

Author Contributions: Conceptualization, A.D.-S., H.S. and W.K.; methodology, A.D.-S.; software, C.M.; validation, C.M., M.A., K.B. and M.L.; formal analysis, A.D.-S., C.M. and M.L.; investigation, M.A. and M.M.; resources, A.D.-S. and M.L.; data curation, A.D.-S. and M.L.; writing—original draft preparation, A.D.-S. and M.L.; writing—review and editing, H.S.; visualization, M.L., A.D.-S. and C.M.; supervision, H.S. and W.K.; project administration, A.D.-S.; funding acquisition, A.D.-S. All authors have read and agreed to the published version of the manuscript.

Funding: A.D.-S. received a research award for the study from the "Mitteldeutsche Gesellschaft für Frauenheilkunde und Geburtshilfe e.V./Middle German Society for Gynecology and Obstetrics e.V." (MGFG). The money was used to support the study.

Institutional Review Board Statement: The study was conducted according to the guidelines of the Declaration of Helsinki and approved by the Ethics Committee of the University of Leipzig (reference number: 086/21-ek; IRB00001750, date of approval: 16 March 2021).

Informed Consent Statement: Informed consent was obtained from all subjects involved in the study.

Data Availability Statement: The data that support the findings of this study are available upon request from the corresponding author. The data are not publicly available due to privacy or ethical restrictions.

Conflicts of Interest: The authors declare no conflict of interest.

Abbreviations

3D	three dimensional
CI	confidence interval
MR(I)	Magnetic resonance imaging
OC	Obstetric conjugate
OR	odds ratio
wog	weeks of gestation

References

1. Ford, J.B.; Roberts, C.L.; Nassar, N.; Giles, W.; Morris, J.M. Recurrence of breech presentation in consecutive pregnancies. *BJOG* **2010**, *117*, 830–836. [CrossRef] [PubMed]
2. Zsirai, L.; Csákány, G.M.; Vargha, P.; Fülöp, V.; Tabák, Á.G. Breech presentation: Its predictors and consequences. An analysis of the Hungarian Tauffer Obstetric Database (1996–2011). *Acta Obstet. Gynecol. Scand.* **2016**, *95*, 347–354. [CrossRef] [PubMed]
3. Hannah, M.E.; Hannah, W.J.; Hewson, S.A.; Hodnett, E.D.; Saigal, S.; Willan, A.R.; Term Breech Trial Collaborative Group. Planned caesarean section versus planned vaginal birth for breech presentation at term: A randomised multicentre trial. *Lancet* **2000**, *356*, 1375–1383. [CrossRef] [PubMed]
4. Vlemmix, F.; Bergenhenegouwen, L.; Schaaf, J.M.; Ensing, S.; Rosman, A.N.; Ravelli, A.C.J.; van der Post, J.A.M.; Verhoeven, A.; Visser, G.H.; Mol, B.W.J.; et al. Term breech deliveries in the Netherlands: Did the increased cesarean rate affect neonatal outcome? A population-based cohort study. *Acta Obstet. Gynecol. Scand.* **2014**, *93*, 888–896. [CrossRef]
5. Hruban, L.; Janků, P.; Ventruba, P.; Oškrdalová, L.; Skorkovská, K.; Hodická, Z.; Tápalová, V.; Mekiňová, L.; Smerek, M. Vaginal breech delivery after 36 week of pregnancy in a selected group of pregnancy—Analysis of perinatal results in years 2008–2011. *Ceska Gynekol.* **2014**, *79*, 343–349.
6. Alarab, M.; Regan, C.; O'Connell, M.P. Singleton vaginal breech delivery at term: Still a safe option. *Obstet. Gynecol.* **2004**, *103*, 407–412. [CrossRef]
7. Sentilhes, L.; Schmitz, T.; Azria, E.; Gallot, D.; Ducarme, G.; Korb, D.; Mattuizzi, A.; Parant, O.; Sananès, N.; Baumann, S.; et al. Breech presentation: Clinical practice guidelines from the French College of Gynaecologists and Obstetricians (CNGOF). *Eur. J. Obstet. Gynecol. Reprod. Biol.* **2020**, *252*, 599–604. [CrossRef]
8. Von Bismarck, A.; Ertl-Wagner, B.; Stöcklein, S.; Schöppe, F.; Hübener, C.; Hertlein, L.; Baron-Tomlinson, D.; Mahner, S.; Delius, M.; Hasbargen, U.; et al. MR Pelvimetry for Breech Presentation at Term- Interobserver Reliability, Incidental Findings and Reference Values. In *RöFo-Fortschritte auf dem Gebiet der Röntgenstrahlen und der Bildgebenden Verfahren*; Georg Thieme Verlag KG: Leipzig, Germany, 2019; Volume 191, pp. 424–432.
9. Klemt, A.-S.; Schulze, S.; Brüggmann, D.; Louwen, F. MRI-based pelvimetric measurements as predictors for a successful vaginal breech delivery in the Frankfurt Breech at term cohort (FRABAT). *Eur. J. Obstet. Gynecol. Reprod. Biol.* **2019**, *232*, 10–17. [CrossRef]
10. Franz, M.; von Bismarck, A.; Delius, M.; Ertl-Wagner, B.; Deppe, C.; Mahner, S.; Hasbargen, U.; Hübener, C. MR pelvimetry: Prognosis for successful vaginal delivery in patients with suspected fetopelvic disproportion or breech presentation at term. *Arch. Gynecol. Obstet.* **2017**, *295*, 351–359. [CrossRef]
11. Van Loon, A.J.; Mantingh, A.; Serlier, E.K.; Kroon, G.; Mooyaart, E.L.; Huisjes, H.J. Randomised controlled trial of magnetic-resonance pelvimetry in breech presentation at term. *Lancet* **1997**, *350*, 1799–1804. [CrossRef]
12. Hoffmann, J.; Thomassen, K.; Stumpp, P.; Grothoff, M.; Engel, C.; Kahn, T.; Stepan, H. New MRI Criteria for Successful Vaginal Breech Delivery in Primiparae. *PLoS ONE* **2016**, *11*, e0161028. [CrossRef] [PubMed]
13. Rath, W.; Gembruch, U.; Schmidt, S. (Eds.) Geburtshilfe und Perinatalmedizin: Pränataldiagnostik–Erkrankungen–Entbindung. In *Klinik der normalen Geburt und Praktisches Vorgehen (II)*, 2nd ed.; Thieme Verlag: Stuttgart, Germany; New York, NY, USA, 2010.
14. Hanzal, E.; Kainz, C.; Hoffmann, G.; Deutinger, J. An analysis of the prediction of cephalopelvic disproportion. *Arch. Gynecol. Obstet.* **1993**, *253*, 161–166. [CrossRef] [PubMed]
15. Tolentino, L.; Yigeremu, M.; Teklu, S.; Attia, S.; Weiler, M.; Frank, N.; Dixon, J.B.; Gleason, R.L. Three-dimensional camera anthropometry to assess risk of cephalopelvic disproportion-related obstructed labour in Ethiopia. *Interface Focus.* **2019**, *9*, 20190036. [CrossRef] [PubMed]
16. Gleason, R.L., Jr.; Yigeremu, M.; Debebe, T.; Teklu, S.; Zewdeneh, D.; Weiler, M.; Frank, N.; Tolentino, L.; Attia, S.; Dixon, J.B.; et al. A safe, low-cost, easy-to-use 3D camera platform to assess risk of obstructed labor due to cephalopelvic disproportion. *PLoS ONE* **2018**, *13*, e0203865. [CrossRef]
17. Poulain, T.; Baber, R.; Vogel, M.; Pietzner, D.; Kirsten, T.; Jurkutat, A.; Hiemisch, A.; Hilbert, A.; Kratzsch, J.; the LIFE Child study team; et al. The Life Child Study: A Population-Based Perinatal and Pediatric Cohort in Germany. *Eur. J. Epidemiol.* **2017**, *32*, 145–158. [CrossRef]
18. Quante, M.; Hesse, M.; Döhnert, M.; Fuchs, M.; Hirsch, C.; Sergeyev, E.; Casprzig, N.; Geserick, M.; Naumann, S.; Koch, C.; et al. The LIFE child study: A life course approach to disease and health. *BMC Public Health* **2012**, *12*, 1021. [CrossRef]
19. Maurer, M. VITUS 3D Body Scanner. In *Asian Workshop on 3D Body Scanning Technologies*; Vitronic GmbH: Wiesbaden, Germany, 2012; Available online: https://www.3dbodyscanning.org/cap/papers/A2012/a12009_08maurer.pdf (accessed on 24 May 2023).

20. Loeffler-Wirth, H.; Vogel, M.; Kirsten, T.; Glock, F.; Poulain, T.; Körner, A.; Loeffler, M.; Kiess, W.; Binder, H. Longitudinal anthropometry of children and adolescents using 3D-body scanning. *PLoS ONE* **2018**, *13*, e0203628. [CrossRef]
21. Steyerberg, E.W.; Vickers, A.J.; Cook, N.R.; Gerds, T.; Gonen, M.; Obuchowski, N.; Pencina, M.J.; Kattan, M.W. Assessing the performance of prediction models: A framework for traditional and novel measures. *Epidemiology* **2010**, *21*, 128–138. [CrossRef]
22. R Core Team. *A Language and Environment for Statistical Computing*; R. Foundation for Statistical Computing: Vienna, Austria, 2021; Available online: https://www.R-project.org/ (accessed on 10 December 2022).
23. Dathan-Stumpf, A.; Hausmann, C.; Thome, U.; Stepan, H. Neonatal admission rate after vaginal breech delivery. *J. Perinat. Med.* **2022**, *50*, 1248–1255. [CrossRef]
24. Kielland-Kaisen, U.; Paul, B.; Jennewein, L.; Klemt, A.; Möllmann, C.J.; Bock, N.; Schaarschmidt, W.; Brüggmann, D.; Louwen, F. Maternal and neonatal outcome after vaginal breech delivery of nulliparous versus multiparous women of singletons at term-A prospective evaluation of the Frankfurt breech at term cohort (FRABAT). *Eur. J. Obstet. Gynecol. Reprod. Biol.* **2020**, *252*, 583–587. [CrossRef]
25. Hofmeyr, G.J.; Hannah, M.; Lawrie, T.A. Planned caesarean section for term breech delivery. *Cochrane Database Syst. Rev.* **2015**, *2015*, CD000166. [CrossRef] [PubMed]
26. Rumbo-Rodríguez, L.; Sánchez-SanSegundo, M.; Ferrer-Cascales, R.; García-D'Urso, N.; Hurtado-Sánchez, J.A.; Zaragoza-Martí, A. Comparison of Body Scanner and Manual Anthropometric Measurements of Body Shape: A Systematic Review. *Int. J. Environ. Res. Public Health* **2021**, *18*, 6213. [CrossRef] [PubMed]
27. Siervogel, R.M.; Roche, A.F.; Himes, J.H.; Chumlea, W.C.; McCammon, R. Subcutaneous fat distribution in males and females from 1 to 39 years of age. *Am. J. Clin. Nutr.* **1982**, *36*, 162–171. [CrossRef] [PubMed]
28. Lia, M.; Martin, M.; Költzsch, E.; Stepan, H.; Dathan-Stumpf, A. Relation between MR pelvimetric measures, obstetrical maneuver rate, active stage of labor and neonatal outcome in vaginal breech deliveries. *Birth* **2023**, in press.
29. Ben-Meir, A.; Elram, T.; Tsafrir, A.; Elchalal, U.; Ezra, Y. The incidence of spontaneous version after failed external cephalic version. *Am. J. Obstet. Gynecol.* **2007**, *196*, 157.e1–157.e3. [CrossRef]
30. Ben-Arie, A.; Kogan, S.; Schachter, M.; Hagay, Z.J.; Insler, V. The impact of external cephalic version on the rate of vaginal and cesarean breech deliveries: A 3-year cumulative experience. *Eur. J. Obstet. Gynecol. Reprod. Biol.* **1995**, *63*, 125–129. [CrossRef]

Disclaimer/Publisher's Note: The statements, opinions and data contained in all publications are solely those of the individual author(s) and contributor(s) and not of MDPI and/or the editor(s). MDPI and/or the editor(s) disclaim responsibility for any injury to people or property resulting from any ideas, methods, instructions or products referred to in the content.

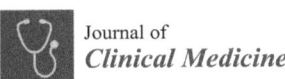 Journal of
Clinical Medicine

Article

Spectrum and Outcome of Prenatally Diagnosed Fetal Primary Cardiomyopathies—A Twenty-Year Overview

Adeline Walter [1,*], Elina Calite [1], Annegret Geipel [1], Brigitte Strizek [1], Florian Recker [1], Ulrike Herberg [2], Christoph Berg [1,3] and Ulrich Gembruch [1]

1. Department of Obstetrics and Prenatal Medicine, University of Bonn, 53127 Bonn, Germany; elina.calite@gmail.com (E.C.); annegret.geipel@ukbonn.de (A.G.); brigitte.strizek@ukbonn.de (B.S.); florian.recker@ukbonn.de (F.R.); prof.berg@icloud.com (C.B.); ulrich.gembruch@ukbonn.de (U.G.)
2. Department of Pediatric Cardiology, University Hospital RWTH Aachen, 52074 Aachen, Germany; uherberg@ukaachen.de
3. Division of Prenatal Medicine, Gynecological Ultrasound and Fetal Surgery, Department of Obstetrics and Gynecology, University of Cologne, 50937 Cologne, Germany
* Correspondence: adeline.walter@ukbonn.de

Abstract: Objective: to assess the course and outcome of fetuses affected by primary cardiomyopathy (CM). Methods: Retrospective study of 21 cases with prenatal diagnosis of a primary CM in one tertiary center over a period of 20 years. Charts were reviewed for echocardiographic findings, pregnancy outcome, and postnatal course. The utility of prenatal evaluation was discussed. Results: The mean gestational age (GA) at diagnosis was 26.7 (±5.1) weeks. A total of 33.3% (7/21) had associated anomalies. Genetic etiology was confirmed in 50.0% (10/20, with one case lost to follow up). The overall survival rate of the entire study population was 40% (8/20) including termination of pregnancy in 20% (4/20) and an intrauterine mortality rate of 5% (1/20). Of the initial survivors ($n = 15$), a neonatal and early infant mortality rate of 46.7% (7/15) was calculated. Prenatal isolated right ventricular involvement was the only identified significant parameter for survival ($p = 0.035$). Four phenotypical groups were identified: 42.9% (9/21) hypertrophic (HCM), 38.1% (8/21) dilated (DCM), 14.3% (3/21) isolated noncompaction (NCCM), and 4.8% (1/21) restrictive CM (RCM). Fetuses assigned to isolated NCCM revealed a 100% survival rate. Conclusion: Prenatal detection is feasible but needs to a introduce classification method for better consulting and management practices. A poor outcome is still observed in many cases, but an increase in examiners' awareness may influence optimal multispecialized care.

Keywords: primary fetal cardiomyopathy; cardiomyopathies; cardiomegaly; fetal echocardiography; prenatal diagnosis

Citation: Walter, A.; Calite, E.; Geipel, A.; Strizek, B.; Recker, F.; Herberg, U.; Berg, C.; Gembruch, U. Spectrum and Outcome of Prenatally Diagnosed Fetal Primary Cardiomyopathies—A Twenty-Year Overview. *J. Clin. Med.* **2023**, *12*, 4366. https://doi.org/10.3390/jcm12134366

Academic Editor: Erich Cosmi

Received: 16 May 2023
Revised: 22 June 2023
Accepted: 23 June 2023
Published: 28 June 2023

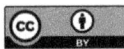

Copyright: © 2023 by the authors. Licensee MDPI, Basel, Switzerland. This article is an open access article distributed under the terms and conditions of the Creative Commons Attribution (CC BY) license (https://creativecommons.org/licenses/by/4.0/).

1. Introduction

Primary cardiomyopathies (CMs) correspond to an important and heterogeneous group of myocardial disorders, which solely or predominantly target the myocardium and affect cardiac filling, contraction, or both [1]. Rarely seen prenatally, they occur as late onset anomalies and account for approximately 2–2.5% of all congenital heart diseases [2,3]. Fetal and neonatal outcomes are extremely poor, with a reported perinatal mortality rate of up to 50–82%, continuing into the neonatal period, with primary CMs being the most common cause of cardiac transplantation in childhood [4–7].

Fetal echocardiography remains the main diagnostic tool in prenatal diagnosis of primary CMs [7]. Based on clinical and anatomical presentation, categorization is most commonly performed into dilated (DCM), hypertrophic (HCM), and restrictive (RCM) cardiomyopathy and might be subdivided into isolated noncompaction cardiomyopathy (NCCM), as published data demonstrated its feasibility in prenatal echocardiographic detection [1,7–11]. Grouping different phenotypes is used to define the underlying cause, which is a significant determinant of neonatal outcome [5]. Clinical presentation, however, is highly variable and fetuses may have perinatal demise in almost one third of affected cases, or may present severe postnatal cardiac failure, or be born with a relatively benign neonatal course with a potential for recurrence [5,12]. Albeit unfavorable, echocardiographic predictors for an intrauterine demise have been defined; previously published data, limited to small study populations and heterogeneous cohorts, have failed to evaluate prognostic criteria for a tailored approach to intrauterine guidance on outcome [5–8].

With contradictory results, consulting and impact on management strategies has to be re-evaluated, especially as rapid increase in clinically available genetic testing facilitated confirmation of an identifiable genetic etiology in 40–80% of neonatal primary CMs, suggesting that not only the demand for prenatal counselling with a known family history will increase in significance, but also that suspecting prenatal primary CM should include targeted screening of the extended family and recurrence-risk counseling for subsequent pregnancies [7,13].

We provided an overview of fetuses diagnosed with primary CM at our center. Prenatal diagnosis was correlated for postnatal course and outcomes were compared to other published data. The utility of prenatal evaluation was discussed.

2. Materials and Methods

2.1. Patients

All cases with a prenatal diagnosis of fetal primary cardiomyopathy (PCM), detected in a 20 years period (2001 to 2021) in a tertiary referral center (University of Bonn, Bonn, Germany), were retrospectively reviewed for course and outcome.

2.2. Definitions

Primary CM was defined according to the American Heart Association (AHA). Based on prenatal phenotype presentation, all cases were further divided into dilated (DCM), hypertrophic (HCM), restrictive (RCM), and isolated noncompaction (NCCM) cardiomyopathy (Figure 1) [1].

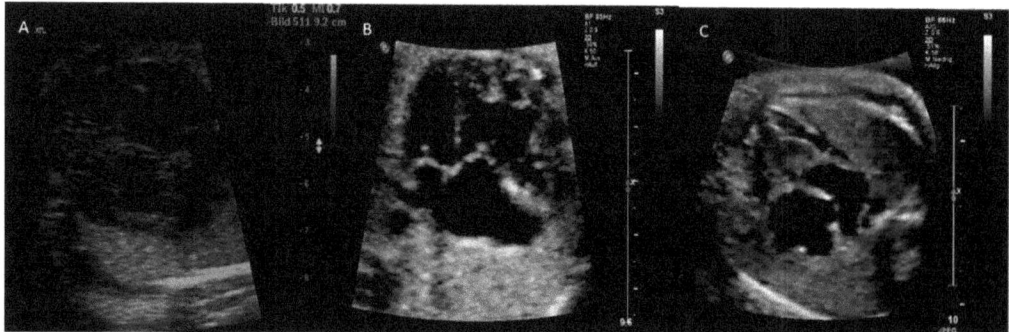

Figure 1. Different phenotypes of PCM illustrating HCM at 32 + 3 weeks gestation (**A**), isolated NCCM affecting only the right ventricle at 28 + 0 weeks (**B**), and RCM 34 + 5 (**C**).

In the presence of two different CM phenotypes, cases were assigned to the dominant subtype. DCM was diagnosed if one or both ventricles had qualitative dilation and there was qualitatively impaired systolic function (Figure 2) [14,15].

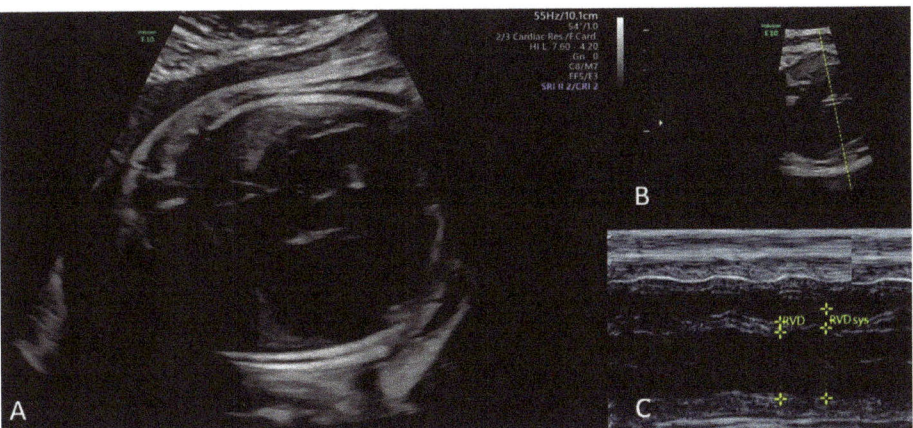

Figure 2. Dilative cardiomyopathy at the four chamber view in a fetus at 34 + 3 weeks gestation (**A**). Corresponding M-Mode cursor through the ventricles in an axial four chamber view of the fetal heart (**B**), with the corresponding M-Mode tracing (**C**). End-diastolic (EDD) (Z-score 3.48) and end-systolic (ESD) (Z-score 6.23) diameter of the right ventricle can be measured accurately to evaluate the shortening fraction (SF) [16]. EDD and ESD are demonstrated to be nearly the same with an SF of less than 5%. Changes in right ventricular diameters during the cardiac cycle are only caused by movement of the interventricular septum (IVS) (**C**).

HCM was defined by the a presence of qualitative hypertrophy in one or both ventricles with an otherwise preserved systolic function [17,18]. Isolated NCCM was suspected in the appearance of an abnormal thick endocardial compact layer with prominent trabeculations best visualized at systole and deep intertrabecular recesses moving with the myocardium and being filled by direct blood flow from the ventricular cavity on color Doppler imaging. Ventricular function was unsuspicious [19]. RCM was defined as one or both atria enlarged compared to ventricles of normal or small size with hemodynamic alterations including a dominant E-wave and a very short-duration A-wave, pulsatile ductus venosus, and atrioventricular-valve regurgitation [1].

Cases in which CM was considered secondary to fetal structural heart diseases (e.g., twin-to-twin transfusion syndrome, maternal diabetes, viral infection, anemia, fetal supraventricular tachyarrhythmias, anti-SSA/anti-SSB antibodies, and for complete fetal heart block) were excluded.

2.3. Ultrasound Assessment

An anatomical survey and fetal echocardiography were performed in a standardized fashion, using a segmental approach with defined anatomical planes incorporating pulsed-wave and color Doppler imaging [20,21]. Multifrequent sector or curved array probes (5 MHz, 7.5 MHz or 9 MHz) were used for all ultrasound examinations (HDI IU22, Phillips, Hamburg, Germany; Voluson E8 and E10, GE Healthcare, Solingen, Germany). Data were retrieved from medical files and stored ultrasound images. Cardiomegaly was defined as a cardiothoracic diameter ratio (CTR) > 0.50 [22]. Cardiac and ventricular sphericity indexes, including ventricular basal and midventricular sphericity indexes, were calculated as described else were [23]. Fetal hydrops was diagnosed in the presence of a fluid accumulation in at least two compartments including polyhydramnios, ascites, generalized skin edema, and pericardial or pleural effusion. All cases included an evaluation of viral myocardial infections (including toxoplasmosis, coxsackievirus, echovirus, cytomegalovirus, and herpes simplex virus) and of maternal antibodies (anti-SSA and anti-SSB).

2.4. Outcome

Outcomes were categorized into five groups: termination of pregnancy (TOP), intrauterine fetal demise (IUFD), neonatal death (NND), death in infancy or childhood (ICHD), and survivors. Neonatal death was defined as death within the first 28 days of life. Postnatal assessment was collected from the neonates' medical records and autopsy findings if available.

2.5. Data Analysis

Statistical analysis was performed using the Statistical Package for Social Sciences (SPSS 25.0, SPSS Inc., Chicago, IL, USA) statistical software. Intergroup comparison were made using one-way ANOVA with a post hoc test, Student's *t*-test, or Fisher's exact test. All values are given as mean ± standard deviation unless indicated otherwise. A *p* value of <0.05 was considered significant. All patients have given written informed consent for data collection, analysis, and their use for research, although the institutional review board of the University of Bonn does not require formal ethical approval for retrospective archived studies.

3. Results

During the study period, we identified 21 pregnancies available for analysis, including two patients with two pregnancies (Figure 3).

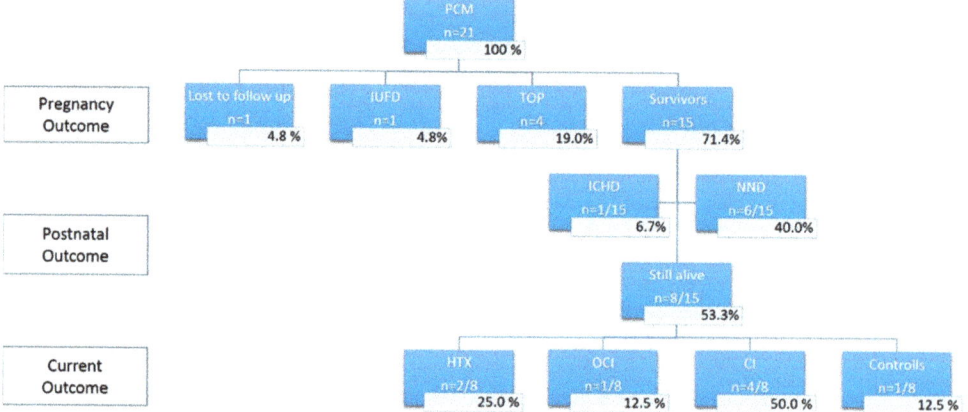

PCM: primary cardiomyopathy, IUFD: intrauterine fetal death, TOP: termination of pregnancy, ICHD: death in infancy or childhood, NND: neonatal death, HTX: heart transplantation, OCI: operative cardiac intervention, CI: cardiac insufficiency.

Figure 3. Flowchart summarizing the outcome of 21 fetuses prenatally diagnosed with primary CM.

Mean maternal age was 31.6 years (±6.2) with a mean body mass index (BMI) of 26.8 kg/m^2 (±5.5). In 19.0% (4/21) parental consanguinity and in 4.8% (1/21) maternal cardiac anomaly (Ebstein anomaly) was known. The gestational age at diagnosis was 26.7 weeks (±5.1), with none of the cases identified in the first trimester. A total of 11/21 (52.4%) fetuses were male. Suspicion of fetal heart disease accounted for 47.6% (10/21) of overall referral reasons. Other indications were family history of primary CM or known genetic mutations in 14.3% (3/21), hydrops fetalis in 14.3% (3/21), and in 23.8% (5/21) no cardiac specific reason. Biventricular involvement was the most common subtype (14/21; 66.7%). In the remaining 33.3% (7/21) predominant right ventricular dysfunction was observed as isolated tricuspid valve regurgitation with a preserved left ventricular function was seen on two-dimensional fetal echocardiography.

3.1. Prenatal CM Phenotype

In 42.9% (9/21) fetuses were assigned to HCM, in 38.1% (8/21) to DCM, in 14.3% (3/21) to isolated NCCM, and in 4.8% (1/21) to RCM. Prenatal cardiac function and echocardiographic characteristics are summarized in Table 1.

Table 1. Cardiac function and echocardiographic characteristics of the different CM phenotypes.

Parameter	Over all $n = 21$	DCM $n = 8$	HCM $n = 9$	Isolated NCCM $n = 3$	RCM $n = 1$	p-Value
Fetal hydrops	9	3	6	0	0	0.141
Arrhythmia	2	1	1	0	0	0.912
FHR	21	146.4 ± 13.4	132.3 ± 8.0	139.7 ± 10.8	137	0.190
EFE	1	1	0	0	0	0.636
TI	13	5	4	3	1	0.234
TI Vmax m/s	1.4 ± 1.4	2.4 ± 1.0	2.4 ± 1.2	1	2.1	0.276
MI	6	1	4	0	1	0.121
CTR	0.55 ± 0.1	0.62 ± 0.1	0.48 ± 0.1	0.57 ± 0.1	0.51	0.323
DV REDF	6	3	2	0	1	0.645
Pulsatile UV flow	7	2	2	2	1	0.329
Associated anomalies	7	2	5	0	0	0.496
Uni-/Bi-ventricular involvement	7/14	5/3	0/9	2/1	0/1	0.023
GSI (LCD/TCD)	1.17 ± 0.10	1.16 ± 0.13	1.12 ± 0.12	1.06 ± 0.12	1.3	0.579
LVLD/LVMTD	2.55 ± 0.96	2.21 ± 0.53	2.64 ± 1.23	2.88 ± 1.17	3.54	0.509
RVLD/RVMTD	2.23 ± 0.96	2.05 ± 0.67	2.63 ± 1.26	1.51 ± 0.22	2.55	0.487
LVLD/LVBD	1.81 ± 0.46	1.72 ± 0.22	1.74 ± 0.57	2.19 ± 0.68	1.91	0.497
RVLD/RVBD	1.66 ± 0.66	1.74 ± 0.36	1.71 ± 0.98	1.37 ± 0.23	1.39	0.843

Abbreviations (in alphabetical order): CTR = cardiothoracic diameter ratio; DV = ductus venosus; DCM = dilated cardiomyopathy; EFE = endocardial fibroelastosis; FHR = fetal heart rate; GSI = global sphericity index; HCM = hypertrophic cardiomyopathy; LCD = longitudinal cardiac diameter; LVBD = left ventricular basal diameter; LVLD = left ventricular longitudinal diameter; LVMTD = left ventricular midtransverse diameter; MI = mitral valve insufficiency, NCCM = noncompaction cardiomyopathy; REDF = reversed end-diastolic flow; RCM = restrictive cardiomyopathy; RVBD = right ventricular basal diameter; RVLD = right ventricular longitudinal diameter; RVMTD = right ventricular midtransverse diameter; TCD = transverse cardiac diameter; TI = tricuspid insufficiency, UV = umbilical vein.

HCM and DCM were diagnosed at an earlier gestational age (24.2 weeks (±4.8) and 26.8 weeks (±3.8)) compared to isolated NCCM and RCM (31.2 weeks (±4.9) and 34.9 weeks), although not reaching significance ($p = 0.080$). Univentricular involvement varied significantly among the different phenotypes ($p = 0.023$), with the most univentricular involvement seen in the isolated NCCM group (66.6%). The global sphericity index (GSI) demonstrated a more globular cardiac shape in general with a mean GSI of 1.17 (±0.1) vs. 1.23 (50th centile) compared to published data by Crispi et al. (Figure 4 A) [23].

Fetuses assigned to the isolated NNCM phenotype revealed the most pronounced globular cardiac shape with the most pronounced globular right ventricular basal sphericity index (SI), although not reaching significance ($p = 0.843$) compared to other subtypes (Figure 4B). In all phenotypes the right basal ventricular sphericity index (SI) was lower compared to the left ventricular SI.

3.2. Additional Cardiac, Extracardiac and Genetic Anomalies

Seven fetuses (33.3%) showed additional anomalies, including two fetuses with a small ventricular septum defect, one fetus with a urogenital disorder, and one fetus of each with vermis hypoplasia, unilateral clubfoot, bilateral hydrothorax, and with lateral cervical cysts.

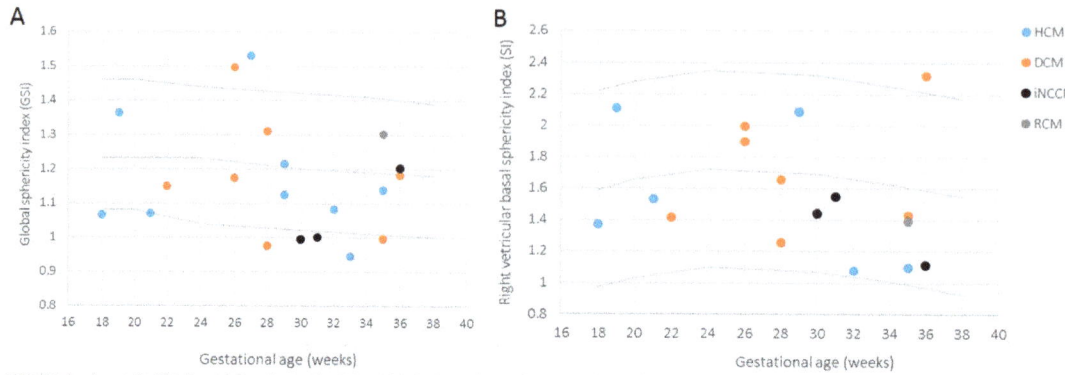

Figure 4. Scatterplot of global sphericity index (GSI) (**A**) and right ventricular basal sphericity index (SI) (**B**), according to gestational age of fetuses affected by primary CM, differentiated by provided phenotypes. Estimated 5th (lower), 50th (middle), and 95th (upper) centile curves are shown.

In total, nonchromosomal and chromosomal syndromes were diagnosed in 10/20 (50.0%) of fetuses (Barth syndrome (BTHS) (*Taffazin* gene mutation) in 2 fetuses; *MYBPC3* gene mutation in 2 fetuses; Noonan syndrome (*RIT1* gene mutation), LEOPARD syndrome (*PTPN11* mutation), Wolf-Hirschhorn syndrome (microdeletion 4p16.3), *KCNH* gene mutation, translocation (1;8) combined with duplication (1p 36.32) and deletion (Xp22.31,x1), and congenital Marfan syndrome in 1 fetus each), of which 60.0% (6/10) were assigned as HCM, and 40.0% (4/10) as DCM. Prenatal CM phenotypes in accordance with postnatal identified syndromes are shown in Table 2.

Table 2. CM Phenotypes in accordance with postnatal syndromes.

	DCM n = 8		HCM n = 9		NCCM n = 3		RCM n = 1
n		n		n		n	
1	Marfan syndrome	2	Barth syndrome	3	none identified	1	none identified
1	Wolf-Hirschhorn syndrome	1	Noonan syndrome				
3	Uhl's anomaly	1	LEOPARD syndrome				
1	Long-QT syndrome	2	*MYBPC3* gene mutation				
2	None identified	3	None identified				

Abbreviations (in alphabetical order): DCM = dilated cardiomyopathy; HCM = hypertrophic cardiomyopathy; NCCM = non-compaction cardiomyopathy; RCM = restrictive cardiomyopathy.

In one case, a mitochondrial myopathy was suspected but muscle biopsy revealed a normal result. Two further cases had an abnormality strongly suspicious for an underlying genetic etiology, resulting in an overall suspected genetic etiology in possibly as high as 60.0% (12/20). Baseline characteristics in comparison to neonatal outcome are displayed in Table 3.

Survivors at last follow up showed a significantly higher proportion of prenatal univentricular myocardial involvement ($p = 0.035$). Other investigated parameters revealed no significant difference, although there was a trend toward further malformations, hydrops fetalis, and a mitral valve regurgitation in the nonsurvivor group.

3.3. Outcome

The postnatal outcome with regard to different CM phenotypes are displayed in Table 4.

Table 3. Comparison neonatal outcome with respect to baseline characteristics.

Parameter	Total (n = 15)	Alive (n = 8)	Death (n = 7)	p-Value
GA at delivery (wks)	35.0 (±3.6)	36.4 (±3.6)	33.8 (±3.4)	0.176
Birth weight (g)	2325.3 (±807.8)	2652.1(±778.4)	2039.2 (±765.2)	0.149
Gender (f/m)	6/9	4/3	2/6	0.315
Univentricular involvement	7	6	1	0.035
Associated anomalies	6	2	4	0.378
Hydrops fetalis	7	2	5	0.214
MI	3	0	3	0.200
TI	9	5	4	0.378
TI vmax m/s	2.0 (±1.2)	1.5 (±0.6)	2.5 (±0.5)	0.207

Abbreviations (in alphabetical order): F = female; GA = gestational age; M = male; MI = mitral valve insufficiency; TI = tricuspid valve insufficiency.

Table 4. Postnatal outcome of the different CM phenotypes.

	Total (%)	IUFD	TOP	ICHD	NND	HTX	Still Alive
HCM	9 (42.9)	0	2	1	3	0	2 *
DCM	8 (38.1)	1	2	0	2	1	3
NCCM	3 (14.3)	0	0	0	0	1	3
RCM	1 (4.8)	0	0	0	1	0	0

Abbreviations (in alphabetical order): DCM = dilated cardiomyopathy; HCM = hypertrophic cardiomyopathy; HTX = heart transplantation; ICHD = infancy or childhood death; IUFD = intrauterine fetal demise; NCCM = non-compaction cardiomyopathy; NND = neonatal death; RCM = restrictive cardiomyopathy; TOP = termination of pregnancy; * one case with lost to follow up excluded.

Figure 3 demonstrates the postnatal outcome of the entire study population. The overall mortality rate at last follow up was 60.0% (12/20, excluding one case lost to follow up. Intrauterine death occurred in one case (5.0%) with hydrops fetalis and severe systolic dysfunction of the right ventricle at 28 weeks; in this case, Barth syndrome was suspected, but postnatal histopathological examination revealed no specific result. In 4/20 cases (20.0%) parents opted for termination of three pregnancy, three of them due to a known genetic mutation and positive family history and one due to severe hydrops fetalis with global systolic cardiac dysfunction at 28 weeks. A total of 15 out of 20 (75.0%) fetuses were live born. In six of the fifteen initial survivors (40%) neonatal death occurred. The mean gestational age within this group at delivery was 32.8 weeks (±4.01). In one case, Uhl's anomaly with severe right ventricular dysfunction including severe tricuspid regurgitation and decreased cardiac output was prenatally seen. Cardiac failure could not be stabilized and NND occurred on the fifth day of life. In one case, left ventricular dysfunction was initially dominant, although prenatally biventricular involvement (RCM) was diagnosed. Multiorgan failure with sepsis led to NND on the 15th day of life. In the remaining four neonates, genetic abnormalities were known (Barth, Noonan, LEOPARD, and Marfan syndrome). Terminal cardiac failure lead to death on the 17th, 12th, 5th, and 10th day of life, respectively. In one neonate being affected by Barth's syndrome, death occurred at an age of three years. As progressive cardiac failure and sepsis due to pneumonia occurred, the parents denied listing for cardiac transplantation and opted for palliative care.

Eight out of fifteen neonates are still alive. In two cases, cardiac transplantation was needed, due to progressive cardiac failure. In one neonate the prenatal diagnosis of a NCCM was changed into small vessel disease via histopathological examination. In the other neonate, long-QT syndrome was detected. Cardiac transplantation was performed at the age of 4 months and of 4 years, respectively.

In two neonates (13.3%; 2/15) phenotypical classification changed. Both were prenatally assigned to NCCM. One of them had a complete recurrence at the age of 8 years. In the other case initial right ventricular hypertrophy and dilation was observed. At the age of 12 years, the right ventricle was unsuspicious; however, the patient is now suffering from a dysplastic aortic valve and short stature. Genetic etiology is highly suspicious as first degree relatives are also suffering from a non-classified heart disease. In one further case, HCM led to severe stenosis of the pulmonary valve, so balloon valvuloplasty was performed at an age of 6 months. In addition, a premature craniosynostosis was seen and surgical procedure was carried out. Although the findings were highly suspicious for Noonan syndrome, no genetic testing was performed until now. In the remaining two out of three cases, Uhl's anomaly was diagnosed. Postnatal genetic evaluation lead to the diagnosis of a genetic mutation in one case with the result of translocation (1;8), combined with duplication (1p 36.32) and deletion (Xp22.31,x1). Both patient are being treated for cardiac failure. In the last case no further cytogenetic description of myopathy was diagnosed, as suspected Pompe disease could not be confirmed via muscle biopsy.

4. Discussion

Fetal cardiomyopathies carry a substantial burden of disease due to the risk of morbidity and mortality and a missing curative therapy. With a still-undefined incidence in prenatal series varying from 0.004% to 7%, compared to 0.001% in our cohort, data remains limited and prenatal diagnosis requires a high level of clinical suspicion [5–7].

4.1. Categorization System

In retrospective studies, primary CMs were categorized either as hypertrophic or nonhypertrophic/dilated phenotypes, with some further differentiating a mixed phenotype, suggesting that a simplifying classification appears to be more accurate and reproducible [5,6,8]. However, increased sophistication in ultrasound technologies has proposed a more detailed classification encompassing RCM and isolated NCCM, taking varying prognostic parameters and adapted prenatal genetic testing into account [7,24,25]. Consequently, in the absence of standardized guidelines and multiple definitions in use, the distribution of fetal phenotypes remains unclear with a prevalence of HCM varying from 18.0% to 60.0% and of DCM from 11.0% to 72.0%, as the most common subgroups [5,6,8]. In accordance to published data, we were able to identify HCM (42.9%) and DCM (38.1%), as the main phenotypes and further differentiated isolated NCCM in 14.3% and RCM as the rarest phenotype. Comparing results for NCCM, the study by Trakmulkichkarn et al., revealed a higher proportion of NCCM (26.0%) [7]. This difference might be explained by the small number of cases in our study, focusing only on the isolated uni-/biventricular NCCM subtype, as well as the recent increase in clinical awareness, leading to the diagnosis of all three cases in a later era. Further, with myocardial compaction occurring to a greater extent in the LV myocardium than in the RV myocardium, it remains difficult to distinguish normal variants of physiologically more trabeculated RV from pathological isolated NCCM, causing a potential underestimation. Data regarding this specific phenotype must, therefore, be treated with caution.

4.2. Echocardiographic Evaluation

Focusing on prenatal echocardiographic predictive parameters, neither the cardiovascular profile score nor the Tei index seem to be able to reliably predict outcomes dealing with primary CM in general, although it might be applied for DCM [6]. Referring to RCM, postnatal research demonstrated an elevated pulmonary vascular resistance, PR prolongation, and the elevation of mitral valve Doppler E/e' ratio being associated with increased mortality, leaving the utility for the prenatal course unproven [26,27]. Regarding NCCM, postnatal data have shown a strong relationship between cardiac phenotype and risk of death or transplantation distinguishing isolated phenotype of NCCM from hypertrophic, dilated, and restrictive, mandating further prenatal research potentially using fetal MRI, as prognostic parameters might be found [28,29]. A possible algorithm for prenatal evaluation in cases of suspicion of a primary CM is demonstrated in Figure 5.

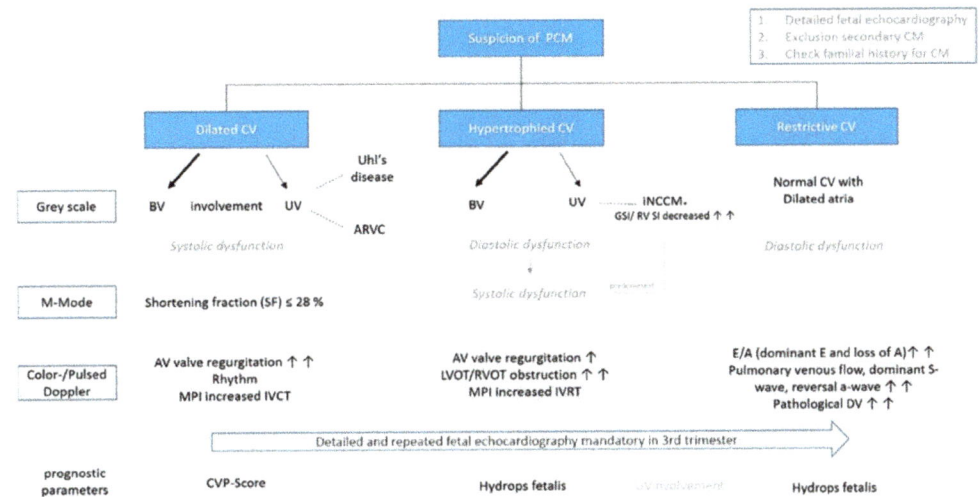

Figure 5. Flowchart illustrating a possible fetal echocardiographic examination in cases of suspected PCM. Mixed phenotypes and new echocardiographic techniques are not listed for better orientation. Arrows represent frequent occurrence (AV = artioventricular; ARVC = Arrhythmogenic right ventricular cardiomyopathy; CV = cardiac ventricles; CVPS = cardiovascular profile score; DV = ductus venosus; GSI = global sphericity index; RV SI = right ventricular basal sphericity index; MPI = myocardial performance index; IVCT = isovolumetric contraction time; IVRT = isovolumetric relaxation time; iNCCM* = may affect also both ventricles or occur with the other phenotypes).

In our study, we identified uni-right ventricular involvement as the only significant parameter for survival ($p = 0.035$), with the most proportion seen in the isolated NCCM phenotype ($p = 0.023$), which might be explained as right ventricular function has the chance to improve after birth [15]. With decreasing postnatal right ventricular afterload, the diseased right side of the heart undergoes physiological unloading and might recover cardiac function. Because in fetal life the right heart is exposed to a greater workload than the left heart, functional analysis of the right ventricle in utero can underestimate its pumping capacity and vice versa. Consequently, biventricular cardiomyopathy may occur prenatally with isolated right ventricular dysfunction and may only be detected after birth. For prenatal evaluation, changed myocardial maturation during gestation and the altered hemodynamic situation from prenatal to postnatal course must, therefore, be taken into account [15].

4.3. Genetic

We observed a genetic etiology in 50.0% (10/20) of patients and suspected it in 60.0% (12/20), which seems to be higher than previously reported [7]. The difference might be explained by including two patients with two pregnancies, with a known gene mutation, but also might be explained by the increasing use of genetic analysis, which will likely further increase the number. However, the interpretation of genetic results needs to be thoughtful, as clinical severity may vary with age for different morphological manifestations of same gene mutation and not all variants identified via genetic testing will be clinically significant or disease-causing [30]. Moreover, Sun et al. identified a distinct genetic spectrum among NCCM in fetal, pediatric, and adult patients, mandating a possible need for different molecular genetic testing/panel and leaving it uncertain whether insights obtained from pediatrics and adult patients can be transferred to fetal primary CMs and vice versa [30–32]. Despite this controversy, there are still several advantages for detailed genetic evaluation, even in the occurrence of an intrauterine fetal demise: (1). Some mutations (*MYH7* gene) have been associated with structural congenital heart disease as well as CM. (2). The outcome and risk for recurrence or subsequent pregnancies might be evaluated. (3). CM may be diagnosed in previously undiagnosed familial members, as demonstrated in our study by identifying a same gene mutation of affected fetuses in 20% (3/15) of the parents.

4.4. Outcome

In a retrospective study, a working group of Toronto found perinatal survival rates of only 18% for fetuses with DCM and 48% for HCM, evaluating CMs in general [8]. In 2014, the same group found improved outcomes in fetuses with dilated compared to hypertrophic CM (45 vs. 47%) [5]. Improvement in outcome was assigned to a better treatment of antibody-mediated CMs [5]. However, nearly 20% of the study population had to be classified as secondary CMs, biasing outcomes [1,5]. Recently published data identified an overall survival rate of 32% (12/38) with a given intrauterine mortality rate of 50% (19/38) [7]. The neonatal and early infant mortality rate was 37% (7/19) [6]. The mortality rate was found to be 71% in those with DCM and 50% in those with HCM [7]. In our study, the overall survival rate was 40.0%, comparable to data by Trakmulkichkarn et al. [7]. The mortality rate was found to be 62.5% (5/8) for DCM and 75.0% for HCM (6/8). The difference in a better survival rate for DCM might be explained by modern perinatal and postnatal management strategies, including improved resuscitation, the growing scope and use of ventricular assist devices, and option for cardiac transplantation. The cardiac transplantation rate of 13.3% was significantly higher compared to previously published data (3.2–6.5%) [5,7,33]. However, as pediatric data provide a similar transplantation rate in the recent era, the earlier recognition of heart failure and medical management seems more likely to cause an improve in outcome [33]. Higher mortality rates of HCM might be explained by a poorer survival in those with a genetic etiology, as extensive life-sustaining interventions might not be offered or opted in to in the context of expected extracardiac manifestations of the underlying disorder. Genetic etiology was known in all cases with neonatal or early infant death assigned to HCM, and 71.4% (5/7) in general, which was higher compared to previous published data with a confirmed genetic etiology in 57% of fetuses assigned to HCM [7]. With a survival rate of 100% (3/3) at last follow up referring to NCCM in our study, the outcome was better compared to reported data on 43% being life born [28]. The difference is highly explained due to the small case load in our study, as well as the missing consensus on the diagnostic criteria and classification of NCCM and the possibility of physiological myocardial maturation being mistaken [19,28,32].

4.5. Limitations

This study has some limitations. The sample size is relatively small, with a particularly limited case number for subgroup analysis of the different CM phenotypes. Intergroup statistical comparisons are, therefore, of relatively limited value. Given the retrospective study design, genetic studies were not available for all fetuses. In addition, no standardized protocol was used, so clinical and echocardiographic evaluated data were not available from all patients. Furthermore, due to being performed at a single institution, a demographic bias cannot be excluded.

5. Conclusions

Prenatal detection of primary CM is desirable as it might change the management and outcome in affected patients. If prenatally suspected, screening and genetic evaluation of other family members should be performed, as primary CM is highly hereditable, resulting in a high risk for recurrence in subsequent pregnancies. In case of a known familial risk, serial monitoring is warranted with evaluations of cardiac function. Although prenatal predictive parameters remain limited, evaluation of ventricular involvement might be seen as a prognostic parameter for survival. Delivery should take place in a perinatal center with multispecialized care.

Nevertheless, future research with a collection of cases to assess outcomes and the impact of management strategies is required and risk factors for adverse outcomes to assist in risk stratification, parental counselling, and appropriated resources at delivery need to be defined.

Author Contributions: Data curation, B.S., A.G., U.H., U.G., F.R. and C.B.; formal analysis, A.W., E.C. and U.G.; writing—review and editing, A.W., U.H. and U.G. All authors have read and agreed to the published version of the manuscript.

Funding: This research received no external funding.

Institutional Review Board Statement: The Ethics Committee of the University of Bonn does not request formal approval for anonymized retrospective analysis of clinical data.

Informed Consent Statement: Informed consent was obtained from all subjects involved in the study.

Data Availability Statement: The data presented in this study are available on request from the corresponding author.

Conflicts of Interest: The authors declare no conflict of interest.

References

1. Maron, B.J.; Towbin, J.A.; Thiene, G.; Antzelevitch, C.; Corrado, D.; Arnett, D.; Moss, A.J.; Seidman, C.E.; Young, J.B. Contemporary definitions and classification of the cardiomyopathies: An American Heart Association Scientific Statement from the Council on Clinical Cardiology, Heart Failure and Transplantation Committee; Quality of Care and Outcomes Research and Functional Genomics and Translational Biology Interdisciplinary Working Groups; and Council on Epidemiology and Prevention. *Circulation* **2006**, *113*, 1807–1816.
2. Davey, B.; Szwast, A.; Rychik, J. Diagnosis and management of heart failure in the fetus. *Minerva Pediatr.* **2012**, *64*, 471–492. [PubMed]
3. Pfitzer, C.; Helm, P.C.; Ferentzi, H.; Rosenthal, L.-M.; Bauer, U.M.M.; Berger, F.; Schmitt, K.R.L. Changing prevalence of severe congenital heart disease: Results from the National Register for Congenital Heart Defects in Germany. *Congenit. Heart Dis.* **2017**, *12*, 787–793. [CrossRef] [PubMed]
4. Aurora, P.; Boucek, M.M.; Christie, J.; Dobbels, F.; Edwards, L.B.; Keck, B.M.; Rahmel, A.O.; Taylor, D.O.; Trulock, E.P.; Hertz, M.I. Registry of the International Society for Heart and Lung Transplantation: Tenth official pediatric lung and heart/lung transplantation report. *J. Heart Lung Transplant.* **2007**, *26*, 1223–1228. [CrossRef] [PubMed]
5. Weber, R.; Kantor, P.; Chitayat, D.; Friedberg, M.; Golding, F.; Mertens, L.; Nield, L.E.; Ryan, G.; Seed, M.; Yoo, S.-J.; et al. Spectrum and outcome of primary cardiomyopathies diagnosed during fetal life. *JACC Heart Fail.* **2014**, *2*, 403–411. [CrossRef]
6. Ezon, D.S.; Ayres, N.A.; Altman, C.A.; Denfield, S.W.; Morris, S.A.; Maskatia, S.A. Echocardiographic parameters and outcomes in primary fetal cardiomyopathy. *J. Ultrasound Med.* **2016**, *35*, 1949–1955. [CrossRef]
7. Trakmulkichkarn, T.; Ghadiry-Tavi, R.; Fruitman, D.; Niederhoffer, K.Y.; Caluseriu, O.; Lauzon, J.L.; Wewala, G.; Hornberger, L.K.; Urschel, S.; Conway, J.; et al. Clinical presentation, genetic etiology and outcome associated with fetal cardiomyopathy: Comparison of two eras. *Ultrasound Obstet. Gynecol.* **2022**, *59*, 325–334. [CrossRef]
8. Pedra, S.R.; Smallhorn, J.F.; Ryan, G.; Chitayat, D.; Taylor, G.P.; Khan, R.; Abdolell, M.; Hornberger, L.K. Fetal cardiomyopathies: Pathogenic mechanisms, hemodynamic findings, and clinical outcome. *Circulation* **2002**, *106*, 585–591. [CrossRef]
9. Honda, T.; Kanai, Y.; Ohno, S.; Ando, H.; Honda, M.; Niwano, S.; Ishii, M. Fetal arrhythmogenic right ventricular cardiomyopathy with double mutations in TMEM. *Pediatr. Int.* **2016**, *58*, 409–411. [CrossRef]
10. Jefferies, J.L.; Wilkinson, J.D.; Sleeper, L.A.; Colan, S.D.; Lu, M.; Pahl, E.; Kantor, P.F.; Everitt, M.D.; Webber, S.A.; Kaufman, B.D.; et al. Cardiomyopathy phenotypes and outcomes for children with left ventricular myocardial noncompaction: Results from the pediatric cardiomyopathy registry. *J. Card. Fail.* **2015**, *21*, 877–884. [CrossRef]
11. McKenna, W.J.; Maron, B.J.; Thiene, G. Classification, Epidemiology, and Global Burden of Cardiomyopathies. *Circ. Res.* **2017**, *121*, 722–730. [CrossRef] [PubMed]
12. Mongiovi, M.; Fesslova, V.; Fazio, G.; Barbaro, G. Pipitone, Diagnosis and prognosis of fetal cardiomyopathies: A review. *Curr. Pharm. Des.* **2010**, *16*, 2929–2934. [CrossRef]
13. Ellepola, C.D.; Knight, L.M.; Fischbach, P.; Deshpande, S.R. Genetic testing in pediatric cardiomyopathy. *Pediatr. Cardiol.* **2018**, *39*, 491–500. [CrossRef]
14. Schmidt, K.G.; Birk, E.; Silverman, N.H.; Scagnelli, S.A. Echocardiographic evaluation of dilated cardiomyopathy in the human fetus. *Am. J. Cardiol.* **1989**, *63*, 599–605. [CrossRef] [PubMed]
15. Crispi, F.; Gratacós, E. Fetal cardiac function: Technical considerations and potential research and clinical applications. *Fetal Diagn. Ther.* **2012**, *32*, 47–64. [CrossRef] [PubMed]
16. Gagnon, C.; Bigras, J.-L.; Fouron, J.-C.; Dallaire, F. Reference values and z scores for pulsed-wave Doppler and M-Mode measurements in fetal echocardiography. *J. Am. Soc. Echocardiogr.* **2016**, *29*, 448–460.e9. [CrossRef] [PubMed]

17. Tan, J.; Silverman, N.H.; Hoffman, J.I.; Villegas, M.; Schmidt, K.G. Cardiac dimensions determined by cross-sectional echocardiography in the normal human fetus from 18 weeks to term. *Am. J. Cardiol.* **1992**, *70*, 1459–1467. [CrossRef]
18. Simpson, J.M.; Cook, A. Repeatability of echocardiographic measurements in the human fetus. *Ultrasound Obstet. Gynecol.* **2002**, *20*, 332–339. [CrossRef]
19. Jenni, R.; Oechslin, E.; Schneider, J.; Jost, C.A.; Kaufmann, P. Echocardiographic and pathoanatomical characteristics of isolated left ventricular non-compaction: A step towards classification as a distinct cardiomyopathy. *Heart* **2001**, *86*, 666–671. [CrossRef]
20. International Society of Ultrasound in Obstetrics and Gynecology; Carvalho, J.S.; Allan, L.D.; Chaoui, R.; Copel, J.A.; DeVore, G.R.; Hecher, K.; Lee, W.; Munoz, H.; Paladini, D.; et al. ISUOG Practice Guidelines (updated): Sonographic screening examination of the fetal heart. *Ultrasound Obstet. Gynecol.* **2013**, *41*, 348–359. [CrossRef]
21. Bhide, A.; Acharya, G.; Baschat, A.; Bilardo, C.M.; Brezinka, C.; Cafici, D.; Ebbing, C.; Hernandez-Andrade, E.; Kalache, K.; Kingdom, J.; et al. ISUOG Practice Guidelines (updated): Use of Doppler velocimetry in obstetrics. *Ultrasound Obstet. Gynecol.* **2021**, *58*, 331–339. [CrossRef]
22. Chaoui, R.; Bollmann, R.; Göldner, B.; Heling, K.; Tennstedt, C. Fetal cardiomegaly: Echocardiographic findings and outcome in 19 cases. *Fetal Diagn. Ther.* **1994**, *9*, 92–104. [CrossRef]
23. García-Otero, L.; Soveral, I.; Sepúlveda-Martínez; Rodriguez-López, M.; Torres, X.; Guirado, L.; Nogué, L.; Valenzuela-Alcaraz, B.; Martínez, J.M.; Gratacós, E.; et al. Reference ranges for fetal cardiac, ventricular and atrial relative size, sphericity, ventricular dominance, wall asymmetry and relative wall thickness from 18 to 41 gestational weeks. *Ultrasound Obstet. Gynecol.* **2021**, *58*, 388–397. [CrossRef]
24. Lopes, L.M.; Pacheco, J.T.; Schultz, R.; Francisco, R.P.V.; Zugaib, M. A prenatal case of arrhythmogenic right ventricular dysplasia. *Arq. Bras. Cardiol.* **2018**, *110*, 201–202. [CrossRef]
25. Rustico, M.; Benettoni, A.; Fontaliran, F.; Fontaine, G. Prenatal echocardiographic appearance of arrhythmogenic right ventricle dysplasia: A case report. *Fetal Diagn. Ther.* **2001**, *16*, 433–436. [CrossRef] [PubMed]
26. Anderson, H.N.; Cetta, F.; Driscoll, D.J.; Olson, T.M.; Ackerman, M.J.; Johnson, J.N. Idiopathic restrictive cardiomyopathy in children and young adults. *Am. J. Cardiol.* **2018**, *121*, 1266–1270. [CrossRef] [PubMed]
27. Weller, R.J.; Weintraub, R.; Addonizio, L.J.; Chrisant, M.R.; Gersony, W.M.; Hsu, D.T. Outcome of idiopathic restrictive cardiomyopathy in children. *Am. J. Cardiol.* **2002**, *90*, 501–506. [CrossRef]
28. Stöllberger, C.; Wegner, C.; Finsterer, J. Fetal ventricular hypertrabeculation/noncompaction: Clinical presentation, genetics, associated cardiac and extracardiac abnormalities and outcome. *Pediatr. Cardiol.* **2015**, *36*, 1319–1326. [CrossRef] [PubMed]
29. Rath, A.; Weintraub, R. Overview of cardiomyopathies in childhood. *Front. Pediatr.* **2021**, *9*, 708732. [CrossRef]
30. Hershberger, R.E.; Givertz, M.M.; Ho, C.Y.; Judge, D.P.; Kantor, P.F.; McBride, K.L.; Morales, A.; Taylor, M.R.G.; Vatta, M.; Ware, S.M.; et al. Genetic evaluation of cardiomyopathy: A clinical practice resource of the American College of Medical Genetics and Genomics (ACMG). *Genet. Med.* **2018**, *20*, 899–909. [CrossRef]
31. Zaban, N.B.; Darragh, R.K.; Parent, J.J. Fetal echocardiography is useful for screening fetuses with a family history of cardiomyopathy. *Pediatr. Cardiol.* **2020**, *41*, 1766–1772. [CrossRef] [PubMed]
32. Sun, H.; Hao, X.; Wang, X.; Zhou, X.; Zhang, Y.; Liu, X.; Han, J.; Gu, X.; Sun, L.; Zhao, Y.; et al. Genetics and clinical features of noncompaction cardiomyopathy in the fetal population. *Front. Cardiovasc. Med.* **2020**, *7*, 617561. [CrossRef] [PubMed]
33. Singh, R.K.; Canter, C.E.; Shi, L.; Colan, S.D.; Dodd, D.A.; Everitt, M.D.; Hsu, D.T.; Jefferies, J.L.; Kantor, P.F.; Pahl, E.; et al. Survival without cardiac transplantation among children with dilated cardiomyopathy. *J. Am. Coll. Cardiol.* **2017**, *70*, 2663–2673. [CrossRef] [PubMed]

Disclaimer/Publisher's Note: The statements, opinions and data contained in all publications are solely those of the individual author(s) and contributor(s) and not of MDPI and/or the editor(s). MDPI and/or the editor(s) disclaim responsibility for any injury to people or property resulting from any ideas, methods, instructions or products referred to in the content.

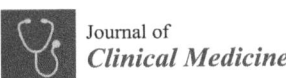

Journal of
Clinical Medicine

Article

Feasibility and Acceptance of Self-Guided Mobile Ultrasound among Pregnant Women in Routine Prenatal Care

Constanza A. Pontones [1,*], Adriana Titzmann [1], Hanna Huebner [1], Nina Danzberger [1], Matthias Ruebner [1], Lothar Häberle [1], Bjoern M. Eskofier [2], Michael Nissen [2], Sven Kehl [1], Florian Faschingbauer [1], Matthias W. Beckmann [1], Peter A. Fasching [1] and Michael O. Schneider [1]

1. Department of Obstetrics and Gynaecology, Universitätsklinikum Erlangen, 91054 Erlangen, Germany; adriana.titzmann@uk-erlangen.de (A.T.); hanna.huebner@uk-erlangen.de (H.H.); nina.danzberger@uk-erlangen.de (N.D.); matthias.ruebner@uk-erlangen.de (M.R.); lothar.haeberle@uk-erlangen.de (L.H.); sven.kehl@uk-erlangen.de (S.K.); florian.faschingbauer@uk-erlangen.de (F.F.); matthias.beckmann@uk-erlangen.de (M.W.B.); peter.fasching@uk-erlangen.de (P.A.F.); michael.schneider@uk-erlangen.de (M.O.S.)
2. Machine Learning and Data Analytics Lab, Friedrich-Alexander-Universität Erlangen-Nürnberg, 91052 Erlangen, Germany; bjoern.eskofier@fau.de (B.M.E.); michael.nissen@fau.de (M.N.)
* Correspondence: constanza.pontones@uk-erlangen.de

Abstract: Background and objectives: Mobile and remote ultrasound devices are becoming increasingly available. The benefits and possible risks of self-guided ultrasound examinations conducted by pregnant women at home have not yet been well explored. This study investigated aspects of feasibility and acceptance, as well as the success rates of such examinations. Methods: In this prospective, single-center, interventional study, forty-six women with singleton pregnancies between 17 + 0 and 29 + 6 weeks of gestation were included in two cohorts, using two different mobile ultrasound systems. The participants examined the fetal heartbeat, fetal profile and amniotic fluid. Aspects of feasibility and acceptance were evaluated using a questionnaire. Success rates in relation to image and video quality were evaluated by healthcare professionals. Results: Two thirds of the women were able to imagine performing the self-guided examination at home, but 87.0% would prefer live support by a professional. Concerns about their own safety and that of the child were expressed by 23.9% of the women. Success rates for locating the target structure were 52.2% for videos of the fetal heartbeat, 52.2% for videos of the amniotic fluid in all four quadrants and 17.9% for videos of the fetal profile. Conclusion: These results show wide acceptance of self-examination using mobile systems for fetal ultrasonography during pregnancy. Image quality was adequate for assessing the amniotic fluid and fetal heartbeat in most participants. Further studies are needed to determine whether ultrasound self-examinations can be implemented in prenatal care and how this would affect the fetomaternal outcome

Keywords: mobile ultrasound; self-guided ultrasound; pregnancy; prenatal care; feasibility; acceptance

1. Introduction

Ultrasound is used in routine prenatal care to monitor fetal growth and to detect fetal abnormalities and other pathologies during pregnancy [1]. Ultrasound examinations are carried out by qualified professionals since the handling of the devices and interpretation of the images are complex and require training and experience [2].

Technology continues to advance worldwide and is becoming more important in the healthcare sector. Mobile and remote medical devices are currently being introduced in prenatal medicine [3,4]. The COVID-19 pandemic might have accelerated this development as alternative designs for prenatal care in accordance with social distancing were needed [5,6]. Various mobile ultrasound devices have been developed and are being used in several countries (mainly for nonmedical self-scanning) as they are becoming more affordable. With an option for remote guidance by professionals, there would also be an opportunity to obtain imaging that might be usable for clinical care [7]. This seems to offer potential advantages, such as enhanced access to healthcare, especially in rural areas, with subsequent reduced visits to outpatient clinics and fewer hospital admissions, which might lead to cost savings in the healthcare system [3].

Although initial research results have shown that mobile health devices are acceptable and feasible for use as home monitoring tools to improve prenatal care [8,9], potential risks for pregnant women and for unborn children should not be disregarded [10].

Purpose

The aim of this study was to investigate the feasibility and acceptance, as well as success rates, of medically supervised self-examinations with mobile ultrasound devices during pregnancy, with the participating women being provided with detailed instructions in advance.

2. Methods

2.1. Study Design and Population

This was an open, prospective, single-center, interventional cohort study. Women with singleton pregnancies aged from 18 to 50 years and in gestational weeks 17 + 0 to 29 + 6 weeks were included. Twin pregnancies were ineligible. The participants were recruited from two settings: women who were hospitalized due to pregnancy-related complications and women presenting for planned antenatal care. The methods were performed in accordance with the relevant guidelines and regulations and approved by the ethics committee of Friedrich-Alexander-Universität Erlangen-Nürnberg (ref. Number 299_20 B). The participants were enrolled into two cohorts, each using one of two different mobile ultrasound devices (cohort A: Instinct, PulseNmore Ltd., Omer, Israel; cohort B: Butterfly iQ, Butterfly Network Inc., Guilford, CT, USA). A total of 47 pregnant women were screened and 46 were enrolled (23 in each cohort), as one patient did not wish to participate in the study.

2.2. Study Procedures and Data Collection

After undergoing a routine ultrasound examination by an experienced examiner assessing the fetal heart rate, biometry, echocardiography, fetal profile and amniotic fluid, pregnant women matching the inclusion criteria were asked to participate in the study. They were given information about the study and written informed consent was obtained. An ultrasound device, a mobile phone and an ultrasound gel were handed to the participant. They received direct instruction on how to use the device and the following tasks were explained over 5–10 min using example images:

- Recording a video of the fetal heartbeat for 30 s;
- Taking a picture and recording a video of the fetal profile for 60 s;
- Taking a picture and recording a 15-s video of the amniotic fluid in each of the four quadrants of the abdomen.

There was only one examination that was completed at the study visit on site. The examination was stopped after 15 min, regardless of whether all of the tasks had been completed. The participants were asked to complete a questionnaire about age, number of pregnancies and parity, demographic background, educational level and experience in using electronic devices. Questions about the feasibility and acceptance of the self-guided ultrasound examination were also included. The study ended with the submission of the questionnaire.

The images and videos obtained were saved on the study phone and then transferred to the study server. The videos were saved as MP4 files and the images were saved as PNG or JPG files. After successful storage, the original recordings were deleted from the study smartphone. The patient data collected were pseudonymized and documented in a database.

2.3. Ultrasound Devices and Settings

Cohort A: Instinct (PulseNmore Ltd.) is a mobile ultrasound system that was developed for home use. It consists of a mobile ultrasound device that can be connected to a mobile phone or tablet (only Android devices are currently applicable). The corresponding app can be downloaded free of charge. The device did not have any preinstalled presets for ultrasound in obstetrics and an individual study setting was therefore created and used uniformly for all participants according to the manufacturer's recommendations: gain 80%, frequency 3 MHz, power 0 dB, focus 50–90 mm, depth 150 mm, frame averaging off, line density 1, rejection 5, dynamic range 60 dB, image enhancement 7, time gain compensation 50% (all), gamma 1.16, speckle reduction 4, contrast 0, map 3, brightness 20%.

Cohort B: Butterfly iQ (Butterfly Network, Inc., Manufacturer: Butterfly Network, city: Burlington, MA, USA) is a mobile ultrasound system that is certified for medical use. It consists of a mobile ultrasound device that can be connected to a mobile phone or tablet by cable (compatible with both Apple and Android devices). The corresponding app can be downloaded free of charge. The cloud function for saving images and videos can be deactivated. The preset for ultrasound in obstetrics was used (frequency 1.7/3.4 MHz, 240 acquired receive lines per frame, dynamic range 32 to 48 dB).

2.4. Evaluation of Image and Video Quality

All images and videos obtained during the self-examination were evaluated by one experienced ultrasound examiner after study recruitment had been completed. Each image or video was assessed individually and was marked as follows:

- Images or videos that showed the required target structure (e.g., heartbeat, fetal profile or amniotic fluid) were marked as "target located."
- Images or videos in which the required target structure was not shown were marked as "target structure not located."
- Images or videos that showed the required target structure, but with poor quality that was not suitable for medical assessment, were marked as "target structure located, but quality low" (e.g., the image quality was blurred, or the target structure was not completely visible).
- If the participant was able to show the fetal heartbeat for at least one second during the video sequence lasting 30 s, it was marked as "target located." For a satisfactory presentation of the fetal profile, the forehead, tip of the nose and chin had to be clearly visible (example in Figure 1). Images and videos taken by the participants in which the fetal profile was also not visible ($n = 18$) were excluded.
- For a satisfactory presentation of images and videos of the amniotic fluid, hypoechoic areas had to be clearly demarcated from parts of the fetus. The four images and four video sequences representing the amniotic fluid were evaluated separately. If the amniotic fluid was clearly displayed in one quadrant, the respective videos or image sequences were marked as "target located." It was also examined whether the women were able to display the amniotic fluid in all four quadrants so that retrospective evaluation of a normal amount of amniotic fluid in a participant would be possible. Accordingly, the videos were marked as "4 out of 4 with sufficient quality" only if the amniotic fluid was visible in all four video sequences.

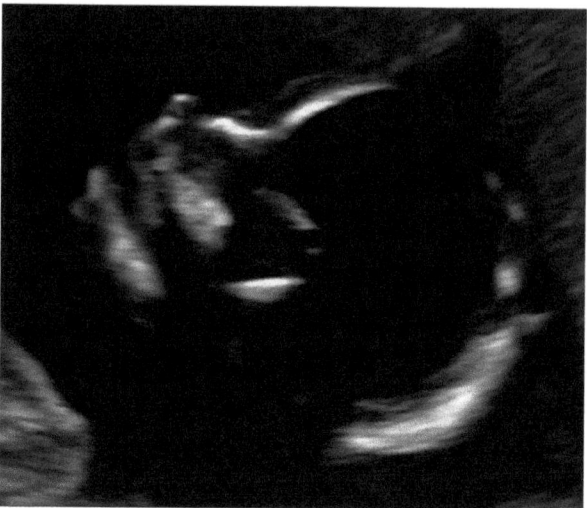

Figure 1. Requirements for satisfactory presentation of fetal profile: the forehead, tip of the nose and chin should be clearly visible.

2.5. Data Analysis

A descriptive statistical analysis of the maternal characteristics and answers given in the questionnaire was carried out. Descriptive statistics (mean, standard deviation, frequency, percentages) were calculated. The success rate in relation to image and video quality in the examinations performed by the pregnant women was also reported using descriptive statistics.

3. Results

All participants completed the required study procedures (self-guided ultrasound examination and questionnaire). They all managed to complete the tasks assigned in ≤15 min. No device-related serious adverse events were noted during the examination.

3.1. General Maternal Characteristics

The participants' characteristics are shown in Table 1. The mean maternal age was 32.6 ± 5.2 years. The mean gestational age was 24.0 ± 3.2 weeks. For more than one third of the patients, it was their first (39.1%) or second pregnancy (34.8%). With regard to educational level, nearly half of the participants (41.3%) had an academic degree and 8.7% had a doctoral degree.

3.2. Evaluation of the Questionnaire on Feasibility and Acceptance

The questionnaire responses are shown in Table 2. Nearly half of the women in cohort B (43.5%) and nearly one third of those in cohort A felt confident using the ultrasound device. A total of 7 of the 46 women (15.2%) felt uncertain when performing the examination. In all, 26.1% of the participants in cohort A and 17.4% of those in cohort B said they would only be willing to carry out the examination with supervision by a physician. Two thirds of the participants (67.4%) could imagine carrying out the self-guided examination at home. A total of 87.0% would like the attending physician to provide live support via video telephony if they were performing the examination at home.

Table 1. Maternal characteristics in 46 participants.

Characteristic	Cohort A and B (n = 46)		Cohort A (n = 23)		Cohort B (n = 23)	
	Mean or n [1]	SD or % [1]	Mean or n [1]	SD or % [1]	Mean or n [1]	SD or % [1]
Maternal age	32.6	5.2	33.8	5.0	31.4	5.1
Gestational week	24.0	3.2	24.1	3.3	23.9	3.0
Pregnancy						
1	18	39.1	8	34.8	10	43.5
2	16	34.8	8	34.8	8	34.8
≥3	12	26.1	7	30.4	5	21.7
Educational level						
No school-leaving qualification	0	0	0	0	0	0
Lower secondary school qualification	1	2.2	0	0	1	4.3
Intermediate school qualification	6	13.0	3	13.0	3	13.0
University entrance qualification	4	8.7	3	13.0	1	4.3
Apprenticeship qualification	12	26.1	5	21.7	7	30.4
Bachelor's/master's degree	19	41.3	10	43.5	9	39.1
Doctoral degree	4	8.7	2	8.7	2	8.7
Smartphone ownership						
No smartphone	0	0	0	0	0	0
iOS	20	43.5	8	34.8	12	52.2
Android	23	50.0	14	60.9	9	39.1
iOS and Android	2	4.3	1	4.3	1	4.3
Unknown	1	2.2	0	0	1	4.3

[1] Mean and standard deviation (SD) are shown for continuous characteristics and frequency (n) and percentage (%) for categorical characteristics.

Table 2. Feasibility and acceptability of self-guided ultrasound among pregnant women.

Questions	Cohort A and B (n = 46)		Cohort A (n = 23)		Cohort B (n = 23)	
	n	%	n	%	n	%
How confident did you feel using the ultrasound probe?						
Very confident	2	4.3	2	8.7	0	0
Confident	17	37.0	7	30.4	10	43.5
Partly/partially	20	43.5	8	34.8	12	52.2
Unsure	7	15.2	6	26.1	1	4.3
Very unsure	0	0	0	0	0	0
Could you imagine doing this examination at home by yourself?						
Yes	31	67.4	14	60.9	17	73.9
No	10	21.7	5	21.7	5	21.7
I do not know	5	10.9	4	17.4	1	4.3
If you were to perform this examination at home, would you like the attending physician to provide live support via video telephony?						
Yes	40	87.0	20	87.0	20	87.0
No	2	4.3	1	4.3	1	4.3
I do not know	4	8.7	2	8.7	2	8.7
If you were doing this examination at home, would it be okay for you if the doctor first had to evaluate and approve the ultrasound image before you could see it?						
Yes	21	45.7	9	39.1	12	52.2
No	16	34.8	9	39.1	7	30.4
I do not know	9	19.6	5	21.7	4	17.4
Do you agree with the following statements?						
The self-examination was fun						
I completely agree	31	67.4	14	60.9	17	73.9
Agree	12	26.1	7	30.4	5	21.7
Neither agree nor disagree	3	6.5	2	8.7	1	4.3
A little	0	0	0	0	0	0
Not at all	0	0	0	0	0	0

Table 2. Cont.

Questions	Cohort A and B (n = 46)		Cohort A (n = 23)		Cohort B (n = 23)	
	n	%	n	%	n	%
	I would like to do the self-examination more often					
I completely agree	18	39.1	8	34.8	10	43.5
Agree	15	32.6	8	34.8	7	30.4
Neither agree nor disagree	5	10.9	3	13.0	2	8.7
A little	8	17.4	4	17.4	4	17.4
Not at all	0	0	0	0	0	0
	The self-examination took too much time					
I completely agree	1	2.2	0	0	1	4.3
Agree	2	4.3	1	4.3	1	4.3
Neither agree nor disagree	1	2.2	0	0	1	4.3
A little	15	32.6	10	43.5	5	21.7
Not at all	27	58.7	12	52.2	15	65.2
	I was afraid of doing something wrong during the self-examination					
I completely agree	1	2.2	1	4.3	0	0
Agree	3	6.5	2	8.7	1	4.3
Neither agree nor disagree	10	21.7	4	17.4	6	26.1
A little	13	28.3	5	21.7	8	34.8
Not at all	19	41.3	11	47.8	8	34.8
	I would only do the self-examination under the supervision of a doctor					
I completely agree	10	21.7	6	26.1	4	17.4
Agree	8	17.4	5	21.7	3	13.0
Neither agree nor disagree	12	26.1	5	21.7	7	30.4
A little	5	10.9	3	13.0	2	8.7
Not at all	11	23.9	4	17.4	7	30.4
	I am concerned that the self-examination may be harmful to me or the child					
I completely agree	0	0	0	0	0	0
Agree	0	0	0	0	0	0
Neither agree nor disagree	2	4.3	2	8.7	0	0
A little	11	23.9	4	17.4	7	30.4
Not at all	33	71.7	17	73.9	16	69.6
	I would like to do the self-examination at home					
I completely agree	18	39.1	7	30.4	11	47.8
Agree	9	19.6	6	26.1	3	13.0
Neither agree nor disagree	11	23.9	6	26.1	5	21.7
A little	7	15.2	4	17.4	3	13.0
Not at all	1	2.2	0	0	1	2.3

The participants were asked whether it would be acceptable for them not to see the images before the evaluation of the scans by a physician, which could take a few hours or days (e.g., using the offline mode five-step scanning procedure). A total of 34.8% said that this would not be acceptable.

With regard to patients' opinions about safety, 33 of the 46 participants (71.7%) did not think that the examinations might be harmful to them or to the unborn child in any way, while 23.9% were slightly concerned about their own safety and that of the child.

3.3. Assessment of Image and Video Quality

The heartbeat was correctly captured by more than half of the participants (n = 24, 52.2%; Table 3) (Figure 2a,b).

Table 3. Evaluation of image and video quality.

Evaluation	Cohort A and B (n = 46)		Cohort A (n = 23)		Cohort B (n = 23)	
	n	%	n	%	n	%
Amniotic fluid—images						
Target structure located	37	80.4	17	73.9	20	87.0
Target structure not located	3	6.5	1	4.3	2	8.7
Target structure located, but quality low	6	13.0	5	21.7	1	4.3
Amniotic fluid—videos						
Target structure located	43	93.5	20	87.0	23	100
Target structure not located	1	2.2	1	4.3	0	0
Target structure located, but quality low	2	4.3	2	8.7	0	0
Amniotic fluid—total images						
4 out of 4 with sufficient quality	20	43.5	8	34.8	12	52.2
Amniotic fluid—total videos						
4 out of 4 with sufficient quality	24	52.2	10	43.5	14	60.9
Heartbeat—videos						
Target structure located	24	52.2	6	26.1	18	78.3
Target structure not located	10	21.7	8	34.8	2	8.7
Target structure located, but quality low	12	26.1	9	39.1	3	13.0
Fetal profile—images	28		13		15	
Target structure located	4	14.3	1	7.7	3	20.0
Target structure not located	23	82.1	11	84.6	12	80.0
Target structure located, but quality low	1	3.6	1	7.7	0	0
Fetal profile—videos	28		13		15	
Target structure located	5	17.9	2	15.4	3	20.0
Target structure not located	23	82.1	11	84.6	12	80.0
Target structure located, but quality low	0	0	0	0	0	0

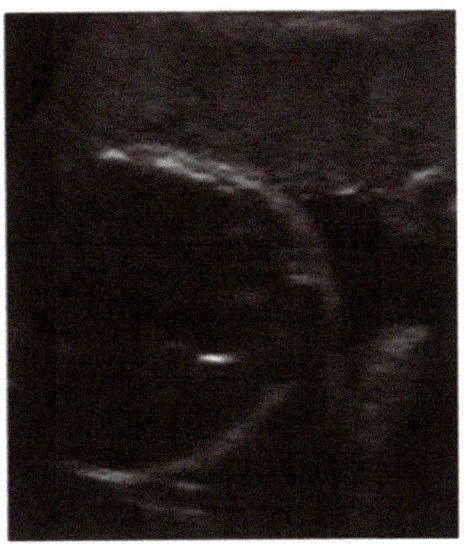 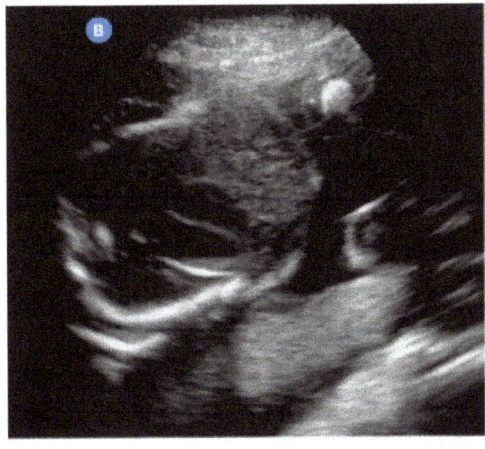

(a) (b)

Figure 2. (a) Example of an image obtained by a study participant in cohort A, showing the heartbeat (satisfactory presentation). (b) Example of an image obtained by a study participant in cohort B, showing the heartbeat (satisfactory presentation).

With regard to identifying the amniotic fluid during the 15-s video, 43 of the 46 participants (93.5%) managed to locate the amniotic fluid correctly in at least one of the four quadrants (Figure 3a,b). A total of 52.2% succeeded in locating the amniotic fluid in all four quadrants in the videos. In relation to capturing still images of the amniotic fluid, the rate of images with sufficient quality was lower than with the videos (80.4% with at least one adequate still image in the four quadrants and 43.5% with sufficient quality in all four quadrants).

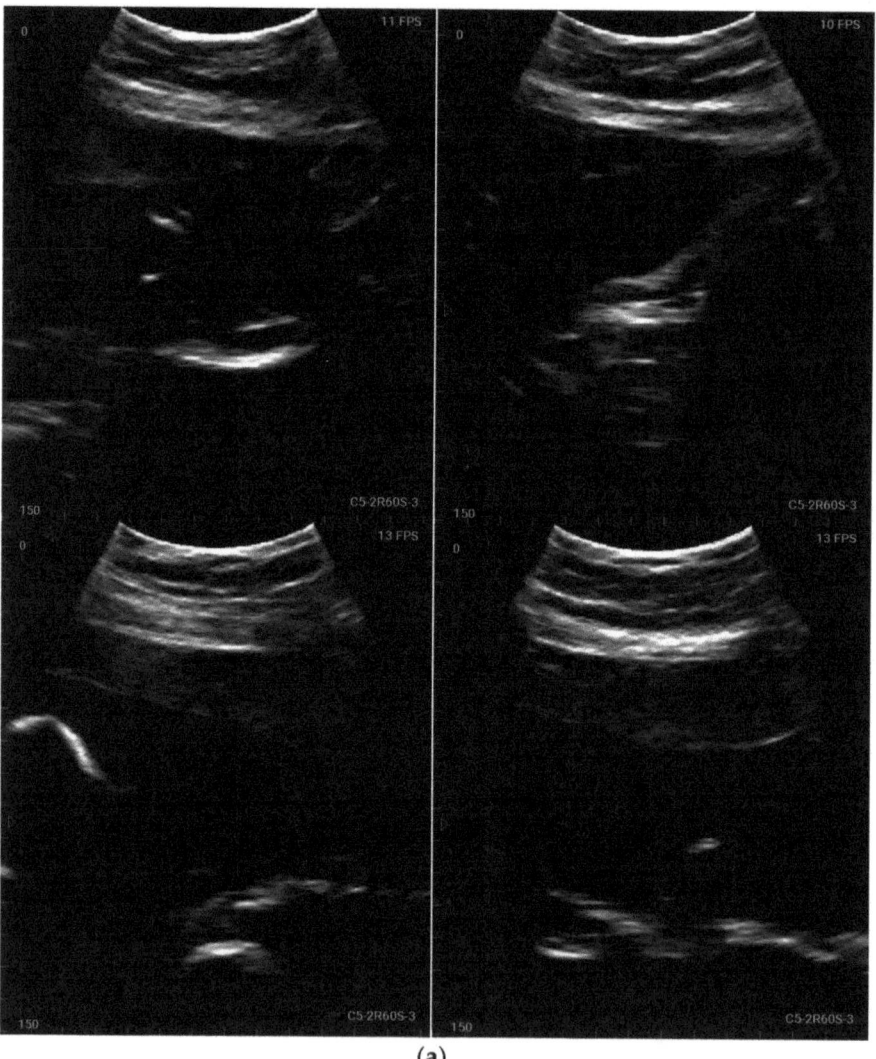

(a)

Figure 3. *Cont.*

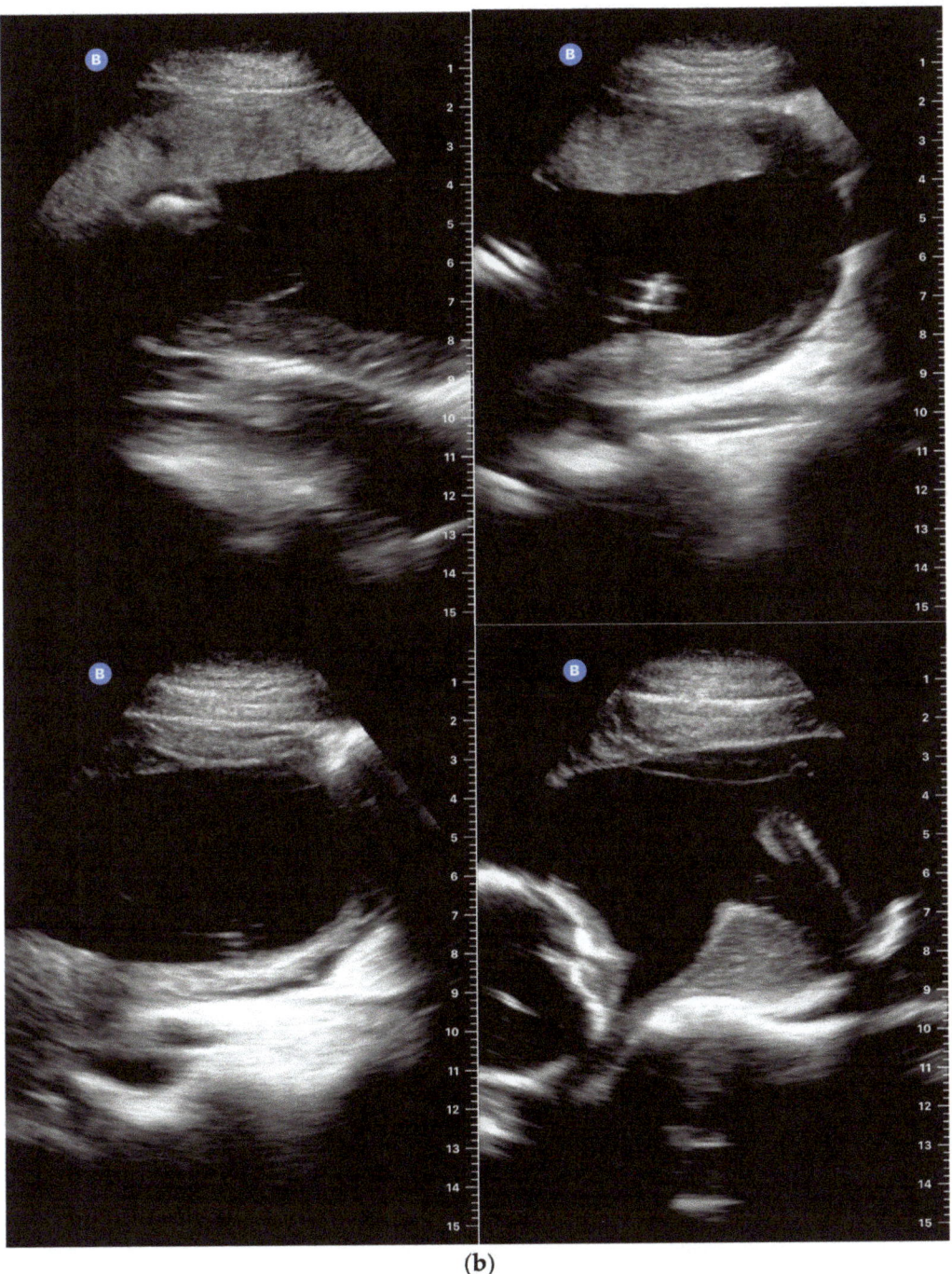

Figure 3. (**a**) Example of an image obtained by a study participant in cohort A, showing the amniotic fluid (satisfactory presentation). (**b**) Example of an image obtained by a study participant in cohort B, showing the amniotic fluid (satisfactory presentation).

The fetal profile was located satisfactorily by 14.3% of the women in still images (an example is shown in Figure 4) and by 17.9% in the videos.

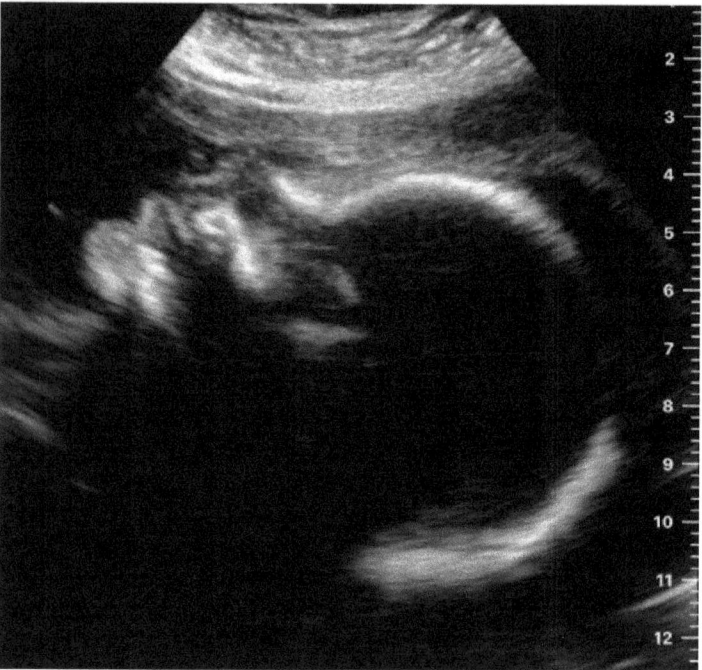

Figure 4. Example of an image obtained by a study participant, showing the fetal profile (satisfactory presentation).

4. Discussion

In this study of the feasibility and acceptability of self-guided mobile ultrasound during pregnancy, two thirds of the pregnant women would be willing to do the self-examination alone at home; however, the majority would prefer the attending physician to provide live support. Nearly half of the women felt confident using the ultrasound device and few women had concerns about their own safety or that of the child. The success rates for locating the target structure were better for the fetal heartbeat and the amniotic fluid than for the fetal profile.

The finding that the majority of the pregnant women (87.0%) would prefer live support during the self-examination is in line with a 2019 survey by Schramm et al. including 509 women, in which skeptical attitudes toward pregnancy self-monitoring were reduced when the procedure was combined with web-based consultation with a physician [11].

With regard to the accuracy of self-examination with ultrasound devices in the present study, the success rate for locating the amniotic fluid (43.5% for images, 52.2% for videos) and fetal heartbeat (52.2% for videos) was good as this was the first time handling the ultrasound device and even trainees in obstetrics and gynecology need more than 24 months of clinical experience to manage ultrasound examinations independently [12]. In particular, displaying the fetal profile is known to be technically demanding [13] and this was accordingly the most challenging task with low success rates (14.3% for images, 17.9% for videos). Depending on factors such as the fetal position, even experienced sonographers cannot always visualize the fetal face sufficiently (frequency of incomplete visualization 6–9% [14,15]).

A similar clinical trial conducted in Israel in 2020–2021 using the Instinct ultrasound system included 100 women with a singleton pregnancy at 14 + 0 to 39 + 6 gestational weeks [16]. In that study, the success rate for detection was 95.3% for fetal heart activity (much higher than in our results in the Instinct cohort, at 26.1%), 88.3% for body movements, 69.4% for tone, 92.2% for normal amniotic fluid volume (similar to our results) and 23.8% for breathing movements. The self-assessed user experience was rated at 4.4/5, whereas device satisfaction was rated at 3.9/5 [16]. As in the present study, each participant received personal face-to-face instruction on how to use the device at the time of recruitment. The first ultrasound scan was performed with guidance from an experienced ultrasound examiner, in contrast to the present study. The women were allowed to perform several scans at home (with a minimum of one and a maximum of three per day, limited to 3 min per scan) over a period of 7–14 days during pregnancy. Before each scan, the women viewed animated video demonstrations of how to move the device across the maternal abdomen. The mean number of scans per participant was 13.6 ± 6.2 each. There were no device-related serious adverse events [16]. There were two additional differences between the study by Hadar et al. and this one: Firstly, the women were allowed to use the mobile device at home up to three times per day, which might influence the stress level and pressure to succeed in performing the self-examination. Secondly, being able to use the device several days in a row might affect the women's learning curve in comparison with a single attempt to perform the examination. It can be assumed that it is much easier to learn how to locate the amniotic fluid than how to detect the fetal heartbeat.

The use of mobile devices in medicine has already been reported to be acceptable and feasible in other investigations, particularly in high-risk groups and specific patient groups. One example is the use of self-operated endovaginal telemonitoring during fertility treatments. In a small pilot study including 15 women, a good correlation was observed between the number of follicles measured in a self-operated ultrasound and in an ultrasound performed by a professional. The procedure also appeared to be more patient-friendly and less time-consuming [17].

Areas in which mobile ultrasound devices may be useful in the prenatal context include situations that require close fetal monitoring. Cuneo et al. investigated the use of mobile devices in pregnant women who have antibodies associated with the risk of a fetal atrioventricular block developing [18]. In the study, which included 315 pregnant women with positive anti-Ro antibodies, fetal heart rate and rhythm were measured twice a day using a portable Doppler device. A total of 87% of the patients completed the monitoring protocol, which did not increase their anxiety levels. Abnormal fetal heart rates and rhythms were detected by 6.7% of the women. No cases of atrioventricular block were missed during home monitoring. Many of the patients managed to reach a hospital within less than 12 h after a fetal atrioventricular block occurred [18]. This example shows that self-monitoring may be able to reduce the number of clinical consultations and even identify fetal pathologies during pregnancy earlier.

Further potential risks during home surveillance of fetal parameters using mobile devices also need to be taken into account. Prospective randomized trials are needed in order to analyze whether self-guided examinations with mobile ultrasound devices reach at least the same levels of sensitivity and specificity as standard-of-care examinations by professionals in the healthcare system. In a retrospective analysis in which 105 cases of fetal gastroschisis were accompanied by daily home monitoring of the fetal heart rate, the false-positive rate of fetal distress at admission was reported to be 58%. A significant increase in the rate of cesarean sections was also observed (50% vs. 24%), without any influence on perinatal outcome parameters such as the Apgar score or umbilical artery pH at birth [19].

Future studies should also investigate whether ultrasound self-monitoring influences anxiety among pregnant women, either positively or negatively. Several studies showed that increased stress and anxiety in pregnancy have been associated with poor birth outcomes and restricted fetal growth [20]. Prenatal anxiety might also have an impact on the number of emergency consultations on the one hand and on postnatal depression on the other. In a survey from 2019, women were asked if they would visit the emergency department less often if smart devices were readily available and only 7.7% affirmed [11]. With regard to depression, it is known that antenatal anxiety is related to postnatal depression [21,22]. Xu et al. found that women who presented to the emergency room during pregnancy were more likely to be admitted to hospital for a diagnosis of postnatal depression [23].

Finally, adverse events due to increased exposure to ultrasonic waves themselves also need to be taken into account. Diagnostic levels of ultrasound can lead to increased temperatures in tissue and nonthermal effects of ultrasound have also been demonstrated in animals. Although no hazardous effects have been demonstrated in humans to date, the European Federation of Societies for Ultrasound in Medicine and Biology (EFSUMB) stated in 2020 that little information is available regarding possible subtle biological effects of ultrasound on the developing human embryo or fetus, so that the exposure time should be limited as much as possible [24].

Strengths and Limitations

Although the study population was small in each cohort in the present study, each of the participants managed to complete all the tasks so that the images and videos could be fully evaluated. The educational level was high, as half of the participants had an academic degree. This may have had a positive influence on the success rate of performing ultrasound self-examinations. The scans were also performed immediately after having a presentation by trained staff—this may also impact the success rate and should be taken into consideration in future studies.

5. Conclusions

Self-examination using mobile systems for fetal ultrasound during pregnancy was generally acceptable for the pregnant women who participated. The analysis showed that the image quality was adequate for assessing amniotic fluid in most participants. Identification of fetal heartbeat and fetal facial profile was more challenging for the women. Further studies are needed to determine whether ultrasound self-examinations can be implemented in prenatal care and what effects this might have on fetomaternal outcomes.

The next step will be to perform a clinical trial using study procedures similar to those in this study, but with the women receiving additional live support from a physician using video telephony.

Author Contributions: C.A.P. provided protocol developments, conceptualized the study, collected and analyzed data and drafted the manuscript. A.T. provided protocol developments, conceptualized the study, collected and analyzed data and drafted the manuscript. H.H. provided research governance and protocol developments, conceptualized the study and analyzed data. N.D. provided protocol developments, conceptualized the study and analyzed data. M.R. analyzed data. L.H. analyzed data. B.M.E. provided research governance and analyzed data. M.N. analyzed data. S.K. collected data. F.F. collected data. M.W.B. provided research governance and protocol developments and drafted the manuscript. P.A.F. provided research governance and protocol developments, conceptualized the study, analyzed data and drafted the manuscript. M.O.S. provided protocol developments, conceptualized the study, collected and analyzed data and drafted the manuscript. All authors have read and agreed to the published version of the manuscript.

Funding: This research was funded by German Research Foundation (DFG) within the framework of the Heisenberg professorship program (grant number ES 434/8-1). The APC was funded by the Friedrich-Alexander-Universität Erlangen-Nürnberg Publication Fund.

Institutional Review Board Statement: The study was conducted in accordance with the Declaration of Helsinki and approved by the ethics committee of Friedrich-Alexander-Universität Erlangen-Nürnberg (ref. Number 299_20 B, date of approval: 28 July 2020).

Informed Consent Statement: Informed consent was obtained from all subjects involved in the study.

Data Availability Statement: The datasets generated during and/or analyzed during this study are available from the corresponding author upon reasonable request.

Acknowledgments: We are grateful to all the pregnant women who took part in this study. The study was supported by the Federal Ministry of Health on the basis of a decision by the German Bundestag.

Conflicts of Interest: The authors declare no conflict of interest.

References

1. Salomon, L.; Alfirevic, Z.; Da Silva Costa, F.; Deter, R.; Figueras, F.; Ghi, T.; Glanc, P.; Khalil, A.; Lee, W.; Napolitano, R.; et al. ISUOG Practice Guidelines: Ultrasound assessment of fetal biometry and growth. *Ultrasound Obstet. Gynecol.* **2019**, *53*, 715–723. [CrossRef] [PubMed]
2. Tolsgaard, M.G. Assessment and learning of ultrasound skills in Obstetrics & Gynecology. *Dan. Med. J.* **2018**, *65*, B5445.
3. Gyselaers, W.; Lanssens, D.; Perry, H.; Khalil, A. Mobile Health Applications for Prenatal Assessment and Monitoring. *Curr. Pharm. Des.* **2019**, *25*, 615–623. [CrossRef] [PubMed]
4. Weichert, J.; Welp, A.; Scharf, J.L.; Dracopoulos, C.; Becker, W.H.; Gembicki, M. The Use of Artificial Intelligence in Automation in the Fields of Gynaecology and Obstetrics—An Assessment of the State of Play. *Geburtshilfe Frauenheilkd.* **2021**, *81*, 1203–1216. [CrossRef] [PubMed]
5. Peahl, A.F.; Smith, R.D.; Moniz, M.H. Prenatal care redesign: Creating flexible maternity care models through virtual care. *Am. J. Obstet. Gynecol.* **2020**, *223*, 389.e1–389.e10. [CrossRef] [PubMed]
6. Stumpfe, F.M.; Titzmann, A.; Schneider, M.O.; Stelzl, P.; Kehl, S.; Fasching, P.A.; Beckmann, M.W.; Ensser, A. SARS-CoV-2 Infection in Pregnancy—A Review of the Current Literature and Possible Impact on Maternal and Neonatal Outcome. *Geburtshilfe Frauenheilkd.* **2020**, *80*, 380–390. [CrossRef] [PubMed]
7. Thorup, T.J.; Zingenberg, H. Use of 'non-medical' ultrasound imaging before mid-pregnancy in Copenhagen. *Acta Obstet. Gynecol. Scand.* **2015**, *94*, 102–105. [CrossRef]
8. Grym, K.; Niela-Vilen, H.; Ekholm, E.; Hamari, L.; Azimi, I.; Rahmani, A.; Liljeberg, P.; Löyttyniemi, E.; Axelin, A. Feasibility of smart wristbands for continuous monitoring during pregnancy and one month after birth. *BMC Pregnancy Childbirth* **2019**, *19*, 34. [CrossRef]
9. Kalafat, E.; Mir, I.; Perry, H.; Thilaganathan, B.; Khalil, A. Is home blood-pressure monitoring in hypertensive disorders of pregnancy consistent with clinic recordings? *Ultrasound Obstet. Gynecol.* **2018**, *52*, 515–521. [CrossRef]
10. Aust, T.; Famoriyo, A. Caution with home fetal Doppler devices. *BMJ* **2009**, *339*, b3220. [CrossRef]
11. Schramm, K.; Grassl, N.; Nees, J.; Hoffmann, J.; Stepan, H.; Bruckner, T.; Haun, M.W.; Maatouk, I.; Haist, M.; Schott, T.C.; et al. Women's Attitudes Toward Self-Monitoring of Their Pregnancy Using Noninvasive Electronic Devices: Cross-Sectional Multicenter Study. *JMIR Mhealth Uhealth* **2019**, *7*, e11458. [CrossRef] [PubMed]
12. Tolsgaard, M.G.; Rasmussen, M.B.; Tappert, C.; Sundler, M.; Sorensen, J.L.; Ottesen, B.; Ringsted, C.; Tabor, A. Which factors are associated with trainees' confidence in performing obstetric and gynecological ultrasound examinations? *Ultrasound Obstet. Gynecol.* **2014**, *43*, 444–451. [CrossRef] [PubMed]
13. Wah, Y.M.; Chan, L.W.; Leung, T.Y.; Fung, T.Y.; Lau, T.K. How true is a 'true' midsagittal section? *Ultrasound Obstet. Gynecol.* **2008**, *32*, 855–859. [CrossRef] [PubMed]
14. Silvestri, M.T.; Pettker, C.M.; Raney, J.H.; Xu, X.; Ross, J.S. Frequency and Importance of Incomplete Screening Fetal Anatomic Sonography in Pregnancy. *J. Ultrasound Med.* **2016**, *35*, 2665–2673. [CrossRef]
15. Chaichanalap, R.; Hanprasertpong, T. Success rate to complete optimal 20 + 2 ISUOG planes for foetal ultrasonographic structural screening during early second trimester pregnancy in Thailand. *Ultrasound J.* **2021**, *13*, 36. [CrossRef]
16. Hadar, E.; Wolff, L.; Tenenbaum-Gavish, K.; Eisner, M.; Shmueli, A.; Barbash-Hazan, S.; Bergel, R.; Shmuel, E.; Houri, O.; Dollinger, S.; et al. Mobile Self-Operated Home Ultrasound System for Remote Fetal Assessment During Pregnancy. *Telemed. J. E. Health* **2021**, *28*, 93–101. [CrossRef]
17. Dalewyn, L.; Deschepper, E.; Gerris, J. Correlation between follicle dimensions recorded by patients at home (SOET) versus ultrasound performed by professional care providers. *Facts Views Vis. Obgyn.* **2017**, *9*, 153–156.
18. Cuneo, B.F.; Sonesson, S.E.; Levasseur, S.; Moon-Grady, A.J.; Krishnan, A.; Donofrio, M.T.; Raboisson, M.-J.; Hornberger, L.K.; Van Eerden, P.; Sinkovskaya, E.; et al. Home Monitoring for Fetal Heart Rhythm During Anti-Ro Pregnancies. *J. Am. Coll. Cardiol.* **2019**, *73*, 1940–1951. [CrossRef]
19. Kuleva, M.; Salomon, L.J.; Benoist, G.; Ville, Y.; Dumez, Y. The value of daily fetal heart rate home monitoring in addition to serial ultrasound examinations in pregnancies complicated by fetal gastroschisis. *Prenat. Diagn.* **2012**, *32*, 789–796. [CrossRef]
20. Wainstock, T.; Anteby, E.; Glasser, S.; Shoham-Vardi, I.; Lerner-Geva, L. The association between prenatal maternal objective stress, perceived stress, preterm birth and low birthweight. *J. Matern.-Fetal Neonatal Med.* **2013**, *26*, 973–977. [CrossRef]
21. Coelho, H.F.; Murray, L.; Royal-Lawson, M.; Cooper, P.J. Antenatal anxiety disorder as a predictor of postnatal depression: A longitudinal study. *J. Affect. Disord.* **2011**, *129*, 348–353. [CrossRef] [PubMed]
22. Austin, M.P.; Tully, L.; Parker, G. Examining the relationship between antenatal anxiety and postnatal depression. *J. Affect. Disord.* **2007**, *101*, 169–174. [CrossRef] [PubMed]

23. Xu, F.; Sullivan, E.A.; Forero, R.; Homer, C.S. The association of Emergency Department presentations in pregnancy with hospital admissions for postnatal depression (PND): A cohort study based on linked population data. *BMC Emerg. Med.* **2017**, *17*, 12. [CrossRef] [PubMed]
24. Kollmann, C.; Jenderka, K.V.; Moran, C.M.; Draghi, F.; Jimenez Diaz, J.F.; Sande, R. EFSUMB Clinical Safety Statement for Diagnostic Ultrasound—(2019 revision). *Ultraschall. Med.* **2020**, *41*, 387–389. [CrossRef] [PubMed]

Disclaimer/Publisher's Note: The statements, opinions and data contained in all publications are solely those of the individual author(s) and contributor(s) and not of MDPI and/or the editor(s). MDPI and/or the editor(s) disclaim responsibility for any injury to people or property resulting from any ideas, methods, instructions or products referred to in the content.

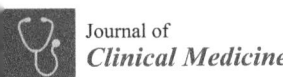

Article

Fetal Cerebellar Area: Ultrasound Reference Ranges at 13–39 Weeks of Gestation

Luigi Manzo [1,2], Giuliana Orlandi [1,2], Olimpia Gabrielli [1,2], Paolo Toscano [1,2], Enrica Di Lella [1,2], Antonia Lettieri [2], Laura Letizia Mazzarelli [1,2], Giordana Sica [3], Letizia Di Meglio [4], Lavinia Di Meglio [5], Gabriele Ruffo [2], Carmine Sica [2], Ferdinando Antonio Gulino [6,*], Giosuè Giordano Incognito [7], Attilio Tuscano [7], Alice Giorno [1] and Aniello Di Meglio [2]

1 Department of Neuroscience, Reproductive Sciences and Dentistry, School of Medicine, University of Naples Federico II, 80138 Naples, Italy; luigimanzo93@libero.it (L.M.); giulianaorlandi@msn.com (G.O.); olimpia.gabrielli3@gmail.com (O.G.); paol.toscano@gmail.com (P.T.); enrica_dilella@hotmail.it (E.D.L.); lauramazzarelli@gmail.com (L.L.M.); giorno.alice@libero.it (A.G.)
2 Diagnostica Ecografica e Prenatale di A. Di Meglio, 80133 Naples, Italy; antonia_lettieri@libero.it (A.L.); gabrieleruffo89@libero.it (G.R.); sicacarmine111@gmail.com (C.S.); aniellodimeglio@gmail.com (A.D.M.)
3 School of Medicine, University of Campania Luigi Vanvitelli, 81031 Caserta, Italy; giordanasica@icloud.com
4 Radiology Department, School of Medicine, University of Milan, 20122 Milan, Italy; letiziadimeglio@gmail.com
5 Pediatric Department, Bambino Gesù Children's Research Hospital IRCCS, 00165 Rome, Italy; laviniadimeglio@gmail.com
6 Department of Obstetrics and Gynaecology, Azienda di Rilievo Nazionale e di Alta Specializzazione (ARNAS) Garibaldi Nesima, 95124 Catania, Italy
7 Department of General Surgery and Medical Surgical Specialties, University of Catania, 95123 Catania, Italy; giordanoincognito@gmail.com (G.G.I.); attiliotuscano@gmail.com (A.T.)
* Correspondence: docferdi@hotmail.it; Tel.: +39-3381111000

Abstract: Background and Objectives: The present study aims to provide prenatal 2-dimensional ultrasonographic (2D-US) nomograms of the normal cerebellar area. Materials and Methods: This is a prospective cross-sectional analysis of 252 normal singleton pregnancies, ranging from 13 to 39 weeks of gestation. The operator performed measurements of the fetal cerebellar area in the transverse plane using 2D-US. The relationship between cerebellar area and gestational age (GA) was determined through regression equations. Results: A significant, strong positive correlation was investigated between the cerebellar area with GA (r-value = 0.89), and a positive correlation indicates that with increasing GA, the cerebellar area increased in all the participants of the study. Several 2D-US nomograms of the normal cerebellar area were provided, and an increase of 0.4% in the cerebellar area each week of GA was reported. Conclusions: We presented information on the typical dimensions of the fetal cerebellar area throughout gestation. In future studies, it could be evaluated how the cerebellar area changes with cerebellar abnormalities. It should be established if calculating the cerebellar area in addition to the routine transverse cerebellar diameter may help in discriminating posterior fossa anomalies or even help to identify anomalies that would otherwise remain undetected.

Keywords: ultrasound; cerebellum; posterior fossa anomalies; biometry

1. Introduction

Without a shadow of a doubt, the realm of obstetric practice presents a complex and multifaceted landscape that ceaselessly evokes fascination and curiosity. Undeniably, at the pulsating heart of this captivating medical discipline, one critical element shines through its pivotal significance—the methodical, meticulous, and precise assessment of the fetal development process. A task of immense gravity and importance, this particular duty is far from being a static or unchanging procedure; instead, it can be more appropriately characterized as a vibrant and dynamic process that constantly evolves, changes, and adapts in line with the unstoppable forward march of technology. In a world where advancements in technology incessantly bring forth new tools, techniques, and methodologies, our understanding of fetal development expands correspondingly. These technological leaps not only deepen our comprehension of the intricate process but also push the boundaries of our explorative capabilities, allowing us to engage in a more thorough, detailed, and comprehensive assessment than ever thought possible in yesteryear. The study of the brain is an important aspect and is based on the definition of its dimensions and the morphology of its components [1]. Among the structures, the assessment of the cerebellum is increasingly debated and evolving [1,2]. Situated within the confines of the posterior cranial fossa, the cerebellum is a key player in the architecture of the hindbrain, boasting the status of being its largest component. It consists of a central part known as the vermis and two convex lateral expansions termed the cerebellar hemispheres. Its external surface has a complicated network of fissures that delimit the flocconodular, anterior, and posterior lobes. Each of these lobes can be further divided into smaller subunits called lobules, the presence of which serves to significantly increase the overall surface area of the cerebellum, thereby enhancing its functional efficiency and capacity. Renowned for its crucial role in controlling and coordinating movement, the cerebellum's capabilities extend much further. In addition to motor control, it profoundly influences a variety of cognitive functions, including but not limited to attention, memory processing, and language comprehension. Furthermore, it plays an instrumental role in regulating emotions, with a particular emphasis on fear and pleasure. The cerebellum is one of the earliest brain structures to differentiate during the embryonic stage, yet it is also one of the last to reach full maturity. This prolonged developmental timeline, spanning both embryonic stages and the postnatal period, leaves the cerebellum vulnerable to a range of potential developmental anomalies. Brain development begins with a fundamental biological process known as neurulation. This process involves the transformation of the neural plate, formed from the ectodermal layer, into encephalic vesicles at its cephalic end, with the remaining part of the neural plate laying the groundwork for the formation of the spinal cord [3]. In the early stages, the brain architecture comprises three primary encephalic vesicles, called the forebrain, the midbrain, and the rhombencephalon. As development advances, these vesicles undergo further diversification. The forebrain splits into two additional vesicles, namely the telencephalon and the diencephalon, while the rhombencephalon divides into the metencephalon and the myelencephalon. The development of the cerebellum involves the alar plate, which is the dorsal part of the metencephalon, and the neural folds, the future rhombic lips. The alar plate, during its lateral expansion, gives birth to structures called rhombomeres. These rhombomeres then undergo a process of medial fusion, which defines the cavity of the fourth ventricle, leading to the formation of a smooth, convex structure known as the rudiment of the cerebellum. Included within this rudiment is the midline vermis, a critical component that plays a vital role in the cerebellum's operation [1]. The cerebellar fissures, initially appearing on the surface of the vermis and the floccular region during the fourth month of development, extend to the level of the hemispheres from the fifth month onward [1,4–6]. After the 19th week of gestation, the mass of the cerebellum undergoes a substantial increase, doubling in size. This remarkable growth continues beyond birth into the postnatal period [1,7–10]. Consequently, the evolution of the cerebellum can provide invaluable insights into the fetus's overall developmental progress [1].

Researchers have conducted numerous studies to understand normal cerebellar growth patterns and establish nomograms of cerebellar dimensions to aid in prenatal diagnosis. For example, Rizzo et al. [11] established reference limits for the cerebellar vermis using three-dimensional ultrasonography images. Alpay et al. [12] constructed nomograms for brainstem structures using two-dimensional ultrasonography (2D-US). A study by Chang et al. [13] demonstrated the effectiveness of three-dimensional ultrasound in assessing fetal cerebellar volume throughout normal gestation, leading to the development of volume-based nomograms. A multitude of ultrasound studies have underscored the clinical significance of transverse cerebellar diameter (TCD) and vermis dimension measurements. These have been proposed as potential alternatives to determining gestational age (GA), providing a fresh perspective compared to the traditional method of measuring the biparietal diameter (BPD) [1,14–17]. Despite the potential clinical significance of these methods in terms of both indicating normal brain development and potentially detecting brain abnormalities, the prenatal ultrasound evaluation of the cerebellar area has yet to be fully explored and understood.

The present study aims to measure the cerebellar area in fetuses exhibiting normal development by utilizing prenatal 2D-US examinations in the transverse plane throughout the gestational period and to provide 2D-US nomograms of the cerebellar area, creating a potentially invaluable tool that could substantially aid future prenatal assessments.

2. Materials and Methods

The current study was designed as a prospective cross-sectional investigation aimed at providing a comprehensive analysis of the intricate relationship between the cerebellar area and GA in a selected cohort of pregnant women. The inclusion criteria included the requirement of a well-documented last menstrual period, serving as an essential reference point for estimating GA. Additionally, crown-rump length (CRL) measurements obtained during first-trimester ultrasound examinations were employed to confirm and accurately determine GA. By employing these standardized methods, the study aimed to establish a solid foundation for accurate GA estimation, which is crucial for investigating the relationship between cerebellar development and GA. Furthermore, fetuses were singleton and non-anomalous to eliminate potential confounding factors associated with multiple gestations. This approach allowed for a more focused investigation into the specific impact of GA on cerebellar development, as it minimized potential variations resulting from differences in the number of fetuses or abnormalities. Moreover, the study considered only pregnancies with the estimated fetal weight falling within the 10th to 90th percentile range, aiming to capture a representative sample of the general population and avoiding any bias towards extreme fetal growth patterns. Moreover, the included participants had negative histories of systemic diseases, normal amniotic fluid volume, intact fetal membranes, and were not in labor at the time of enrollment.

The evaluation of the cerebellar area was conducted during routine ultrasound examinations, performed for first-, second-, and third-trimester screening. This multidimensional approach allowed for a comprehensive analysis of cerebellar development throughout pregnancy, capturing the dynamic changes that occur across different periods.

To ensure consistency and facilitate meaningful comparisons, a standardized approach was adopted for categorizing GA. Fractions of weeks were rounded to the nearest whole week, providing a uniform system for characterizing GA across the study population. Weeks with a GA of ≤ 4 days were assigned to the lower week, while weeks with >5 days were assigned to the higher week. This systematic categorization ensured the accurate representation of GA and allowed for the exploration of cerebellar development at various stages of pregnancy.

Only healthy neonates with no evidence of growth disturbances (such as growth restriction or macrosomia) were included. This approach aimed to establish a baseline understanding of cerebellar development in the absence of significant deviations from the norm. Adhering to the principles of cross-sectional studies, each fetus was included only once to ensure the independence of data points and prevent potential duplication, further strengthening the study's validity and reliability.

The 2D-US examinations were performed using standard Aloka (Aloka Co., Ltd., Tokyo, Japan) and Voluson E10 (GE Healthcare Ultrasound, Milwaukee, WI, USA) machines equipped with a curved linear array transabdominal transducer (2–5 MHz) and a transvaginal 4–8 MHz probe. The fetal cerebellum was assessed in the transverse plane of the fetal brain, including the cavum septum pellucidum, cerebellum, and cisterna magna, during fetal and maternal rest using a transabdominal acquisition angle of 45–60°, depending on GA. By focusing on this specific plane, the study ensured a standardized approach and consistent measurement technique across all participants. Freeze-frame capabilities allowed for the capture of static images at specific moments, enabling detailed analysis and precise measurements of the cerebellar area. Additionally, an electronic on-screen manual trace was employed to outline the boundaries of the cerebellar structures (Figure 1).

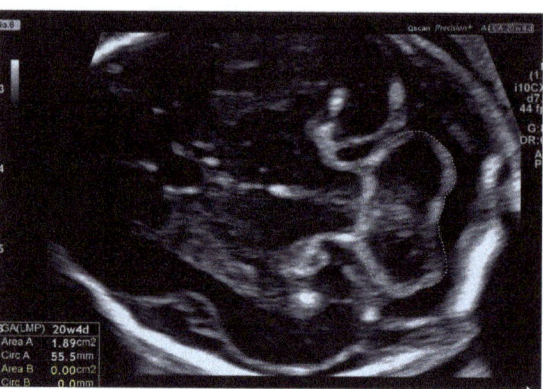

Figure 1. Assessment of the fetal cerebellar area by 2D-US transabdominal approach.

The decision was made not to incorporate color Doppler imaging into the examination protocol. By excluding the color Doppler, the focus remained solely on measuring the cerebellar area without the potential influence of vascular dynamics. This approach ensured that the measured cerebellar area was specific to the cerebellar structures of interest and minimized potential confounding factors related to blood flow patterns.

The cerebellar area was acquired in cross-section with a hand trace, involving a systematic tracing process guided by specific anatomical landmarks. The tracing started at the anterior border of the posterior wall of the spinal cord bridge, followed by the tracing along the contours of the two cerebellar hemispheres. Subsequently, the tracing continued along the posterior margin of the cerebellar vermis, capturing the entirety of the cerebellar area of interest. In cases where the transabdominal route did not provide a clear transverse view of the fetal brain, the transvaginal approach was utilized. It was often due to the fetal position or maternal habitus, which could impact the optimal visualization of the cerebellum. By incorporating this approach, the study aimed to ensure accurate cerebellar measurements, regardless of any potential imaging challenges. The cerebellar area was assessed during the routine scan and obtained by means of two measurements.

The statistical analysis was carried out using GraphPad Prism version 8.4.2 for Windows (GraphPad Software, San Diego, CA, USA) and IBM® SPSS® statistical software version 21.0 (SPSS Inc., Chicago, IL, USA). Only cases with GA between 13 and 39 weeks were included in the analysis. The clinical characteristics of the participants were expressed as the mean and standard deviation. These descriptive statistics provided a comprehensive overview of the central tendency and variability within the study population, offering insights into the overall characteristics of the sample. The clinical characteristics of the participants were expressed as mean and standard deviation, and the normal distribution of the data was assessed using the Kolmogorov-Smirnov test. Spearman's rank correlation coefficient and scatter plots were drawn to explore the relationship between the cerebellar area and the GA. A linear regression analysis equation was calculated to highlight how the increase in GA accelerated the progression of the cerebellar area. A p-value less than 0.05 was considered statistically significant, indicating meaningful associations between variables.

3. Results

The study comprised 283 pregnant women who fulfilled the inclusion criteria.

Measurements of the cerebellar area were performed on all 283 fetuses between 13 and 39 weeks of gestation.

The cerebellum appeared as a "butterfly image", with two symmetrically curved hemispheres conjoined by a hyperechoic structure, known as the cerebellar vermis. There appeared to be no change in its sonolucency between 13 and 39 weeks of gestation.

We obtained satisfactory cerebellar area measurements in the large majority of cases. Precisely, in 89.9% of the instances, which equates to 252 out of the total 283 cases, we considered the measurements to be adequately accurate. We adopted a dual approach in our measurement methodology, which involved either a transabdominal technique, applied in 225 cases, or a transvaginal technique, utilized in 32 cases. The choice of technique was determined by the unique specifics of each case. In a small subset of cases, representing approximately 10.1% of the total cohort, the measurements could not be included in our analysis. In these specific cases, factors such as fetal position and certain attributes of the maternal body structure hindered an optimal evaluation of the fetal cerebellum. More specifically, these factors resulted in our inability to capture a satisfactory transverse plane image, including the cavum septum pellucidum, the cerebellum, and the cisterna magna.

To encapsulate the clinical characteristics of the study population, we compiled these details into Table 1. This compilation provides an account of the Hadlock Ultrasound measurements used in our study.

Table 1. Clinical characteristics of the study population using Hadlock Ultrasound measurements.

Characteristics	Value
BPD (mm)	54.90 ± 16.42
BPD (percentile)	55.53 ± 27.17
HC (mm)	204.7 ± 60.89
HC (percentile)	59.84 ± 25.61
AC (mm)	184 ± 60.33
AC (percentile)	60.80 ± 24.43
FL (mm)	39.52 ± 14.32
FL (percentile)	61.02 ± 22.51
EFW (g)	778.4 ± 802.1

AC, abdominal circumference; BPD, biparietal diameter; EFW, estimated fetus weight; FL, femur length; HC, head circumference. Data are presented as mean and standard deviation.

In Table 2, the predicted 10th, 50th, and 90th percentiles of the cerebellar area, expressed in square centimeters (cm^2), as a function of the GA, expressed in weeks, were reported.

Table 2. Predicted 10th, 50th, and 90th percentiles of the cerebellar area (cm^2) by gestational age (weeks).

Gestational Age	Number of Cases	10th Percentile	50th Percentile	90th Percentile
13	2	0.2	0.22	0.24
14	4	0.35	0.435	0.49
15–16	2	0.55	0.575	0.6
17	3	0.87	1.06	1.07
18	5	0.95	1.16	1.6
19	7	1.3	1.54	1.88
20	48	1.444	1.775	2.162
21	57	1.618	1.89	2.262
22–24	50	1.893	2.265	2.939
25–27	8	1.95	3.57	4.46

Table 2. Cont.

Gestational Age	Number of Cases	10th Percentile	50th Percentile	90th Percentile
28–30	14	3.61	5.005	6.655
31–33	24	5.4	7.04	8.135
34–39	24	6.105	8.545	11.21

One of the outcomes of our study was the discovery of a positive correlation between GA and the cerebellar area. This correlation suggests that as the GA advances, there is a corresponding increase in the cerebellar area. This finding was consistent across all participants in the study (Table 3) (Figure 2).

Table 3. Correlation between the cerebellar area with gestation age.

	Gestation Age (r-Value)	p-Value
Cerebellar area (cm^2)	0.89	<0.0001

r-value, correlation value; Spearman's Rank correlation test.

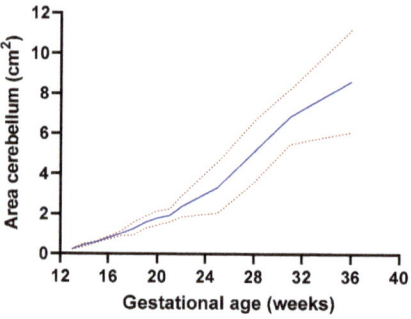

Figure 2. Plot showing the cerebellar area observed measurements and the fitted 10th (lower line), 50th (median line), and 90th (higher line) percentiles for gestational age.

Our research conclusions were further reinforced by the regression equations we derived. These equations encapsulate the relationship between the mean cerebellar area (represented by y) and GA (represented by x). This relationship is captured by the equation: y = 0.4176x − 6.692. Additionally, to gain a comprehensive understanding of the data, we derived a second equation, which defines the relationship between the standard deviation of the cerebellar area (represented by y') and GA: y' = 0.009x + 0.215. Collectively, these equations suggest a steady increase of approximately 0.4% in the cerebellar area for each week of GA progression.

4. Discussion

Cerebellum development occurs over a long period of time, so it has a high susceptibility to experiencing various disorders [18]. One of the most common posterior fossa anomalies is the Chiari malformation. This malformation manifests as an extension of the lower part of the cerebellum into the spinal canal. This can lead to compression of the brain tissue and obstruct the flow of cerebrospinal fluid, leading to potential complications. There are four types of Chiari malformations. Type I is the most common variant, where the lower part of the cerebellum extends into the opening at the base of the skull. This type often does not cause any symptoms and may be discovered incidentally during imaging performed for another reason. Type II, on the other hand, is usually associated with spina bifida, a birth defect where the spinal cord does not develop properly. This type results in both the cerebellum and the brainstem being displaced into the spinal canal, leading to compromised breathing and swallowing functions. Type III is a rare and severe form where the cerebellum and brainstem extend into a sac that protrudes through an opening at the back of the skull. This can result in severe neurological symptoms and is often diagnosed shortly after birth. Finally, type IV is the rarest and most severe of all, where the cerebellum fails to develop properly. This malformation is often fatal before or shortly after birth. In Dandy-Walker malformation (DWM) [19], the cerebellar vermis does not fully develop, resulting in an enlarged posterior fossa and fourth ventricle. This is accompanied by an upward displacement of the lateral sinuses, tentorium, and torcular [19,20]. In this pathology, the TCD can be normal. Vermis hypoplasia is a cerebellar malformation difficult to diagnose prenatally due to the normal vermis position or minimal upward rotation (without tentorium elevation). The fluid collection behind the cerebellum is typically minor and is directly connected to the fourth ventricle [21]. Another category of cerebellar malformations includes cerebellar hypoplasia, characterized by a reduction in cerebellar volume. This group of disorders presents heterogeneity in its manifestations, and the TCD is usually small when measured in the axial or coronal plane. The diagnosis of cerebellar hypoplasia typically occurs late in pregnancy or after delivery due to its late onset and the fact that the TCD is not routinely evaluated during the third trimester [19]. Among the rare cerebellar malformations is pontocerebellar hypoplasia (PCH), which is characterized by the prenatal onset of cerebellar hypoplasia with superimposed atrophy [19]. Fetuses with PCH are very infrequently diagnosed. According to Leibovitz et al. [22], there were only two cases of PCH diagnosed at 29 gestational weeks, and both cases exhibited reduced midbrain and hindbrain measurements. The authors concluded that relying solely on prenatal imaging for the diagnosis of this disorder could prove unreliable. Another rare congenital cerebellar defect is rhombencephalosynapsis (RES), characterized by a complete or partial absence of the vermis along with fused cerebellar hemispheres, middle cerebellar peduncles, and dentate nuclei [23]. Usually, the transcerebellar diameter in these cases is smaller than average. The typical fissure between the hemispheres is indistinguishable on the axial plane, and the dorsal part of the cerebellum displays a circular shape and does not show the typical "butterfly" shape; transverse cerebellar folias appear continuous and cross the midline. In the sagittal view of the brain, the fourth ventricle takes on a circular shape, and the main fissure is imperceptible [19]. The detection of RES using ultrasound before 22 weeks of gestation is infrequent, and patients are typically referred for fetal ventriculomegaly [24,25]. Generally, the TCD in such cases is smaller than expected. Joubert syndrome is a rare autosomal recessive genetic disease associated with syndromic retinitis pigmentosa and characterized by the absence or underdevelopment of the cerebellar vermis and a brainstem malformation that gives a typical "molar tooth" appearance [19,26]. A prenatal diagnosis is extremely difficult in such cases. On the transcerebellar plane, the vermis appears hypoplastic, missing the inferior part and producing a midline cleft connecting the 4th ventricle to the cisterna magna [27]. Prenatal diagnosis has been described following a positive family history or when associated with other typical anomalies, such as renal malformations [28]. The visualization of the molar tooth is difficult and requires ultrasound scans performed by experienced operators. Axial magnetic resonance imaging (MRI) scans usually aid in the diagnosis by allowing the visualization of the pathognomonic "molar tooth sign" [27,29].

Ultrasound serves as an essential diagnostic instrument for a multitude of obstetric and gynecological conditions [30–35]. A crucial application of this technology is the examination of the fetal brain. In particular, the evaluation of the fetal posterior fossa using ultrasound typically involves visualizing axial planes, including coronal and sagittal planes, via the transabdominal approach. The axial plane enables the assessment of the vermis and the cerebellar hemispheres, the TCD, the fourth ventricle size, and the cerebellar peduncle thickness [19]. TDC measurement is part of the second-trimester routine scan [36] and part of the assessment of the fetal brain [37]. This involves measuring the cerebellar diameter in the transcerebellar plane, which is a plane passing through the thalamus and cavum septum pellucidum. In this section, it is possible to identify the occipital horns of the lateral ventricles, the thalami, the interhemispheric fissure, and the cerebellum [38], which, in cross-section, appears as a butterfly-shaped structure, with the vermis recognizable as being slightly more echogenic than the two cerebellar hemispheres [27]. Among the coronal planes, the only one that can be acquired via the posterior fontanelle is the transcerebellar plane [37]. The vermis can also be measured in the same plane as TDC. The length, width, and thickness of the vermis can be measured to assess its size and growth. There is a lot of research about the TDC, correct vermis measurement, and nomograms to use during the ultrasound for each GA. For example, at 20 weeks of gestation, the average TCD measurement range is between 16.3 mm and 22.1 mm, and at 32 weeks of gestation, the average TCD measurement range is between 31.1 mm and 40.7 mm. These ranges can vary slightly depending on the specific nomogram used in the measurement. [19,22,39,40].

Yet, there are no reports comparing the cerebellar area to nomograms to define abnormal growth. Therefore, we suggest that the cerebellar area might be a useful parameter for its actual size. We provided prenatal 2D-US nomograms of the normal cerebellar area and reported an increase of 0.4% in the cerebellar area each week of GA.

Moreover, both TDC and vermis measurements can be used to detect a range of fetal abnormalities. Posterior fossa anomalies can be suspected during the first-trimester screening ultrasound, but they must be confirmed in a second-trimester scan [19]. Anomalies during the second and third trimesters are typically detected when a small cerebellum, morphological anomalies, or communication between the fourth ventricle and the cisterna magna are visualized during routine screening [19,41]. Although most of the cerebellar anomalies can present with a reduced TCD, any of these can show only a morphological anomaly in association with a normal TDC. In these cases, an untrained operator may fail in its recognition, and using the cerebellar area assessment for biometric evaluation could be supportive in the differential diagnosis of posterior fossa abnormalities or even help identify abnormalities. The transcerebellar plane is the landmark also used for the measurement of the cerebellar area. The technique used to measure the cerebellar area is the hand trace, following anteriorly the posterior wall of the spinal cord bridge, continuing along the two cerebellar hemispheres, and finally passing posteriorly along the posterior margin of the cerebellar vermis. Using the cerebellar area measurement may be helpful to suspect the presence of cerebellar and posterior fossa anomalies and refer the patient to a second-third level center if further studies are necessary.

While TCD measurement can be easily evaluated by sonographers, the morphological assessment of the cerebellum may be challenging for less trained operators. We could not obtain the cerebellar area measurement in 10.1% of cases because an adequate transverse plane could not be obtained due to the fetal position or the maternal habitus. However, the transcerebellar plane is the same one used for the measurement of both TDC and vermis measurements, whose evaluations would be inadequate in the same percentage of cases as the cerebellar area.

A limitation of the present study is the small population sample. Larger population studies will be necessary to demonstrate the feasibility of this measurement. Moreover, the data about the first-trimester cerebellar area are limited, and more studies are necessary. The TCD measurement has not been reported, and it would be useful to compare the cerebellar area to this already known and used parameter in future research.

5. Conclusions

We presented information on the typical dimensions of the fetal cerebellar area throughout gestation, providing normograms and reporting an increase of 0.4% in the cerebellar area each week of GA. In future studies, it could be evaluated how the cerebellar area changes with cerebellar abnormalities. It should be established if calculating the cerebellar area in addition to the routine TCD may help in discriminating posterior fossa anomalies or even help to identify anomalies that would otherwise remain undetected. In this study, we presented information regarding the typical dimensions of the fetal cerebellar area at various stages of gestation. We constructed nomograms that illustrate the expected growth patterns of the cerebellar area throughout the course of pregnancy, providing healthcare professionals with a valuable reference tool. Moreover, our findings revealed a consistent and remarkable increase of 0.4% in the cerebellar area per week of GA. In order to further advance our knowledge in this field, it is imperative to conduct future research endeavors focusing on comprehensively evaluating how the cerebellar area changes in the presence of various cerebellar abnormalities. By systematically examining and quantifying these abnormalities, we can gain valuable insights into their impact on cerebellar growth patterns and determine whether calculating the cerebellar area, in addition to routine TCD measurements, can serve as an indispensable diagnostic modality for discriminating and precisely characterizing posterior fossa anomalies. The potential clinical implications of integrating cerebellar area calculations into routine screening protocols are highly promising. By augmenting the existing diagnostic arsenal, we may be able to effectively identify and categorize anomalies that might otherwise elude detection. Given the complex nature of cerebellar development and the diverse spectrum of cerebellar abnormalities, we advocate for further investigations in this domain to unravel the intricate mechanisms underpinning cerebellar growth and to delineate the diagnostic accuracy of incorporating cerebellar area measurements in clinical practice.

Author Contributions: Conceptualization, L.M.; methodology, G.O.; software, O.G.; validation, P.T.; formal analysis, E.D.L.; formal analysis, A.L.; investigation, L.L.M.; resources, G.S.; data curation, L.D.M. (Letizia Di Meglio) and L.D.M. (Lavinia Di Meglio); writing—original draft preparation, L.M. and C.S.; writing—review and editing, F.A.G., G.G.I., and A.T.; visualization, G.R. and A.G.; supervision and writing-review and editing, A.D.M. All authors have read and agreed to the published version of the manuscript.

Funding: This research received no external funding.

Institutional Review Board Statement: This study was approved by the ethics board of the Diagnostica Ecografica Di Meglio srl on 1 February 2023. All of the patients signed a written informed consent form to perform the ultrasounds.

Informed Consent Statement: Informed consent was obtained from all subjects involved in this study.

Data Availability Statement: Data are unavailable due to privacy restrictions.

Conflicts of Interest: The authors declare no conflict of interest.

References

1. Vulturar, D.; Fărcăşanu, A.; Turcu, F.; Boitor, D.; Crivii, C. The volume of the cerebellum in the second semester of gestation. *Clujul Med.* **2018**, *91*, 176–180. [CrossRef] [PubMed]
2. Schmahmann, J.D.; Sherman, J.C. Cerebellar Cognitive Affective Syndrome. *Int. Rev. Neurobiol.* **1997**, *41*, 433–440. [CrossRef] [PubMed]
3. Spinelli, M.; Sica, C.; Meglio, L.D.; Bolla, D.; Raio, L.; Surbek, D. Fetal Cerebellar Vermis Circumference Measured by 2-Dimensional Ultrasound Scan: Reference Range, Feasibility and Reproducibility. *Ultrasound Int. Open* **2016**, *2*, E124–E128. [CrossRef] [PubMed]
4. Marzban, H.; Del Bigio, M.R.; Alizadeh, J.; Ghavami, S.; Zachariah, R.M.; Rastegar, M. Cellular commitment in the developing cerebellum. *Front. Cell. Neurosci.* **2015**, *8*, 450. [CrossRef]
5. Ito, M. Cerebellar circuitry as a neuronal machine. *Prog. Neurobiol.* **2006**, *78*, 272–303. [CrossRef]
6. Leto, K.; Arancillo, M.; Becker, E.B.; Buffo, A.; Chiang, C.; Ding, B.; Dobyns, W.; Dusart, I.; Haldipur, P.; Hatten, M.E.; et al. Consensus Paper: Cerebellar Development. *Cerebellum* **2015**, *15*, 789–828. [CrossRef]
7. Guihard-Costa, A.-M.; Larroche, J.-C. Differential growth between the fetal brain and its infratentorial part. *Early Hum. Dev.* **1990**, *23*, 27–40. [CrossRef]
8. Guihard-Costa, A.-M.; Larroche, J. Growth velocity of some fetal parameters. I. Brain weight and brain dimensions. *Biol. Neonate* **1992**, *62*, 309–316. [CrossRef]
9. Co, E.; Raju, T.N.; Aldana, O. Cerebellar dimensions in assessment of gestational age in neonates. *Radiology* **1991**, *181*, 581–585. [CrossRef]
10. Triulzi, F.; Parazzini, C.; Righini, A. MRI of fetal and neonatal cerebellar development. *Semin. Fetal Neonatal Med.* **2005**, *10*, 411–420. [CrossRef] [PubMed]

11. Rizzo, G.; Pietrolucci, M.E.; Mammarella, S.; Dijmeli, E.; Bosi, C.; Arduini, D. Assessment of cerebellar vermis biometry at 18–32 weeks of gestation by three-dimensional ultrasound examination. *J. Matern. Neonatal Med.* **2011**, *25*, 519–522. [CrossRef]
12. Alpay, V.; Davutoglu, E.A.; Kaymak, D.; Madazli, R. Establishment of nomograms for fetal vermis and brainstem structures in the midsagittal cranial plane by ultrasonography. *J. Clin. Ultrasound* **2021**, *49*, 947–955. [CrossRef]
13. Chang, C.-H.C.; Chang, F.-M.; Yu, C.-H.; Ko, H.-C.; Chen, H.-Y. Assessment of fetal cerebellar volume using three-dimensional ultrasound. *Ultrasound Med. Biol.* **2000**, *26*, 981–988. [CrossRef]
14. Júnior, E.A.; Martins, W.P.; Nardozza, L.M.M.; Pires, C.R.; Filho, S.M.Z. Reference Range of Fetal Transverse Cerebellar Diameter Between 18 and 24 Weeks of Pregnancy in a Brazilian Population. *J. Child Neurol.* **2014**, *30*, 250–253. [CrossRef]
15. Leung, T.N.; Pang, M.W.; Daljit, S.S.; Poon, C.F.; Wong, S.M.; Lau, T.K. Fetal biometry in ethnic Chinese: Biparietal diameter, head circumference, abdominal circumference and femur length. *Ultrasound Obstet. Gynecol.* **2008**, *31*, 321–327. [CrossRef]
16. Vinkesteijn, A.; Mulder, P.; Wladimiroff, J. Fetal transverse cerebellar diameter measurements in normal and reduced fetal growth. *Ultrasound Obstet. Gynecol.* **2000**, *15*, 47–51. [CrossRef]
17. Serhatlioglu, S.; Kocakoc, E.; Kiris, A.; Sapmaz, E.; Boztosun, Y.; Bozgeyik, Z. Sonographic measurement of the fetal cerebellum, cisterna magna, and cavum septum pellucidum in normal fetuses in the second and third trimesters of pregnancy. *J. Clin. Ultrasound* **2003**, *31*, 194–200. [CrossRef] [PubMed]
18. Andescavage, N.N.; Du Plessis, A.; McCarter, R.; Serag, A.; Evangelou, I.; Vezina, G.; Robertson, R.; Limperopoulos, C. Complex Trajectories of Brain Development in the Healthy Human Fetus. *Cereb. Cortex* **2016**, *27*, 5274–5283. [CrossRef] [PubMed]
19. Lerman-Sagie, T.; Prayer, D.; Stöcklein, S.; Malinger, G. Fetal cerebellar disorders. *Handb. Clin. Neurol.* **2018**, *155*, 3–23. [CrossRef]
20. Li, L.; Fu, F.; Li, R.; Xiao, W.; Yu, Q.; Wang, D.; Jing, X.; Zhang, Y.; Yang, X.; Pan, M.; et al. Genetic tests aid in counseling of fetuses with cerebellar vermis defects. *Prenat. Diagn.* **2020**, *40*, 1228–1238. [CrossRef] [PubMed]
21. Parisi, M.A.; Dobyns, W.B. Human malformations of the midbrain and hindbrain: Review and proposed classification scheme. *Mol. Genet. Metab.* **2003**, *80*, 36–53. [CrossRef] [PubMed]
22. Leibovitz, Z.; Shkolnik, C.; Haratz, K.K.; Malinger, G.; Shapiro, I.; Lerman-Sagie, T. Assessment of fetal midbrain and hindbrain in mid-sagittal cranial plane by three-dimensional multiplanar sonography. Part 2: Application of nomograms to fetuses with posterior fossa malformations. *Ultrasound Obstet. Gynecol.* **2014**, *44*, 581–587. [CrossRef]
23. Truwit, C.L.; Barkovich, A.J.; Shanahan, R.; Maroldo, T.V. MR imaging of rhombencephalosynapsis: Report of three cases and review of the literature. *Am. J. Neuroradiol.* **1991**, *12*, 957–965.
24. Miller, E.; Orman, G.; Huisman, T.A. Fetal MRI assessment of posterior fossa anomalies: A review. *J. Neuroimaging* **2021**, *31*, 620–640. [CrossRef]
25. Pasquier, L.; Marcorelles, P.; Loget, P.; Pelluard, F.; Carles, D.; Perez, M.-J.; Bendavid, C.; de La Rochebrochard, C.; Ferry, M.; David, V.; et al. Rhombencephalosynapsis and related anomalies: A neuropathological study of 40 fetal cases. *Acta Neuropathol.* **2009**, *117*, 185–200. [CrossRef]
26. Valente, E.M.; Logan, C.V.; Mougou-Zerelli, S.; Lee, J.H.; Silhavy, J.L.; Brancati, F.; Iannicelli, M.; Travaglini, L.; Romani, S.; Illi, B.; et al. Mutations in TMEM216 perturb ciliogenesis and cause Joubert, Meckel and related syndromes. *Nat. Genet.* **2010**, *42*, 619–625. [CrossRef]
27. De Catte, L.; De Keersmaecker, B.; Joyeux, L.; Aertsen, M. *Sonography of the Fetal Central Nervous System*; Elsevier BV: Amsterdam, The Netherlands, 2020.
28. Poretti, A.; Brehmer, U.; Scheer, I.; Bernet, V.; Boltshauser, E. Prenatal and Neonatal MR Imaging Findings in Oral-Facial-Digital Syndrome Type VI. *Am. J. Neuroradiol.* **2008**, *29*, 1090–1091. [CrossRef]
29. Saleem, S.N.; Zaki, M.S.; Soliman, N.A.; Momtaz, M. Prenatal Magnetic Resonance Imaging Diagnosis of Molar Tooth Sign at 17 to 18 Weeks of Gestation in Two Fetuses at Risk for Joubert Syndrome and Related Cerebellar Disorders. *Neuropediatrics* **2011**, *42*, 35–38. [CrossRef]
30. Leanza, V.; D'urso, V.; Gulisano, M.; Incognito, G.G.; Palumbo, M. Bulging of both membranes and fetal lower limbs: Conservative management. *Minerva Obstet. Gynecol.* **2021**, *73*, 654–658. [CrossRef] [PubMed]
31. Leanza, V.; Incognito, G.G.; Gulino, F.A.; Tuscano, A.; Cimino, M.; Palumbo, M. Cesarean Scar Pregnancy and Successful Ultrasound-Guided Removal after Uterine Artery Ligation. *Case Rep. Obstet. Gynecol.* **2023**, *2023*, 6026206. [CrossRef] [PubMed]
32. Orlandi, G.; Toscano, P.; Gabrielli, O.; Di Lella, E.; Lettieri, A.; Manzo, L.; Mazzarelli, L.L.; Sica, C.; Di Meglio, L.; Di Meglio, L.; et al. Prenatal Diagnosis of an Intrathoracic Left Kidney Associated with Congenital Diaphragmatic Hernia: Case Report and Systematic Review. *J. Clin. Med.* **2023**, *12*, 3608. [CrossRef]
33. Leanza, V.; Incognito, G.; Gulisano, M.; Incognito, D.; Correnti, S.; Palumbo, M. Herlyn-Werner-Wunderlich syndrome and central placenta previa in a COVID-19 positive pregnant woman: A case report. *Ital. J. Gynaecol. Obstet.* **2023**, *35*, 136. [CrossRef]
34. Di Guardo, F.; Incognito, G.G.; Lello, C.; D'Urso, G.; Genovese, F.; Palumbo, M. Efficacy of sonohysterography and hysteroscopy for evaluation of endometrial lesions in tamoxifen treated patients: A systematic review. *Eur. J. Gynaecol. Oncol.* **2022**, *43*, 78–86.
35. Incognito, G.G.; D'urso, G.; Incognito, D.; Lello, C.; Miceli, A.; Palumbo, M. Management of a giant uterine smooth muscle tumor of uncertain malignant potential in a 32-year-old woman: Case report and review of the literature. *Minerva Obstet. Gynecol.* **2022**, *74*, 466–470. [CrossRef]
36. Salomon, L.J.; Alfirevic, Z.; Berghella, V.; Bilardo, C.M.; Chalouhi, G.E.; Costa, F.D.S.; Hernandez-Andrade, E.; Malinger, G.; Munoz, H.; Paladini, D.; et al. ISUOG Practice Guidelines (updated): Performance of the routine mid-trimester fetal ultrasound scan. *Ultrasound Obstet. Gynecol.* **2022**, *59*, 840–856. [CrossRef] [PubMed]

37. Paladini, D.; Malinger, G.; Birnbaum, R.; Monteagudo, A.; Pilu, G.; Salomon, L.J.; Timor-Tritsch, I.E. ISUOG Practice Guidelines (updated): Sonographic examination of the fetal central nervous system. Part 2: Performance of targeted neurosonography. *Ultrasound Obstet. Gynecol.* **2021**, *57*, 661–671. [CrossRef] [PubMed]
38. Tan, S.; Ipek, A. Detailed ultrasound screening in the second trimester: Pictorial essay of normal fetal anatomy. *J. Clin. Ultrasound* **2012**, *40*, 280–300. [CrossRef] [PubMed]
39. Ginath, S.; Lerman-Sagie, T.; Krajden, K.H.; Lev, R.; Cohen-Sacher, B.; Bar, J.; Malinger, G. The Fetal vermis, pons and brainstem: Normal longitudinal development as shown by dedicated neurosonography. *J. Matern. Neonatal Med.* **2013**, *26*, 757–762. [CrossRef]
40. Leibovitz, Z.; Shkolnik, C.; Haratz, K.K.; Malinger, G.; Shapiro, I.; Lerman-Sagie, T. Assessment of fetal midbrain and hindbrain in mid-sagittal cranial plane by three-dimensional multiplanar sonography. Part 1: Comparison of new and established nomograms. *Ultrasound Obstet. Gynecol.* **2014**, *44*, 575–580. [CrossRef]
41. Malinger, G.; Lev, D.; Lerman-Sagie, T. Normal and abnormal fetal brain development during the third trimester as demonstrated by neurosonography. *Eur. J. Radiol.* **2006**, *57*, 226–232. [CrossRef]

Disclaimer/Publisher's Note: The statements, opinions and data contained in all publications are solely those of the individual author(s) and contributor(s) and not of MDPI and/or the editor(s). MDPI and/or the editor(s) disclaim responsibility for any injury to people or property resulting from any ideas, methods, instructions or products referred to in the content.

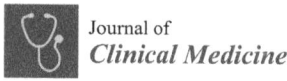

Article

Predicting Preterm Birth with Strain Ratio Analysis of the Internal Cervical Os: A Prospective Study

Alina-Madalina Luca [1,†], Raluca Haba [1,†], Luiza-Maria Cobzeanu [2,†], Dragos Nemescu [1,*], Anamaria Harabor [3,*], Raluca Mogos [1], Ana-Maria Adam [3], Valeriu Harabor [3], Aurel Nechita [3], Gigi Adam [4], Alexandru Carauleanu [1], Sadiye-Ioana Scripcariu [1], Ingrid-Andrada Vasilache [1], Tudor Gisca [1] and Demetra Socolov [1]

[1] Department of Obstetrics and Gynecology, 'Grigore T. Popa' University of Medicine and Pharmacy, 700115 Iasi, Romania
[2] Surgical Department, Faculty of Medicine, University of Medicine and Pharmacy "Grigore T. Popa", 700115 Iasi, Romania
[3] Clinical and Surgical Department, Faculty of Medicine and Pharmacy, 'Dunarea de Jos' University, 800216 Galati, Romania
[4] Department of Pharmaceutical Sciences, Faculty of Medicine and Pharmacy, 'Dunarea de Jos' University, 800216 Galati, Romania; gigi.adam@ugal.ro
* Correspondence: dragos.nemescu@umfiasi.ro (D.N.); ana.harabor@ugal.ro (A.H.)
† These authors contributed equally to this work.

Abstract: (1) Background: Cervical elastography is a new concept that could allow clinicians to assess cervical consistency in various clinical scenarios. We aimed to evaluate the predictive performance of the strain ratio (SR) at the level of the internal os, either individually or in combination with other parameters, in the prediction of spontaneous preterm birth (PTB) at various gestational ages. (2) Methods: This prospective study included 114 pregnant patients with a high-risk profile for PTB who underwent cervical elastography during the second trimester. Clinical and paraclinical data were assessed using univariate analysis, logistic regression, and sensitivity analysis. (3) Results: The SR achieved an area under the receiver operating curve (AUROC) value of 0.850, a sensitivity of 85.71%, and a specificity of 84.31% in the prediction of PTB before 37 weeks of gestation. The combined model showed superior results in terms of accuracy (AUROC = 0.938), sensitivity (92.31%), and specificity (95.16%). When considering PTB subtypes, the highest AUROC value (0.80) and accuracy (95.61%) of this marker were achieved in the prediction of extremely preterm birth, before 28 weeks of gestation. (4) Conclusions: The SR achieved an overall good predictive performance in the prediction of PTB and could be further evaluated in various cohorts of patients.

Keywords: cervix; elastography; preterm birth; prediction; performance

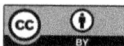

1. Introduction

The uterine cervix plays a crucial role in supporting pregnancy until delivery. The cervix's ability to adapt to the expanding volume of the uterine contents and increasing pressure is contingent on its length and firmness, and the closure of its internal orifice. The mechanical characteristics of the cervix undergo modifications during the course of pregnancy. Preceding parturition, the cervix undergoes a process of ripening, followed by effacement and dilation in response to uterine contractions. Inadequate cervical ripening can lead to premature delivery, with important consequences for neonatal outcomes.

Recently, cervical elastography has emerged as a new concept that can allow clinicians to assess cervical consistency. The theoretical basis of elastography is founded on the measurement of the displacement between two points within an organ when external pressure is applied [1]. The tissue can be characterized as hard and rigid when there is either no alteration in distance or a negligible change. Soft and dilatable tissue exhibits notable alterations [2]. The determination of tissue consistency is denoted as strain, whereby an increase in strain is indicative of lower tissue firmness, and conversely, a decrease in strain is associated with higher tissue firmness.

Several studies have outlined the applicability of cervical elastography for the prediction of preterm birth (PTB) [3–5]. A prospective study by Woźniak et al., on 109 pregnant patients with a short cervix evaluated during the second trimester scan, showed that preterm birth was associated with softening of the internal cervical orifice [6]. Moreover, Hernandez-Andrade et al. reported comparable findings in a cross-sectional study of 545 patients with a low risk of preterm birth that evaluated the values of the strain ratio for quartiles of the endocervical region and whole cervix [7]. Specifically, the authors reported a positive correlation between an increased strain ratio in the internal os region and the risk of preterm delivery, but without significant correlations between elastography parameters of the complete cervix or external os and preterm birth.

Several algorithms for the prediction of preterm birth, based on maternal risk factors, ultrasound markers, and serum biomarkers, have been evaluated in the current literature [8,9]. Among the most commonly associated maternal risk factors for PTB are the following: age, ethnicity, obesity, smoking during pregnancy, assisted reproductive techniques, genital and urinary tract infections, autoimmune disorders, thrombotic disorders, gestational diabetes and preeclampsia, and personal history of adverse pregnancy outcomes (recurrent pregnancy loss, history of PTB, etc.) [10–14]. The predictive performance of algorithms that are solely based on maternal risk factors is modest, with an area under the curve (AUC) value of 0.67, as reported by Damaso et al. [10].

Ultrasound parameters such as a short cervical length and the pulsatility index of the uterine artery have also been assessed from the perspective of PTB, but the results have been conflicting [15–17]. In a secondary analysis conducted by Grobman and colleagues, a short cervical length (<30 mm) on transvaginal ultrasound in the second trimester, between 16 and 22 weeks of gestation, achieved an AUC value of only 0.63 in the prediction of spontaneous PTB before 34 weeks of gestation [18].

Recently, some authors have questioned the predictive performance of a short cervical length of less than 30 mm compared to that of less than 25 mm and suggested that a cut-off of 30 mm in the second trimester of pregnancy may more accurately predict the risk of PTB before 35 and 37 weeks of gestation (AUC: 0.70) [19]. However, the majority of observational studies reported a cut-off of 2.5 cm [20–22], which demonstrated a moderate predictive performance.

Finally, numerous biomarkers have been studied for the prediction of PTB, but only a few, such as cervical fetal fibronectin, alpha fetoprotein, C-reactive protein, and interleukin 6, have obtained good results in terms of the predictive performance in spontaneous preterm birth [23,24].

A recent study by Jung et al. demonstrated that the addition of cervical elastography parameters to the cervical length determined via transvaginal ultrasound can improve the overall prediction of spontaneous preterm birth before 32 weeks of gestation [3]. The aim of this study was to evaluate the predictive performance of the strain ratio measured at the level of the internal os in the prediction of spontaneous preterm birth. A secondary aim of this study was to evaluate the predictive performance of this parameter in combination with the cervical length and clinical risk factors for PTB and its subtypes.

2. Materials and Methods

This prospective study included 114 pregnant patients who attended the Clinical Hospital of Obstetrics and Gynecology "Cuza-Voda", Iasi, Romania, between July 2021 and January 2023, with a high-risk profile for PTB either due to a short cervical length (less than 2.5 cm) or due to the presence of at least two risk factors for PTB. The patients were enrolled in this study during the second trimester anatomy scan, between 18 and 24 weeks of gestation. Informed consent was obtained from all participants, and ethical approval for this study was obtained from the Institutional Ethics Committee of the University of Medicine and Pharmacy "Grigore T. Popa" (No. 101/8 July 2021).

The inclusion criteria were as follows: patients aged between 18 and 45 years with singleton pregnancies, between 18 and 24 weeks of gestation at enrollment, who had a history of adverse pregnancy outcomes (history of preterm birth, recurrent pregnancy loss, stillbirth, ischemic placental disease, or cervical insufficiency) or a cervical length less than 2.5 cm as determined via transvaginal ultrasound, and who offered their informed consent to participate in this study. The exclusion criteria comprised underage patients, twin pregnancies, fetal chromosomal and structural abnormalities, history of cervical surgery such as cervical conization or loop electrosurgical excision procedures, diagnosis of placenta accreta spectrum disorders, incomplete medical data, or inability to provide informed consent.

The patients were subjected to a detailed assessment of their medical history and current medical conditions, along with a thorough clinical examination. The study documented several variables, including age, medium, body mass index (BMI), smoking status, gestational age at enrollment, parity, adverse pregnancy outcomes (such as preterm birth, preeclampsia, intrauterine growth restriction, and stillbirth), and comorbidities.

The patients underwent standard anatomy scans as well as transvaginal ultrasounds performed by experienced obstetricians, with at least a level 2 qualification in ultrasound examination, using an E10 scanner with a 4.8 MHz transabdominal probe, and a 5–15 MHz intravaginal probe (GE Medical Systems, Milwaukee, WI, USA).

The participants were instructed to empty their bladders and to adopt the lithotomy position for the cervical elastography examination. A transvaginal probe was inserted into the anterior vaginal fornix to locate the bladder as a reference point. Subsequently, a conventional sagittal image of the cervix was acquired, and the cervical length was determined as the distance between the internal cervical os and external cervical os. The probe was utilized to generate a maximum of five compression and decompression cycles while operating in elastography mode. We obtained a sagittal section of the cervix and marked the regions of interest (ROIs) at the level of the internal cervical os as reported by Hernandez-Andrade et al. [7]: region of interest on the anterior lip of the internal cervical os, region of interest on the posterior lip of the internal cervical os, reference region on the anterior lip of the external cervical os, and reference region on the posterior lip of the external cervical os (see examples in Figures 1 and 2). The Elastography Analysis program was used to calculate numerical values for the strain ratio based on the selected regions during 5 cycles of compression–decompression, and the mean recorded values of the strain ratios in the regions of interest corresponded to mean recorded value of the internal cervical os strain ratio.

The patients were followed up until delivery, and pregnancy outcomes were recorded. Depending on the gestational age at delivery, the patients were segregated into the following groups: group 1 (n = 63 patients) comprised patients who delivered before term (before 37 completed weeks of gestation), and group 2 (n = 51 patients) comprised patients who delivered at term and were considered controls.

The evaluated pregnancy outcomes were gestational age at birth, type of birth, newborn's gender, Apgar score, neonatal intensive care unit (NICU) admission, fetal death, and the need for mechanical ventilation.

In the first stage of the statistical analysis, categorical variables were evaluated with chi-squared and Fisher exact tests, which are presented as frequencies with the corresponding percentages, and continuous variables were evaluated with t-tests, which are presented as means and standard deviations (SD).

In the second stage of the analysis, we evaluated and compared the predictive performance of the strain ratio and a combined algorithm using logistic regression and ROC analysis. Cut-off values, adjusted to gestational age at diagnosis, were identified according to the Youden index. The combined algorithm comprised the values of the strain ratio, cervical length, and maternal characteristics recorded during the prenatal visit in the second trimester (maternal age, BMI, smoking status, previous history of preterm birth, gestational diabetes, pregnancy-induced hypertension, vaginal or urinary tract infections).

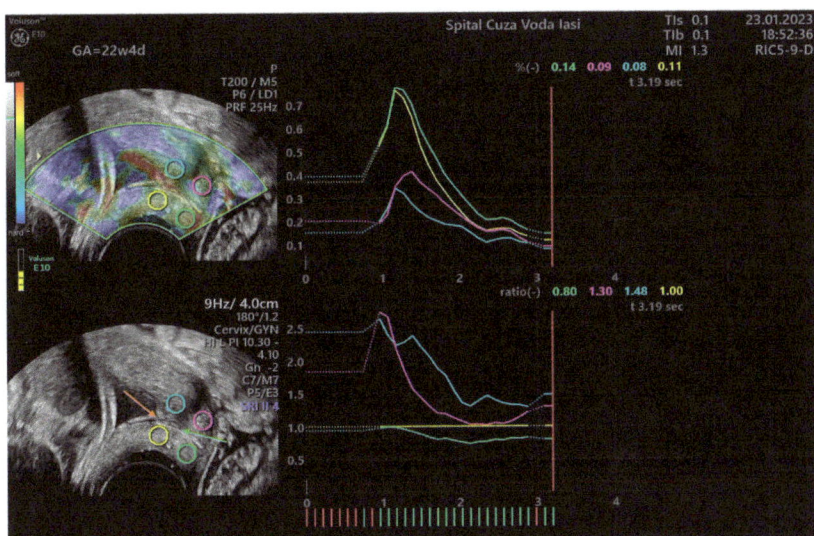

Figure 1. Cervical elastography with the dynamic measurement of the strain ratio in the first 3 cycles of compression–decompression (first example). Legend: orange arrow—internal cervical os; green arrow—cervical canal; blue ring—region of interest on the anterior lip of the internal cervical os; yellow ring—region of interest on the posterior lip of the internal cervical os; pink ring—reference region on the anterior lip of the external cervical os; green ring—reference region on the posterior lip of the external cervical os.

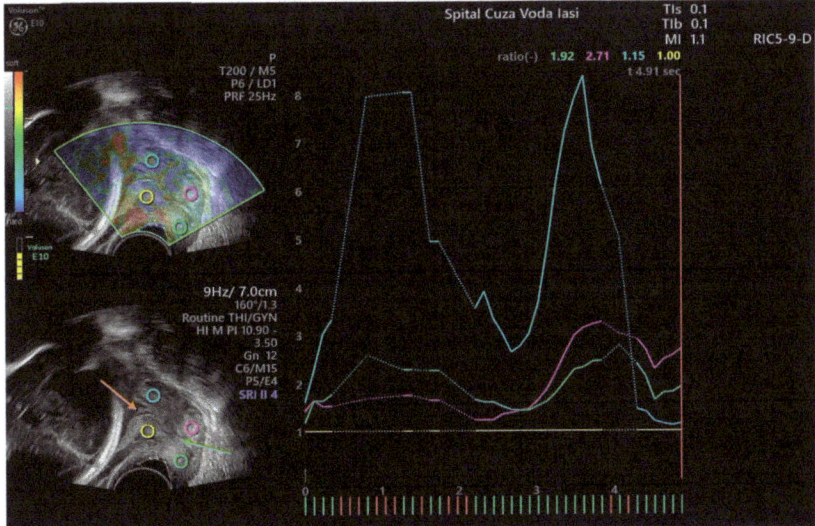

Figure 2. Cervical elastography with the measurement of the strain ratio after 5 cycles of compression–decompression (second example). The mean strain ratio of the internal cervical os was considered for further analysis. Legend: orange arrow—internal cervical os; green arrow—cervical canal; blue ring—region of interest on the anterior lip of the internal cervical os; yellow ring—region of interest on the posterior lip of the internal cervical os; pink ring—reference region on the anterior lip of the external cervical os; green ring—reference region on the posterior lip of the external cervical os.

The classification systems for PTB are heterogeneously reported in the literature [25]. The WHO classifies this concept as follows: extremely PTB (<28 weeks of gestation), very PTB (between 28 and 31 + 6 weeks of gestation), moderate PTB (between 32 and 33 + 6 weeks of gestation), and late PTB (between 34 and 36 + 6 weeks of gestation) [26]. Since our cohort of patients was small, we decided to evaluate the predictive performance of the SR and combined model considering the following subtypes of preterm birth: late preterm birth (between 34 and 37 weeks of gestation), early preterm birth (between 28 and 34 weeks of gestation), and extremely preterm birth (before 28 completed weeks of gestation).

The statistical analyses were performed using STATA SE (version 17, 2022, StataCorp LLC, College Station, TX, USA). A p value less than 0.05 was considered statistically significant.

3. Results

A total of 114 pregnant patients were included in this prospective study, segregated into the following groups: group 1 (n = 63 patients, preterm birth) and group 2 (n = 51 patients, controls). Their clinical and demographic characteristics are presented in Table 1. The pregnant patients who delivered prematurely presented a significant personal history of preterm birth ($p < 0.001$) and other adverse pregnancy outcomes ($p < 0.001$), as well as a shorter cervical length ($p = 0.03$), in comparison with controls.

Table 1. Clinical and demographic characteristics of the patients included in the evaluated groups.

Patient's Characteristics	Group 1 (PTB, n = 63)	Group 2 (Controls, n = 51)	p Value
Age, years (mean ± SD)	30.23 ± 4.16	30.43 ± 4.63	0.48
Medium (n/%)	Urban = 29 (46%) Rural = 34 (54%)	Urban = 25 (49%) Rural = 26 (51%)	0.75
BMI, kg/m^2 (mean ± SD)	22.77 ± 4.98	22.06 ± 3.76	0.28
Smoking (n/%)	Yes = 5 (8.2%)	Yes = 6 (12.8%)	0.43
Parity	Nulliparity = 12 (19%) Primiparity = 30 (47.6%) Multiparity = 21 (33.3%)	Nulliparity = 0 (0%) Primiparity = 42 (82.4%) Multiparity = 9 (17.6%)	<0.001
Personal history of preterm birth (n/%)	Yes = 12 (19%)	Yes = 0 (0%)	<0.001
Confirmed vaginal infection (n/%)	Yes = 21 (33.3%)	Yes = 19 (37.3%)	0.66
Confirmed urinary tract infection (n/%)	Yes = 11 (17.5%)	Yes = 10 (19.6%)	0.76
Hypertension (n/%)	Yes = 9 (14.3%)	Yes = 3 (5.9%)	0.14
Diabetes (n/%)	Yes = 6 (9.5%)	Yes = 3 (5.9%)	0.47
Personal history of adverse pregnancy outcomes (n/%)	Yes = 12 (19%)	Yes = 0 (0%)	<0.001
Cervical length, cm (mean ± SD)	1.97 ± 0.67	2.01 ± 0.88	0.03
Cervical funneling (n/%)	Yes = 8 (12.69%)	Yes = 0 (0%)	0.03

Table legend: PTB—preterm birth; SD—standard deviation; BMI—body mass index.

Cervical funneling was discovered in eight patients who delivered before term (12.69%, $p = 0.03$). On the other hand, the control group had a significantly higher primiparity rate in comparison with the first group ($p < 0.001$).

Regarding pregnancy and neonatal outcomes, we determined significantly higher rates of NICU admission ($p = 0.02$) and invasive ventilation ($p = 0.03$) in the preterm group compared to controls (Table 2). Moreover, the birthweight ($p < 0.001$) and Apgar score at 1 min ($p = 0.003$) were significantly lower compared with controls. Two neonatal deaths were recorded in this cohort of patients due to extreme prematurity.

Table 2. Pregnancy and neonatal outcomes in preterm deliveries.

Outcome	Group 1 (PTB, $n = 63$)	Group 2 (Controls, $n = 51$)	p Value
Cesarean delivery (n/%)	Yes = 9 (14.28%)	Yes = 1 (1.96%)	0.68
Apgar score at 1 min (mean ± SD)	7.07 ± 2.34	8.70 ± 1.22	0.003
Birthweight, g (mean ± SD)	2516.13 ± 407.28	2911.20 ± 683.04	<0.001
Gender (n/%)	Male = 31 (49.2%) Female = 32 (50.8%)	Male = 24 (47.1%) Female = 27 (52.9%)	0.82
NICU admission (n/%)	Yes = 9 (14.3%)	Yes = 1 (1.96%)	0.02
Invasive ventilation (n/%)	Yes = 8 (12.6%)	Yes = 0 (0%)	0.03
Neonatal death (n/%)	Yes = 2 (3.2%)	Yes = 0 (0%)	0.19

Table legend: PTB—preterm birth; SD—standard deviation; NICU—neonatal intensive care unit.

The sensitivity analysis revealed an area under the receiver operating curve (ROC) value of 0.850 (Figure 3), considering a determined cut-off of 0.93 for the SR (Figure 4). The corresponding values for sensitivity, specificity, and precision were 85.71%, 84.31%, and 87.10%, respectively (Table 3). Cervical length achieved a modest value for the AUROC: 0.55 (Figure 5). The combined model, which comprised SR values, cervical length, and the presence of maternal risk factors, showed superior results in terms of accuracy (area under ROC = 0.9388), sensitivity (92.31%), specificity (95.16%), and precision (94.12%) (Figure 5 and Table 3).

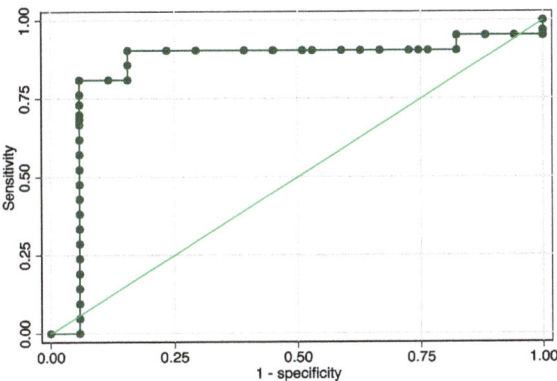

Figure 3. Graphical representation of area under the ROC for the SR at the internal cervical os.

Table 3. Predictive performance of simple and combined approaches for the prediction of preterm birth.

Types of PTB	Approach Used	Sensitivity	Specificity	Precision	NPV	FPR	FDR	FNR	Accuracy
PTB before 37 weeks of gestation	SR (cut-off: 0.93)	85.71	84.31	87.10	82.69	15.6	12.9	14.2	85.09
	Combined model	92.31	95.16	94.12	93.65	4	5	7	93.86
PTB between 34 and 37 weeks of gestation	SR (cut-off: 2.56)	5.2	98.9	50	83.9	1	50	94.7	83.3
	Combined model	96.15	24.42	52.63	89.4	72.58	47.37	3.8	58.1
PTB between 28 and 34 weeks of gestation	SR (cut-off: 1.66)	33.33	81.33	48.15	70.11	18.67	51.85	66.6	64.91
	Combined model	98.08	61.29	68	97.44	38.71	32	1	78.07
PTB at less than 28 weeks of gestation	SR (cut-off: 1.96)	20	99	50	96.43	0.9	50	80	95.61
	Combined model	98	6	46.79	80	93.55	53.21	1	48.25

Table legend: PTB—preterm birth; SR—strain ratio at the level of the internal os; NPV—negative predictive value; FPR—false positive rate; FDR—false detection rate; FNR—false negative rate.

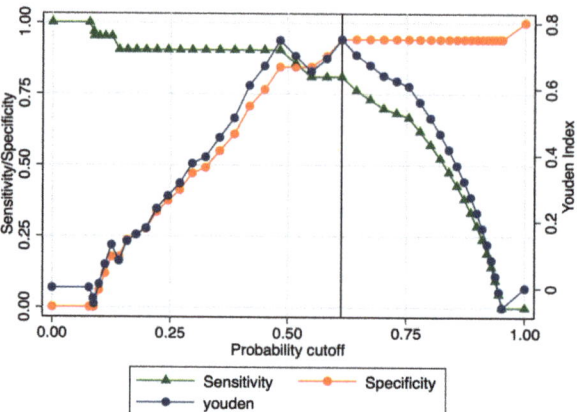

Figure 4. Graphical representation of the Youden Index for the SR at the internal cervical os.

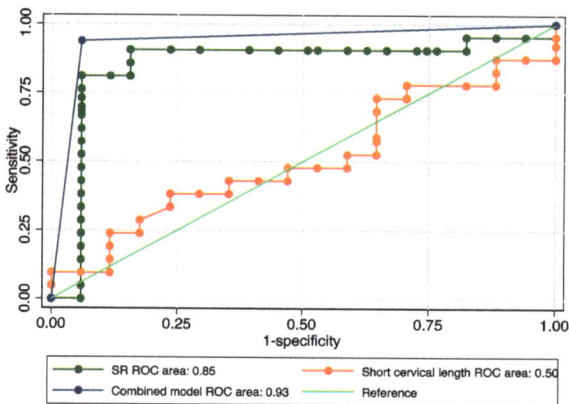

Figure 5. Graphical representation of the comparison between ROC curves for the SR, short cervical length, and combined model.

When evaluating the predictive performance of the strain ratio considering the subtypes of preterm birth, our results revealed an AUROC value of 0.69 in the prediction of late preterm birth (Figure 6). The calculated probability cut-off using the Youden index was 0.58 (Figure 7), and the determined cut-off for this elastography marker using sensitivity analysis was 2.56 (Table 3). The corresponding values for sensitivity, specificity, and precision were 5.2%, 98.9%, and 50%, indicating a poor overall predictive performance (Table 3). The combined model showed slightly better results in terms of the AUROC (0.71), sensitivity (96.15%), specificity (24.42%), and precision (52.63%), but the overall accuracy was low (58.1%) (Figure 8 and Table 3).

When evaluating the predictive performance of the strain ratio at the level of the internal cervical os in the prediction of early preterm birth, it achieved an AUROC value of 0.70 (Figure 9). The calculated probability cut-off using the Youden index was 0.53 (Figure 10), and the determined cut-off for this elastography marker using sensitivity analysis was 1.66 (Table 3). The corresponding values for sensitivity, specificity, and precision were 33.33%, 81.33%, and 48.15%, respectively (Table 3). The combined model showed an improved performance in terms of the AUROC (0.82), sensitivity (98.08%), specificity (61.29%), and precision (68%), with a good overall accuracy (78.07%) (Figure 11 and Table 3).

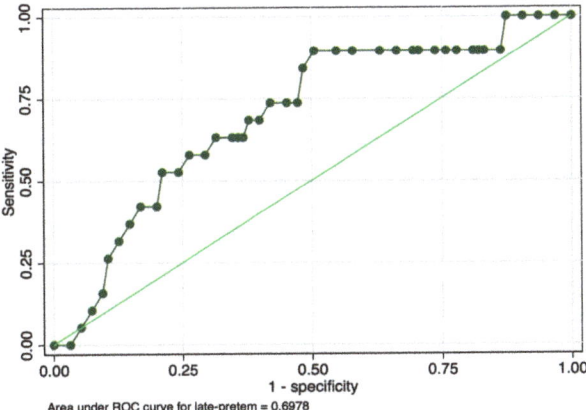

Figure 6. Graphical representation of the area under the ROC for the SR at the internal cervical os considering the late preterm category.

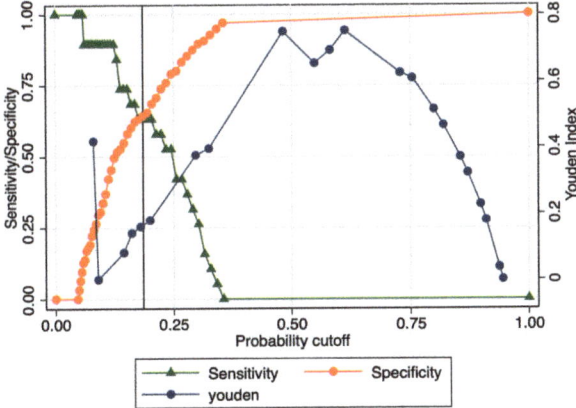

Figure 7. Graphical representation of the Youden Index for the SR at the internal cervical os considering the late preterm category.

When evaluating the predictive performance of the elastography marker in the prediction of extremely preterm birth, we obtained an AUROC value of 0.800 (Figure 12). The calculated probability cut-off using the Youden index was 0.63 (Figure 13), and the determined cut-off for this elastography marker using sensitivity analysis was 1.96 (Table 3). The corresponding values for sensitivity, specificity, and precision were 20%, 99%, and 50%, respectively (Table 3). In this context, its negative predictive value (NPV) was high (96.43%), which led to a good overall accuracy (95.61%). The combined model, however, showed a modest performance in terms of the AUROC (0.630), specificity (46.79%), and overall accuracy (48.25%) (Figure 14 and Table 3).

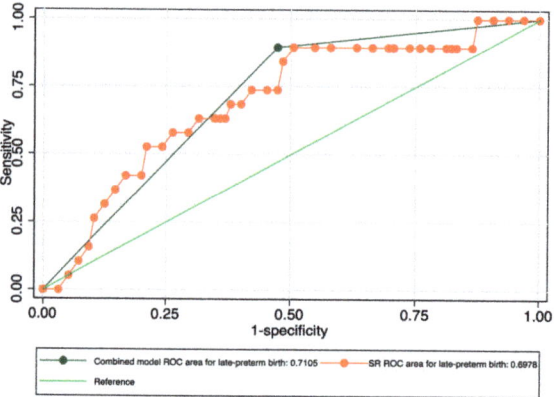

Figure 8. Graphical representation of the comparison between ROC curves for the SR and combined model considering the late preterm category.

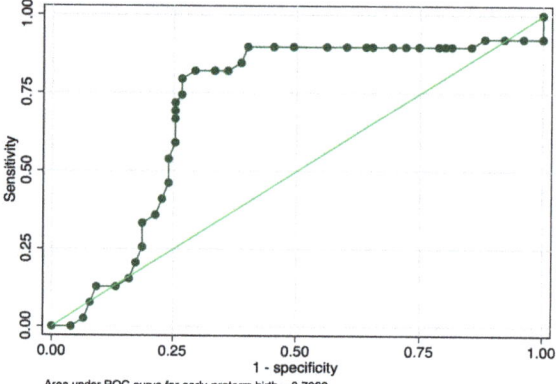

Figure 9. Graphical representation of the area under the ROC for the SR at the internal cervical os considering the early preterm category.

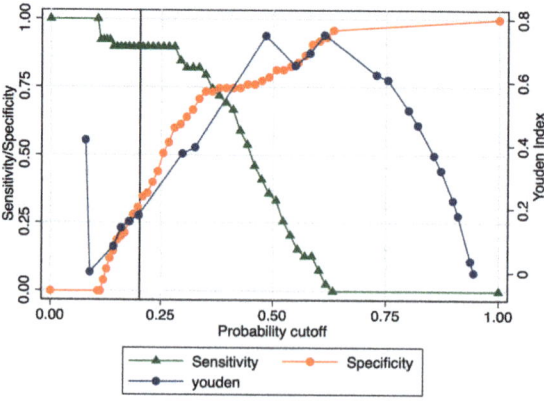

Figure 10. Graphical representation of the Youden Index for the SR at the internal cervical os considering the early preterm category.

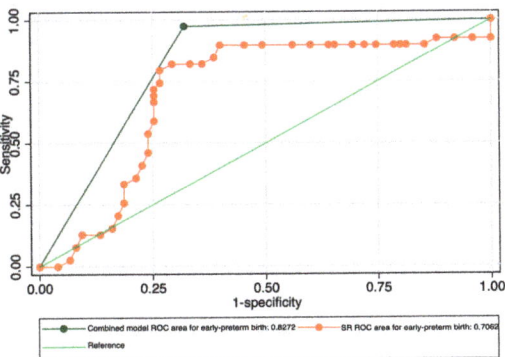

Figure 11. Graphical representation of the comparison between ROC curves for the SR and combined model considering the early preterm category.

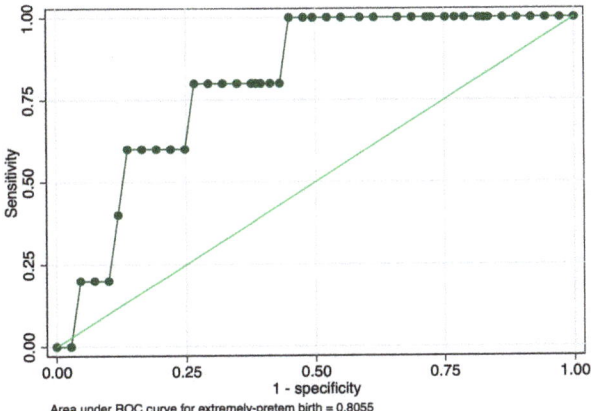

Figure 12. Graphical representation of the area under the ROC for the SR at the internal cervical os considering the extremely preterm category.

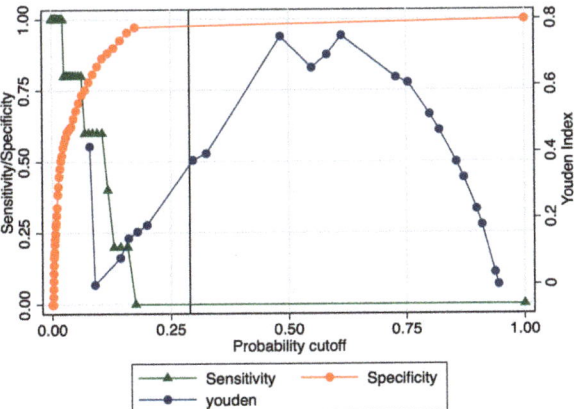

Figure 13. Graphical representation of the Youden Index for the SR at the internal cervical os considering the extremely preterm category.

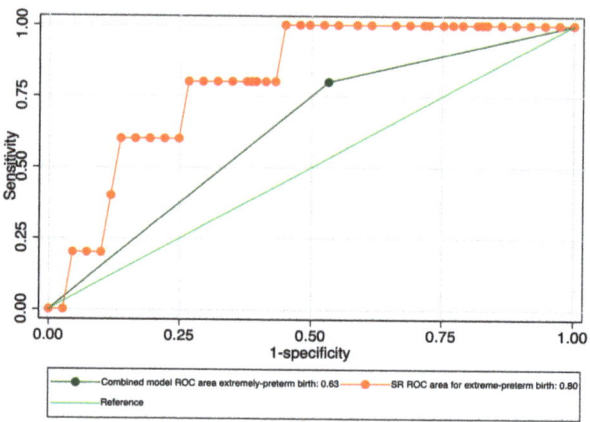

Figure 14. Graphical representation of the comparison between ROC curves for the SR and combined model considering the extremely preterm category.

4. Discussion

One of the issues facing contemporary obstetricians is identifying pregnant patients who are really at risk of PTB. The predictive performance of current individual markers and combined algorithms is modest, and more in-depth studies on elastography assessment of the uterine cervix, particularly the internal os stiffness, will lead to the eventual adoption of this technique by local hospitals. Cervical elastography has the potential to reduce the need for therapeutic interventions in patients whose risk of PTB is low. This will lessen the needless financial burden involved in managing pregnancies while also improving the comfort of pregnant women.

In this study, we evaluated 114 pregnant patients with a high-risk profile of PTB considering the cervical length and personal comorbidities, who were followed up until birth. Our univariate analysis indicated that women who later delivered prematurely had a shorter cervical length, as well as a personal history of preterm birth, in comparison with controls. All these risk factors were included in the regression analysis of the combined algorithm. Moreover, adverse neonatal outcomes such as rates of NICU admission, need for mechanical ventilation, low birthweight, and low Apgar scores were significantly more prevalent in this group.

The results from our univariate analysis regarding maternal risk factors for PTB and the neonatal outcomes confirm many of the findings published in the current literature. A personal history of PTB is one of the most important risk factors for the recurrence of this event, as demonstrated in a recent analysis of a database comprising 213,335 women [27].

In the second stage of the analysis, we evaluated and compared the predictive performance of the strain ratio at the level of the internal cervical os considering the occurrence of preterm birth and its subtypes. Moreover, we compared its performance to that achieved by a combined algorithm as described above. Our results indicated a good predictive performance of this elastography marker in the prediction of preterm birth before 37 weeks of gestation, and its addition to the combined algorithm resulted in an increase in the overall performance.

When evaluating the predictive performance of this marker in relation to PTB subtypes, we obtained mixed results. Specifically, this marker achieved a low sensitivity and high specificity when taken individually, which indicates that it can correctly identify most patients who will not deliver prematurely. This aspect is extremely important because it can help reduce unnecessary interventions.

On the other hand, the highest AUROC value and accuracy of this marker were achieved in the prediction of extremely preterm birth, which is another important aspect to be taken into consideration because this group of neonates is susceptible to numerous serious complications associated with prematurity and need the most expensive and time-consuming therapeutic interventions. When used in combination with the cervical length and maternal risk factors, the overall accuracy was improved only in the prediction of preterm birth before 37 weeks of gestation, and early preterm birth.

In a prospective nested case–control study by Du et al. that assessed cervical elastography parameters and cervical length during the three trimesters of pregnancy, the authors demonstrated that the strain ratio of the internal os measured in the second trimester of pregnancy was the best predictor of spontaneous PTB, with an AUC value of 0.73, while the cervical length measured in any trimester did not achieve a statistical association with this event [28]. These aspects were confirmed in other observational studies in low- and high-risk populations of pregnant patients [6,29,30].

Similar results were obtained using shear wave elastography in singletons and twin pregnancies. Sun et al. conducted a prospective study that evaluated the predictive performance of this type of elastography in the prediction of PTB in dichorionic diamniotic twin pregnancies [31]. For the mean shear wave elastography of the anterior cervical lip, the authors reported a sensitivity of 83.3%, with a specificity of 57.9%, which confirmed its potential use for the prediction of the evaluated outcome. Another study by Yang et al. assessed the predictive performance of shear wave elastography and cervical length in the prediction of spontaneous PTB in singleton pregnancies, obtaining an AUROC value of 0.98 [32].

A recent systematic review and meta-analysis evaluated the diagnostic accuracy of cervical elastography (both strain and shear wave elastography) in the prediction of PTB [33]. The results indicated an overall AUC value of 0.90 for cervical elastography and 0.60 for cervical length in the prediction of PTB. Therefore, this meta-analysis confirmed the superior predictive performance of cervical elastography and its possible implementation in routine clinical practice.

The majority of previous studies were performed using the semiautomatic tool E-Cervix, while very few studies used the General Electric elastography module. One of these tools was used in a cross-sectional study of 116 pregnant women at 18 to 40 weeks of gestation that assessed the factors affecting the cervical tissue strain [34]. The authors outlined a positive correlation between the cervical strain values at the level of the internal os and gestational age, as well as a negative correlation of this parameter with the cervical length. Another multicentric observational study by Jiang et al. [35], which evaluated the performance and capability of various elastography parameters determined in the second trimester of pregnancy, demonstrated that the strain in the anterior lip of the internal os was an independent predictor of spontaneous preterm birth.

An important problem with elastography is represented by the lack of standardization of the procedure due to the multiple types of analytic software, the lack of associated normograms validated in specific populations, various techniques of transvaginal probe manipulation, strategies for the selection of regions of interest, etc. [36]. For this cohort of patients, we adjusted the strain ratio values to the gestational age at enrollment and calculated specific cut-offs using statistical modeling.

The results of this study must be evaluated considering the following limitations: a small sample size, a lack of specific cut-offs and normograms for the studied population, and a lack of correlation with histological data. On the other hand, its prospective design, the evaluation of the predictive performance of this elastography marker in relation to preterm birth and its subtypes, and the integration of this marker into a combined algorithm constitute strong points of this research. Furthermore, these data can contribute to the limited knowledge in the current literature regarding the applications of the General Electric elastography module for the prediction of preterm birth.

Our results support the idea of external validation of a combined model that includes the values of the strain ratio, cervical length, and maternal characteristics in larger cohorts of patients. Such an approach can help to better quantify the predictive performance of a combined model in heterogenous populations. Moreover, this model could be included in pilot studies for further evaluation, and if its predictive performance is confirmed, it could be implemented in clinical practice, thus reducing costs and unnecessary interventions.

5. Conclusions

The strain ratio at the internal cervical os is a reliable tool for the prediction of spontaneous preterm birth before 37 completed weeks of gestation and has a good ability to discriminate most patients who will not deliver prematurely, thus limiting unnecessary therapeutic interventions.

This elastography marker achieved a good predictive performance in the prediction of extremely preterm birth, before 28 weeks of gestation, thus indicating its potential for risk stratification in selected cohorts of patients.

Further studies, on larger cohorts of patients, will be needed to confirm the predictive accuracy of the strain ratio at the internal cervical os in the prediction of preterm birth at various gestational ages.

Author Contributions: Conceptualization, A.-M.L., D.N., A.H., R.H., R.M., A.C., S.-I.S., L.-M.C. and D.S.; methodology, A.-M.A., V.H., A.N., G.A., I.-A.V. and T.G.; software, T.G. and I.-A.V.; validation, A.-M.A., V.H., A.N. and G.A.; formal analysis, A.-M.L.; investigation, A.-M.L., D.N., A.H., R.H., R.M., A.C., S.-I.S., L.-M.C. and D.S.; resources, A.-M.A., V.H., A.N. and G.A.; data curation, T.G. and I.-A.V.; writing—original draft, A.-M.L., D.N., A.H., R.H., R.M., A.C., S.-I.S., L.-M.C. and D.S.; writing—review and editing, A.-M.L., D.N., A.H., R.H., R.M., A.C., S.-I.S., L.-M.C. and D.S.; visualization, I.-A.V.; supervision, D.S.; project administration, A.-M.L. All authors have read and agreed to the published version of the manuscript.

Funding: This research received no external funding.

Institutional Review Board Statement: This study was conducted according to the guidelines of the Declaration of Helsinki and approved by the Institutional Ethics Committee of the University of Medicine and Pharmacy "Grigore T. Popa" (No. 101/8 July 2021).

Informed Consent Statement: Informed consent was obtained from all subjects involved in the study.

Data Availability Statement: The data presented in this study are available on request from the corresponding author. The data are not publicly available due to local policies.

Conflicts of Interest: The authors declare no conflict of interest.

References

1. Oturina, V.; Hammer, K.; Möllers, M.; Braun, J.; Falkenberg, M.K.; De Murcia, K.O.; Schmitz, R. Assessment of cervical elastography strain pattern and its association with preterm birth. *J. Perinat. Med.* **2017**, *45*, 925–932. [CrossRef] [PubMed]
2. Mazza, E.; Parra-Saavedra, M.; Bajka, M.; Gratacos, E.; Nicolaides, K.; Deprest, J. In vivo assessment of the biomechanical properties of the uterine cervix in pregnancy. *Prenat. Diagn.* **2014**, *34*, 33–41. [CrossRef] [PubMed]
3. Jung, Y.J.; Kwon, H.; Shin, J.; Park, Y.; Heo, S.J.; Park, H.S.; Oh, S.-Y.; Sung, J.-H.; Seol, H.-J.; Kim, H.M.; et al. The Feasibility of Cervical Elastography in Predicting Preterm Delivery in Singleton Pregnancy with Short Cervix Following Progesterone Treatment. *Int. J. Environ. Res. Public. Health* **2021**, *18*, 2026. [CrossRef] [PubMed]
4. Gesthuysen, A.; Hammer, K.; Möllers, M.; Braun, J.; Oelmeier de Murcia, K.; Falkenberg, M.K.; Köster, H.A.; Möllmann, U.; Fruscalzo, A.; Bormann, E.; et al. Evaluation of Cervical Elastography Strain Pattern to Predict Preterm Birth. *Ultraschall Med.* **2020**, *41*, 397–403. [CrossRef] [PubMed]
5. Nazzaro, G.; Saccone, G.; Miranda, M.; Crocetto, F.; Zullo, F.; Locci, M. Cervical elastography using E-cervix for prediction of preterm birth in singleton pregnancies with threatened preterm labor. *J. Matern. Fetal Neonatal Med.* **2022**, *35*, 330–335. [CrossRef]
6. Woźniak, S.; Czuczwar, P.; Szkodziak, P.; Wrona, W.; Paszkowski, T. Elastography for predicting preterm delivery in patients with short cervical length at 18–22 weeks of gestation: A prospective observational study. *Ginekol. Pol.* **2015**, *86*, 442–447. [CrossRef]
7. Hernandez-Andrade, E.; Garcia, M.; Ahn, H.; Korzeniewski, S.J.; Saker, H.; Yeo, L.; Chaiworapongsa, T.; Hassan, S.S.; Romero, R. Strain at the internal cervical os assessed with quasi-static elastography is associated with the risk of spontaneous preterm delivery at ≤34 weeks of gestation. *J. Perinat. Med.* **2015**, *43*, 657–666. [CrossRef]
8. Beta, J.; Akolekar, R.; Ventura, W.; Syngelaki, A.; Nicolaides, K.H. Prediction of spontaneous preterm delivery from maternal factors, obstetric history and placental perfusion and function at 11–13 weeks. *Prenat. Diagn.* **2011**, *31*, 75–83. [CrossRef]
9. Celik, E.; To, M.; Gajewska, K.; Smith, G.C.; Nicolaides, K.H. Cervical length and obstetric history predict spontaneous preterm birth: Development and validation of a model to provide individualized risk assessment. *Ultrasound Obs. Gynecol.* **2008**, *31*, 549–554. [CrossRef]

10. Damaso, E.L.; Rolnik, D.L.; Cavalli, R.C.; Quintana, S.M.; Duarte, G.; da Silva Costa, F.; Marcolin, A. Prediction of Preterm, B.irth by Maternal Characteristics and Medical History in the Brazilian Population. *J. Pregnancy* **2019**, *2019*, 4395217. [CrossRef]
11. Vicoveanu, P.; Vasilache, I.A.; Nemescu, D.; Carauleanu, A.; Scripcariu, I.S.; Rudisteanu, D.; Burlui, A.; Rezus, E.; Socolov, D. Predictors Associated with Adverse Pregnancy Outcomes in a Cohort of Women with Systematic Lupus Erythematosus from Romania—An Observational Study (Stage 2). *J. Clin. Med.* **2022**, *11*, 1964. [CrossRef] [PubMed]
12. Vicoveanu, P.; Vasilache, I.A.; Scripcariu, I.S.; Nemescu, D.; Carauleanu, A.; Vicoveanu, D.; Covali, A.R.; Filip, C.; Socolov, D. Use of a Feed-Forward Back Propagation Network for the Prediction of Small for Gestational Age Newborns in a Cohort of Pregnant Patients with Thrombophilia. *Diagnostics* **2022**, *12*, 1009. [CrossRef] [PubMed]
13. Radu, V.D.; Vasilache, I.A.; Costache, R.C.; Scripcariu, I.S.; Nemescu, D.; Carauleanu, A.; Nechifor, V.; Groza, V.; Onofrei, P.; Boiculese, L.; et al. Pregnancy Outcomes in a Cohort of Patients Who Underwent Double-J Ureteric Stenting—A Single Center Experience. *Medicina* **2022**, *58*, 619. [CrossRef]
14. Săndulescu, M.S.; Văduva, C.C.; Siminel, M.A.; Dijmărescu, A.L.; Vrabie, S.C.; Camen, I.V.; Tache, D.E.; Neamțu, S.D.; Nagy, R.D.; Carp-Velișcu, A.; et al. Impact of COVID-19 on fertility and assisted reproductive technology (ART): A systematic review. *Rom. J. Morphol. Embryol.* **2022**, *63*, 503–510. [CrossRef] [PubMed]
15. Van Zijl, M.D.; Koullali, B.; Mol, B.W.J.; Snijders, R.J.; Kazemier, B.M.; Pajkrt, E. The predictive capacity of uterine artery Doppler for preterm birth-A cohort study. *Acta Obs. Gynecol. Scand.* **2020**, *99*, 494–502. [CrossRef]
16. Camen, I.V.; Manolea, M.M.; Vrabie, S.C.; Sandulescu, M.S.; Serbanescu, M.S.; Boldeanu, M.V.; Novac, M.B. The Ability of Doppler Uterine Artery Ultrasound to Predict Premature Birth. *Curr. Health Sci. J.* **2022**, *48*, 277–283.
17. Bernad, S.E.; Barbat, T.; Barbu, D.; Albulescu, V. Assessment of the placental blood flow in the normally developing and growth-restricted fetus. In *Advances in Perinatal Medicine*; Springer: Berlin/Heidelberg, Germany, 2010; pp. 127–130. ISBN 978-88-6521-027-7. Accession Number: WOS:000281970400019.
18. Grobman, W.A.; Lai, Y.; Iams, J.D.; Reddy, U.M.; Mercer, B.M.; Saade, G.; Tita, A.T.; Rouse, D.J.; Sorokin, Y.; Wapner, R.J.; et al. Prediction of Spontaneous Preterm Birth among Nulliparous Women with a Short Cervix. *J. Ultrasound Med.* **2016**, *35*, 1293–1297. [CrossRef] [PubMed]
19. Guerby, P.; Girard, M.; Marcoux, G.; Beaudoin, A.; Pasquier, J.C.; Bujold, E. Midtrimester Cervical Length in Low-Risk Nulliparous Women for the Prediction of Spontaneous Preterm Birth: Should We Consider a New Definition of Short Cervix? *Am. J. Perinatol.* **2023**, *40*, 187–193. [CrossRef]
20. Singh, P.K.; Srivastava, R.; Kumar, I.; Rai, S.; Pandey, S.; Shukla, R.C.; Verma, A. Evaluation of Uterocervical Angle and Cervical Length as Predictors of Spontaneous Preterm Birth. *Indian J. Radiol. Imaging* **2022**, *32*, 10–15. [CrossRef]
21. O'Hara, S.; Zelesco, M.; Sun, Z. Cervical length for predicting preterm birth and a comparison of ultrasonic measurement techniques. *Australas. J. Ultrasound Med.* **2013**, *16*, 124–134. [CrossRef]
22. Suresh, S.; MacGregor, C.; Dude, A.; Hirsch, E. Single second-trimester cervical length is predictive of preterm delivery among patients with prophylactic cerclage. *Am. J. Obstet. Gynecol.* **2022**, *227*, 910–911.e1. [CrossRef] [PubMed]
23. Lucaroni, F.; Morciano, L.; Rizzo, G.; Antonio, F.D.; Buonuomo, E.; Palombi, L.; Arduini, D. Biomarkers for predicting spontaneous preterm birth: An umbrella systematic review. *J. Matern. Fetal Neonatal Med.* **2018**, *31*, 726–734. [CrossRef] [PubMed]
24. Hornaday, K.K.; Wood, E.M.; Slater, D.M. Is there a maternal blood biomarker that can predict spontaneous preterm birth prior to labour onset? A systematic review. *PLoS ONE* **2022**, *17*, e0265853. [CrossRef] [PubMed]
25. Vogel, J.P.; Chawanpaiboon, S.; Moller, A.B.; Watananirun, K.; Bonet, M.; Lumbiganon, P. The global epidemiology of preterm birth. *Best Pract. Res. Clin. Obs. Gynaecol.* **2018**, *52*, 3–12. [CrossRef]
26. Karnati, S.; Kollikonda, S.; Abu-Shaweesh, J. Late preterm infants–Changing trends and continuing challenges. *Int. J. Pediatr. Adolesc. Med.* **2020**, *7*, 38–46. [CrossRef]
27. Tingleff, T.; Vikanes, Å.; Räisänen, S.; Sandvik, L.; Murzakanova, G.; Laine, K. Risk of preterm birth in relation to history of preterm birth: A population-based registry study of 213,335 women in Norway. *BJOG Int. J. Obstet. Gynaecol.* **2022**, *129*, 900–907. [CrossRef]
28. Du, L.; Zhang, L.H.; Zheng, Q.; Xie, H.N.; Gu, Y.J.; Lin, M.F.; Wu, L. Evaluation of Cervical Elastography for Prediction of Spontaneous Preterm Birth in Low-Risk Women: A Prospective Study. *J. Ultrasound Med.* **2020**, *39*, 705–713. [CrossRef]
29. Światkowska-Freund, M.; Traczyk-łoś, A.; Preis, K.; łukaszuk, M.; Zielińska, K. Prognostic value of elastography in predicting premature delivery. *Ginekol. Pol.* **2014**, *85*, 204–207. [CrossRef]
30. Wozniak, S.; Czuczwar, P.; Szkodziak, P.; Milart, P.; Wozniakowska, E.; Paszkowski, T. Elastography in predicting preterm delivery in asymptomatic, low-risk women: A prospective observational study. *BMC Pregnancy Childbirth* **2014**, *14*, 238. [CrossRef]
31. Sun, J.; Li, N.; Jian, W.; Cao, D.; Yang, J.; Chen, M. Clinical application of cervical shear wave elastography in predicting the risk of preterm delivery in DCDA twin pregnancy. *BMC Pregnancy Childbirth* **2022**, *22*, 202. [CrossRef]
32. Yang, X.; Ding, Y.; Mei, J.; Xiong, W.; Wang, J.; Huang, Z.; Li, R. Second-Trimester Cervical Shear Wave Elastography Combined with Cervical Length for the Prediction of Spontaneous Preterm Birth. *Ultrasound Med. Biol.* **2022**, *48*, 820–829. [CrossRef] [PubMed]
33. Wang, B.; Zhang, Y.; Chen, S.; Xiang, X.; Wen, J.; Yi, M.; Hu, B. Diagnostic accuracy of cervical elastography in predicting preterm delivery A systematic review and meta-analysis. *Medicine* **2019**, *98*, e16449. [CrossRef] [PubMed]
34. Wongsaroj, P.; Moungmaithong, S. Cervical Strain Values Measured by Ultrasonographic Elastography in Pregnant Women between 18 and 40 Weeks' Gestation. *J. Med. Assoc. Thai* **2017**, *100*, 825.

35. Jiang, L.; Peng, L.; Rong, M.; Liu, X.; Pang, Q.; Li, H.; Wang, Y.; Liu, Z. Nomogram Incorporating Multimodal Transvaginal Ultrasound Assessment at 20 to 24 Weeks' Gestation for Predicting Spontaneous Preterm Delivery in Low-Risk Women. *Int. J. Womens Health* **2022**, *14*, 323–331. [CrossRef] [PubMed]
36. Swiatkowska-Freund, M.; Preis, K. Cervical elastography during pregnancy: Clinical perspectives. *Int. J. Womens Health* **2017**, *9*, 245–254. [CrossRef] [PubMed]

Disclaimer/Publisher's Note: The statements, opinions and data contained in all publications are solely those of the individual author(s) and contributor(s) and not of MDPI and/or the editor(s). MDPI and/or the editor(s) disclaim responsibility for any injury to people or property resulting from any ideas, methods, instructions or products referred to in the content.

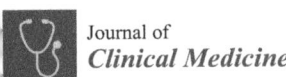 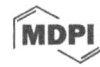

Article

Prediction of Neonatal Respiratory Morbidity Assessed by Quantitative Ultrasound Lung Texture Analysis in Twin Pregnancies

Ana L. Moreno-Espinosa [1,2,3,*], Ameth Hawkins-Villarreal [1,2,3], David Coronado-Gutierrez [1,4], Xavier P. Burgos-Artizzu [1,4], Raigam J. Martínez-Portilla [1,3,5], Tatiana Peña-Ramirez [6,7], Dahiana M. Gallo [6,7], Stefan R. Hansson [8,9], Eduard Gratacòs [1,10,11] and Montse Palacio [1,10,11]

1. BCNatal-Fetal Medicine Research Center, Hospital Clínic and Hospital Sant Joan de Déu, Universitat de Barcelona, 08028 Barcelona, Spain
2. Department of Obstetrics and Gynecology, Hospital Santo Tomás, Universidad de Panamá, Panama City 07096, Panama
3. Iberoamerican Research Network in Obstetrics, Gynecology and Translational Medicine, Mexico City 06720, Mexico
4. Transmural Biotech SL, 08021 Barcelona, Spain
5. Clinical Research Branch, National Institute of Perinatology, Mexico City 11000, Mexico
6. School of Medicine, Universidad del Valle, Cali 760032, Colombia
7. Department of Obstetrics and Gynecology, Hospital Universitario del Valle Evaristo García E.S.E., Cali 760043, Colombia
8. Department of Obstetrics and Gynecology, Institute of Clinical Sciences Lund, Lund University, 221 00 Lund, Sweden
9. Skåne University Hospital, 214 28 Malmö, Sweden
10. Centre for Biomedical Research on Rare Diseases (CIBERER), 28029 Madrid, Spain
11. Institut d'Investigacions Biomèdiques August Pi i Sunyer, 08036 Barcelona, Spain
* Correspondence: analisbeth22@yahoo.com; Tel.: +34-932-27-54-00 (ext. 7281)

Abstract: The objective of this study was to evaluate the performance of quantitative ultrasound of fetal lung texture analysis in predicting neonatal respiratory morbidity (NRM) in twin pregnancies. This was an ambispective study involving consecutive cases. Eligible cases included twin pregnancies between 27.0 and 38.6 weeks of gestation, for which an ultrasound image of the fetal thorax was obtained within 48 h of delivery. Images were analyzed using quantusFLM® version 3.0. The primary outcome of this study was neonatal respiratory morbidity, defined as the occurrence of either transient tachypnea of the newborn or respiratory distress syndrome. The performance of quantusFLM® in predicting NRM was analyzed by matching quantitative ultrasound analysis and clinical outcomes. This study included 166 images. Neonatal respiratory morbidity occurred in 12.7% of cases, and it was predicted by quantusFLM® analysis with an overall sensitivity of 42.9%, specificity of 95.9%, positive predictive value of 60%, and negative predictive value of 92.1%. The accuracy was 89.2%, with a positive likelihood ratio of 10.4, and a negative likelihood ratio of 0.6. The results of this study demonstrate the good prediction capability of NRM in twin pregnancies using a non-invasive lung texture analysis software. The test showed an overall good performance with high specificity, negative predictive value, and accuracy.

Keywords: fetal lung maturity; quantitative lung texture analysis; twin pregnancies; neonatal respiratory morbidity

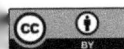

1. Introduction

The reported rates of neonatal respiratory morbidity (NRM) in twins are variable. Overall rates of 13.5% [1] to 19% [2] have been addressed in different studies. In addition, rates of 5.34% have been described for late preterm twins [3]. Gender [4], birth order [5], chorionicity [3], and birthweight discordance [6,7] are some of the factors which may affect the risk of NMR. In twin pregnancies, there is usually disparity between twins, so the risk of respiratory morbidity may be different for each infant in each twin pair [8].

Non-invasive prediction of fetal lung maturity by ultrasound has been under research for many years now. The method used by quantusFLM® is based on a combination of machine learning and texture extraction, which have shown a strong correlation with gestational age [9], and a test to predict fetal lung maturation (FLM), previously widely performed on amniotic fluid [10]. The prediction of NRM was also addressed in a single-center [11] and a multicenter study [12], in which pregnancies with different co-morbidities were recruited, including multiple pregnancies.

The prevalence of twins born at <37 weeks is almost invariably reported to be around 50%, with 32% of births prior to 35 weeks, between 15 and 20% at <34 weeks, and 9 to 11.4% at <32 weeks [13–17].

Publications on NRM and its prediction in twin pregnancies are scarce and present mixed outcomes, with twin pregnancies frequently being an exclusion criterion to evaluate results in diagnostic tests. Some studies have evaluated fetal lung maturity in twin pregnancies [18–20]; however, none of these studies have focused on predicting NRM or reporting the performance of the tests used. We hypothesized that the performance of quantusFLM® in predicting NRM in neonates from twin pregnancies would be comparable to that previously reported in the general population.

The objective of this study was to evaluate the performance of quantitative ultrasound fetal lung texture analysis in predicting NRM in twin pregnancies.

2. Materials and Methods

2.1. Patient Recruiting

This was an ambispective study involving twin pregnancies. Prospective cases were recruited at the Hospital Clinic, Barcelona, Spain, in collaboration with Hospital Universitario del Valle, "Evaristo García" E.S.E., Cali, Colombia. Patients were recruited from January 2018 to February 2020. Retrospective cases were identified from a database designed for a multicenter study [12] (recruited from June 2011 to December 2014), and the information was added to the present study for the analysis. Eligible cases included consecutive cases of twin pregnancies between 25.0 and 38.6 weeks of gestation, for which an ultrasound image of the fetal thorax was obtained within 48 h of delivery. Every ultrasound image of the fetal thorax included in the study for analysis corresponded to a fetus from a twin pregnancy. When the image of one twin could not be obtained or was discarded after quality control, the image of the remaining twin was included. Fetal position was the main factor that did not allow for obtainment of the image, regardless of the presentation or whether it was the first or second fetus. Images were discarded after image quality control when the following were present: insufficient magnification, blurred images, calipers within the area of analysis, and acoustic shadows. Cases of twin pregnancies in which fetal death occurred spontaneously or secondary to procedures such as placental laser due to twin-to-twin transfusion syndrome, cord occlusion due to fetal malformation, or selective intrauterine growth restriction were also included.

Cases were excluded in two scenarios: (i) if steroids for fetal lung maturity had been used between the image acquisition and delivery, and (ii) fetuses with known congenital malformations or chromosomal abnormalities. Additionally, in the postnatal period, we excluded: neonates with sepsis, umbilical artery pH < 7.00, symptomatic anemia, postnatal diagnosis of chromosomal abnormalities, and meconium aspiration syndrome, which could explain respiratory difficulties due to reasons other than lung immaturity.

2.2. Image Processing

Ultrasound images were obtained following an acquisition protocol as detailed previously [12]. Images fulfilling the quality criteria were uploaded via the Internet by the engineers at the coordinating center through restricted access to a commercial software website (www.quantusflm.com (accessed on 26 February 2021); Transmural Biotech, Barcelona, Spain) and analyzed using the new quantusFLM® version 3.0 [21]. This software automatically delineates a region of interest (ROI) in the fetal lung and calculates an NRM risk score, defined as the occurrence of either respiratory distress syndrome (RDS) or transient tachypnea of the newborn (TTN), as a continuous variable. To evaluate the risk of NRM, continuous output NRM risk scores were binarized using the optimal cut-off point threshold, computed as that which maximizes accuracy in the test images, thereby obtaining a categorical result (i.e., high or low risk). The optimal cut-off threshold was computed as that which maximizes the F1-Score using the entire dataset. The F1-Score is an accuracy metric which balances sensitivity and positive predictive values (PPV) to better judge the real usefulness of the prediction. It measures the harmonic average between sensitivity and PPV and is defined as (2 × True Positives)/(2 × True positives + False Positives + False Negatives).

2.3. Reference Standard

The primary outcome of the study was the development of NRM defined as the occurrence of either TTN or RDS. Perinatal and neonatal characteristics and outcomes were recorded from clinical charts in databases designed for the study. RDS was defined based on the typical chest radiography findings and admission to the neonatal intensive care unit for respiratory support, or the need for supplemental oxygen, together with clinical criteria, including grunting, nasal flaring, tachypnea, and chest wall retraction. Transient tachypnea of the newborn was diagnosed based on a chest X-ray showing hyperaeration of the lungs and prominent pulmonary vascular patterns, together with the clinical criteria of early and short-lived respiratory distress (isolated tachypnea, rare grunting, minimal retraction).

2.4. Ethical Approval

All patients included in the study provided written informed consent for the use of ultrasound images and perinatal data. The study was approved by the Institutional Review Board of the Hospital Clinic of Barcelona (HCB/2017/0642), and Hospital Universitario del Valle, "Evaristo García" E.S.E. (008-2019).

2.5. Statistical Analysis

Quantitative variables were assessed using the Shapiro–Wilk test for normality, and normally distributed variables were expressed as the mean and standard deviation (SD). Non-normally distributed quantitative variables were expressed as the median and interquartile range (IQR: p25–75). Qualitative variables were reported as frequencies and percentages. The performance of quantusFLM® in predicting NRM was analyzed by cross-tabulation of the results of the test against those of the reference standard, in this case the neonatal diagnosis of TTN or RDS. Contingency tables were used to estimate accuracy measurements. Fagan nomograms were constructed to show the pre-test probabilities of NRM in twins at different gestational ages, positive and negative likelihood ratios, and post-test probabilities. The data were analyzed using STATA, v.15.0 (College Station, TX, USA).

3. Results

3.1. Patient and Sample Characteristics

Prospective data: A total of 102 images were acquired, 10 (9.8%) of which were discarded after image quality control and 13 (12.7%) of which were excluded due to the use of antenatal steroids between the image acquisition and delivery. The remaining 79 images were included in the study. **Retrospective data**: A total of 87 images already chosen in the selection process of a previous study were added for analysis. This study included 166 images from 166 fetuses which were stratified into three groups: from 25.0 to 33.6 weeks [35/166 (21.1%)], from 34.0 to 36.6 weeks [48/166 (28.9%)], and from 37.0 to 38.6 weeks [83/166 (50.0%)]. The flowchart of the eligible cases according to the Standards for Reporting of Diagnostic Accuracy Studies (STARD) guidelines is shown in Figure 1. The excluded cases with the quantusFLM® results and perinatal outcomes are shown in Table S1.

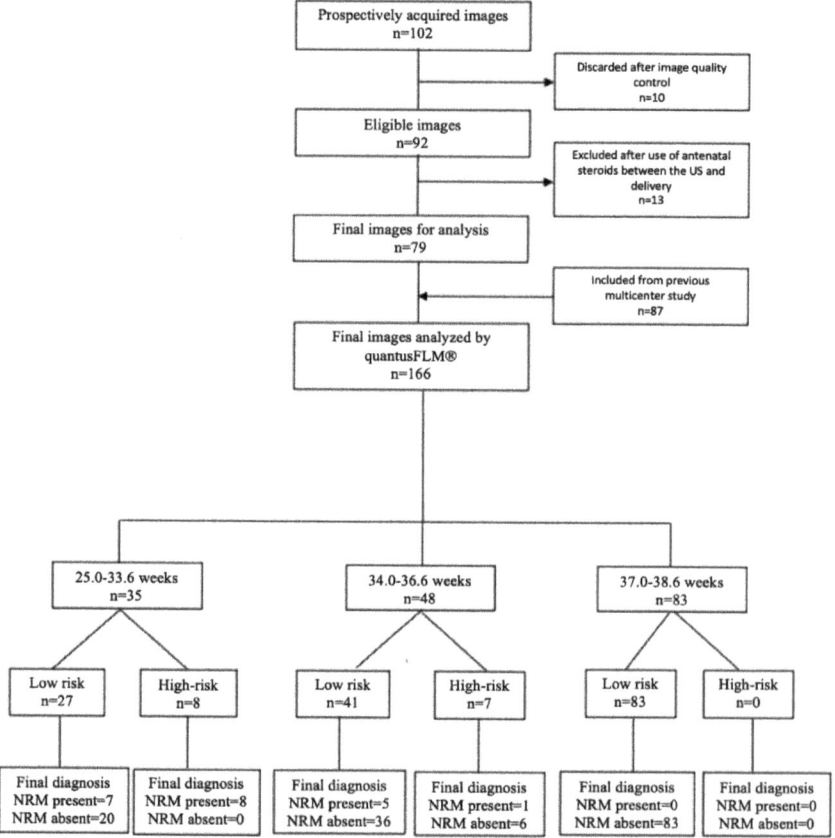

Figure 1. Flowchart of the eligible cases according to STARD guidelines.

The baseline and clinical characteristics of the women included in the study are described in Table 1. This study included 1 woman at <28.0 weeks; 20 women at 28.0 to <34.0 weeks; 32 women at 34.0 to <37.0 weeks; and 52 women at ≥37.0 weeks of gestation. Perinatal and neonatal characteristics are shown in Table 2. The overall prevalence of NRM was 12.7% (21/166), of which 61.9% (13/21) was diagnosed as TTN and 38.1% (8/21) as RDS. The prevalence of NRM was 42.9% (15/35) in the group from 25.0 to 33.6 weeks, and 12.5% (6/48) from 34.0 to 36.6 weeks, while in the group > 37.0 weeks, we found no cases of NRM. The newborns diagnosed with TTN received continuous positive airway pressure (CPAP) [92.3% (12/13)], oxygen ≥ 40% [23.1% (3/13)], or non-invasive ventilation/bilevel positive airway pressure (NIV/BIPAP) [15.4% (2/13)] up to 48 h. While newborns diagnosed with RDS were treated with invasive ventilation [62.5% (5/8)] or a combination of CPAP, NIV/BIPAP, and oxygen ≥ 40% [37.5% (3/8)], almost all received at least one dose of surfactant [87.5% (7/8)] and all were born below 34.0 weeks.

Table 1. Baseline characteristics of women included in the study.

		Gestational Age at US Scan, Weeks		
	Total (n = 105)	25.0–33.6 (n = 21)	34.0–36.6 (n = 32)	37.0–38.6 (n = 52)
Maternal age, mean (SD)	34.6 (4.3)	33.8 (4.8)	34.4 (3.6)	35.0 (4.4)
Nulliparity, n (%)	72 (68.6)	14 (66.7)	23 (71.9)	35 (67.3)
BMI, median (IQR)	22.7 (20.8–24.7)	22.4 (21.0–25.0)	22.7 (19.8–23.7)	23.0 (21.2–25.5)
Ethnicity, n (%)				
Caucasian, n (%)	87 (83.7)	14 (66.7)	30 (93.8)	43 (84.3)
Black	0 (0)	0 (0)	0 (0)	0 (0)
Asian	3 (2.9)	0 (0)	2 (3.1)	2 (3.9)
Hispanic	9 (8.7)	6 (28.6)	0 (0)	3 (5.9)
Other	5 (4.7)	1 (4.7)	1 (3.1)	3 (5.9)
Chorionicity, n (%)				
Dichorionic	61 (66.3)	8 (40.0)	17 (63.0)	36 (80.0)
Monochorionic	31 (33.7)	12 (60.0)	10 (37.0)	9 (20.0)
Antenatal steroids, n (%)	32 (31.4)	21 (100)	8 (25.0)	4 (7.7)
Relevant maternal–fetal conditions, n (%)				
IVF	38 (36.2)	5 (23.8)	13 (40.6)	20 (38.5)
Preeclampsia	15 (14.3)	5 (23.8)	9 (28.1)	1 (2.0)
IUGR [a]	16 (15.2)	4 (19.1)	9 (28.1)	3 (5.8)
Diabetes	9 (8.6)	4 (19.1)	2 (6.3)	3 (5.8)
Preterm labor/PPROM	15 (14.3)	9 (42.9)	5 (15.6)	1 (2.0)

Data are presented as the mean (SD: standard deviation), number (%: percentage), or median (IQR: interquartile range) when appropriate. US: ultrasound; BMI: body mass index; IUGR: intrauterine growth restriction; IVF: in vitro fertilization; PPROM: preterm premature rupture of membranes. [a] IUGR in 16 mothers corresponds to 23/166 (13.9%) fetuses.

Table 2. Perinatal and neonatal outcomes.

		Gestational Age at US Scan, Weeks		
	Total (n = 166)	25.0–33.6 (n = 35)	34.0–33.6 (n = 48)	37.0–38.6 (n = 83)
GA at delivery, median (IQR)	36.8 (34.6–37.5)	33 (32.1–33.4)	36.3 (35.4–36.4)	37.5 (37.2–38.1)
US-to-delivery time days, mean (SD)	0.7 (0.8)	0.9 (0.7)	0.8 (0.8)	0.5 (0.8)
Mode of delivery, n (%)				
Spontaneous vaginal delivery	34 (20.5)	6 (17.1)	16 (33.3)	12 (14.5)
Operative vaginal delivery	9 (5.4)	0 (0)	5 (10.4)	4 (4.8)
Non-elective cesarean delivery	26 (15.7)	7 (20.0)	6 (12.5)	13 (15.7)
Elective cesarean delivery	97 (58.4)	22 (62.9)	21 (43.8)	54 (65.0)
Birthweight, mean (SD)	2313 (510)	1665 (333)	2199 (359)	2653 (319)
Female sex, n (%)	89 (53.9)	18 (51.4)	30 (62.5)	41 (50.0)
Apgar at 5 min < 7, n (%)	0 (0)	0 (0)	0 (0)	0 (0)
pH UA < 7.10, n (%)	3 (1.8)	0 (0)	3 (6.3)	0 (0)
Phototherapy, n (%)	26 (15.7)	14 (40)	10 (20.8)	2 (2.4)
NICU admission, n (%)	36 (21.7)	26 (74.3)	9 (18.8)	1 (1.2)
NICU length of stay, mean (SD)	15.3 (13.3)	17.9 (14.2)	8.8 (6.2)	1 (1.0)
Neonatal death, n (%)	0 (0)	0 (0)	0 (0)	0 (0)
Characteristics of the respiratory morbidity and support, n (%)				
Neonatal respiratory morbidity	21 (12.7)	15 (42.9)	6 (12.5)	0 (0)

Table 2. Cont.

	Total (n = 166)	Gestational Age at US Scan, Weeks		
		25.0–33.6 (n = 35)	34.0–33.6 (n = 48)	37.0–38.6 (n = 83)
Respiratory distress syndrome	8 (4.8)	8 (22.9)	0 (0)	0 (0)
Transient tachypnea	13 (7.8)	7 (20.0)	6 (12.5)	0 (0)
Respiratory support	21 (12.7)	16 (45.7)	5 (10.4)	0 (0)
Oxygen therapy ≥ 40%	9 (5.4)	7 (20.0)	2 (4.2)	0 (0)
CPAP	20 (12.1)	15 (42.9)	5 (10.4)	0 (0)
NIV/BiPAP	6 (3.6)	4 (11.4)	2 (4.2)	0 (0)
Invasive ventilation	5 (3.0)	5 (14.3)	0 (0)	0 (0)
High-frequency ventilation	0 (0)	0 (0)	0 (0)	0 (0)
Surfactant use	7 (4.2)	7 (20.0)	0 (0)	0 (0)

Data are presented as the mean (SD: standard deviation) or number n (%: percentage) when appropriate. GA: gestational age; US: ultrasound; pH UA: pH umbilical artery; NICU: neonatal intensive care unit; CPAP: continuous positive airway pressure; NIV/BiPAP: non-invasive/bilevel positive airway pressure.

3.2. Performance of the Test

The occurrence of NRM was predicted by the quantusFLM® analysis in the overall population with a sensitivity of 42.9% (9/21), specificity of 95.9% (139/145), positive predictive value (PPV) of 60% (9/15), and negative predictive value (NPV) of 92.1% (139/151). The accuracy was 89.2% (148/166), the positive likelihood ratio (LR+) was 10.4, and the negative likelihood ratio (LR-) was 0.6. Table 3 shows the performance of the tests by groups of gestational age. A summary of the overall performance of quantusFLM® described in the general population in previous studies and in twin pregnancies is shown in Table S2.

Table 3. Performance of quantusFLM in predicting neonatal respiratory morbidity in twin pregnancies.

	Total (n = 166)	Gestational Age at US Scan, Weeks		
		25.0–33.6 (n = 35)	34.0–36.6 (n = 48)	37.0–38.6 (n = 83)
Neonatal respiratory morbidity, n (%)	21 (12.7)	15 (42.9)	6 (12.5)	0 (0)
Sensitivity, % (95% CI)	42.9 (24.5–63.5)	53.1 (30.1–75.2)	16.7 (3.0–56.4)	n/a
Specificity, % (95% CI)	95.9 (91.3–98.1)	97.6 (83.9–100)	85.7 (72.2–93.3)	99.9 (95.6–100)
True positives (n)	9	8	1	0
True negatives (n)	139	20	36	83
False positives (n)	6	0	6	0
False negatives (n)	12	7	5	0
Positive predictive value, % (95% CI)	60.0 (35.7–80.2)	94.4 (67.6–100)	14.3 (2.6–51.3)	n/a
Negative predictive value, % (95% CI)	92.1 (86.6–95.4)	73.4 (55.3–86.8)	87.8 (75.0–97.8)	99.9 (95.6–100)
Accuracy, % (95% CI)	89.2 (83.5–93.0)	78.4 (64.1–90.0)	77.1 (63.5–86.7)	n/a
F1-Score (%)	50.0	68.0	15.4	n/a
Positive likelihood ratio (95% CI)	10.4 (4.1–26.1)	22.3 (19.0–26.2)	1.2 (0.2–8.1)	n/a
Negative likelihood ratio (95% CI)	42.9 (24.5–63.5)	53.1 (30.1–75.2)	16.7 (3.0–56.4)	n/a

Data are presented as the percentage (%) when appropriate. CI: confidence interval. Continuity correction factor of 0.5 for cells with cero values. n/a: not applicable. US: ultrasound.

Figure 2 depicts the Fagan nomogram analysis to evaluate the clinical utility of the prediction of neonatal respiratory morbidity by quantusFLM® in twin pregnancies. Table S3 shows the pre-test and post-test risk and probabilities of neonatal respiratory morbidity in twins.

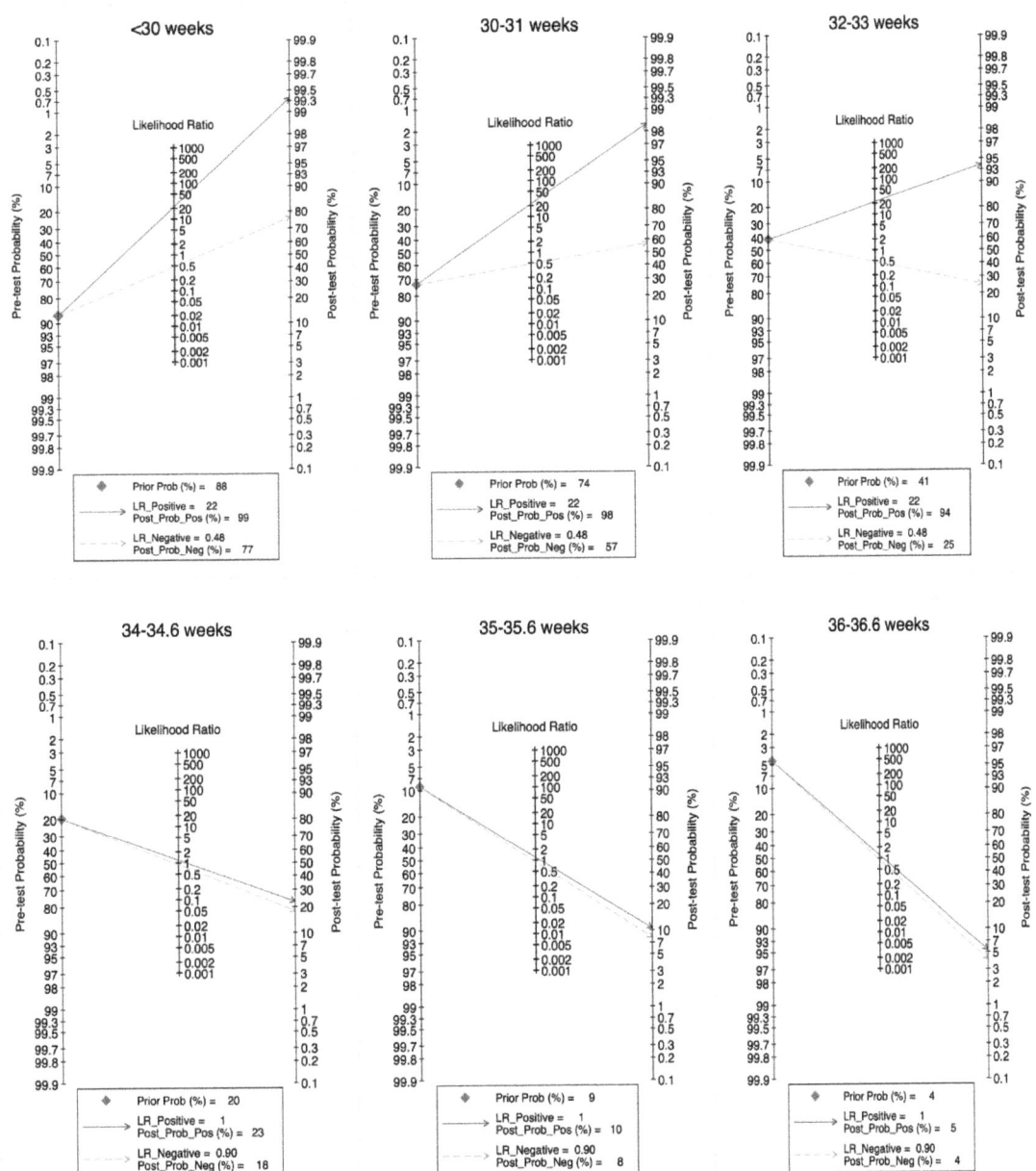

Figure 2. Fagan nomogram analysis to evaluate the clinical utility of the prediction of neonatal respiratory morbidity by quantusFLM® in twin pregnancies. Pre-test probabilities of neonatal respiratory morbidity in twins were obtained from Clin Chim Acta 484 (2018) 293–297 for <30.0 up to 33.6 weeks [22] and from BMJ 2016;354: i4353 for 34.0 up to 36.6 weeks of gestation [3].

4. Discussion

In this study, we explored, for the first time, the performance of a non-invasive lung texture analysis in predicting NRM in twin pregnancies. Considering different ranges of gestational age, we found better performance below 34.0 weeks with a specificity of 97.6%, an NPV of 73.4%, and an LR+ of 22.3, allowing for the identification of fetuses at high risk of NRM, with an accuracy of 78.4%. A high-risk result is accurate in predicting the presence of NRM because the LR for this result generates large changes in the pre-test probabilities of NRM. In the group between 34.0 and 36.6 weeks, we found a specificity of 85.7%, an NPV of 87.8%, and an LR+ of 1.2, albeit with a low sensitivity of 16.7%. A high-risk result generates fewer changes in the pre-test probabilities, and a low-risk result is less accurate in predicting the absence of NRM, as shown in the Fagan plots. Above 37 weeks, there was no case of RDS/TTN, precluding the calculation of all the parameters. All images were classified as having a low risk of NRM. Therefore, the ability of the test to correctly identify a fetus without NRM with a negative result is effective at any gestational age.

Compared to the results previously reported for the test in the general population, the twin results showed a similar performance in the overall specificity, with 94.7% and 95.9%, respectively. The negative predictive value (NPV) and accuracy changed from 95.4% to 92.1% and 91.5% to 89.2%, respectively. A more pronounced decrease was noted in the sensitivity from 71.0% to 42.9%, the PPV from 67.9 to 60%, and the F1-Score from 69.4 to 50.0%.

These findings are in line with those reported by Tsuda et al. [23], who evaluated a model combining gestational age and lamellar body count (LBC) to predict NRM in twins. They reported a sensitivity of 69.0% and a specificity of 88.0% for the best cut-off value, which is in line with our results in the gestational age group <32 weeks, and obtained a specificity of 97.0% for predicting RDS/TTN, although in the gestational age group >37 weeks, the diagnostic accuracy decreased compared to the preterm period. Gestational age is the strongest factor associated with FLM and should therefore be considered in the interpretation of a false positive and/or a false negative result.

The overall prevalence of NRM in our population was 12.7%, which is in line with that reported by Tsuda et al., using the amniotic lamellar body count (LBC) as a predictive tool in different series of twin pregnancies [1,23]. Other studies have reported prevalence of up to 19% including TTN and RDS [2].

The management of twin pregnancies remains challenging, even more so when the delivery of preterm fetuses is indicated due to medical conditions. As 32% of twins have been reported to be born prior to 35 weeks, in this scenario, more than 30% of twins would receive antenatal steroids, considering that the most widespread use of antenatal steroids is up to 34.0/34.6 weeks. However, harmful effects should be considered. Many studies have shown that the administration of corticosteroids in twin pregnancies does not improve neonatal morbidity and mortality [24], but rather can cause higher rates of hypoglycemia [25] or reduced fetal biometry [26]. It should also be noted that nearly 75% of women with twins deliver outside the optimal window for either the initial or rescue corticosteroid courses [27].

Given the controversial data that do not clearly show the same benefits of corticosteroids in twin pregnancies compared to singletons, and the increasing data showing that there may even be harmful effects [28,29], the prediction of NRM may play a role in the decision-making process. Its usefulness could also be tested in clinical protocols when corticosteroids have already been administered and an attempt is made to avoid repeated doses. Additionally, the technique can be used in any center in the world, and reliable results can be obtained if good-quality images are sent via the web for analysis.

The main strength of our study is that the prediction of NRM of fetuses from twin pregnancies was evaluated with a non-invasive, machine learning-based technology. This technology has proven to be robust in the general population and has the advantages of being accessible and easy to use. In the present study, only 10 images were discarded after image quality control. The method tested herein is an indirect approach to predict

NRM, and it is largely related to gestational age, but not to other factors influencing lung maturity status. Our study had a limited number of cases with NRM in some gestational ages compared to late gestational ages, in which NRM is a rarer event. However, the Fagan plots showed that, although there were fewer changes compared to the pre-test probability, the method can provide useful information if needed, and the NPV supports the strategy in ruling out NRM. Additionally, the algorithms have not been designed for each specific gestational age, precluding assessment of the performance of the software in each gestational age. However, the gestational age range is a widely used measure to drive clinical decisions in the field of maternal–fetal medicine.

In summary, the results of this study show that NRM in twins can be predicted by a non-invasive lung texture analysis with an overall good specificity, NPV, and accuracy. QuantusFLM® may be useful in planning indicated delivery of twin pregnancies because of medical conditions and may help to avoid repeated doses of corticosteroids when the fetuses have already been exposed and the risk of preterm delivery is still present. Therefore, in adequate facilities, this technology can be incorporated into protocols according to gestational age and may be helpful in the decision-making process when delivery is planned.

Supplementary Materials: The following supporting information can be downloaded at: https://www.mdpi.com/article/10.3390/jcm11164895/s1, Table S1: Summary of excluded cases due to administration of antenatal steroids after image acquisition and before delivery; Table S2: Summary of performance of quantusFLM® in the general population and in twin pregnancies to predict neonatal respiratory morbidity; Table S3: Pre-test risk and probabilities, positive and negative likelihood ratios and a post-test probabilities and risk of the neonatal respiratory morbidity in twin pregnancies.

Author Contributions: Conceptualization, M.P. and A.L.M.-E.; methodology, M.P. and A.L.M.-E.; software, X.P.B.-A. and D.C.-G.; formal analysis, A.L.M.-E., A.H.-V., D.C.-G and R.J.M.-P.; investigation, A.L.M.-E., A.H.-V., D.M.G. and T.P.-R.; resources, A.L.M.-E. and T.P.-R.; data curation, X.P.B.-A. and D.C.-G.; writing—original draft preparation, A.L.M.-E. and A.H.-V.; writing—review and editing, M.P. and S.R.H.; visualization, A.L.M.-E.; supervision, M.P., D.M.G. and S.R.H.; project administration, M.P. and E.G.; funding acquisition, E.G. and A.L.M.-E. All authors have read and agreed to the published version of the manuscript.

Funding: This research was partially funded with the support of the *Erasmus + Programme of the European Union* (Framework Agreement No. 2013-0040) and Transmural Biotech SL. This publication reflects the views of the authors only, and the Commission cannot be held responsible for any use which may be made of the information contained herein. Additionally, A.L.M.-E. and A.H.-V. have received financial support from the *Secretaría Nacional de Ciencia y Tecnología de Panamá* (SENACYT) grant No. 270-2017-294 and *Instituto Nacional para la formación y aprovechamiento de Recursos Humanos de Panamá* (IFARHU), respectively. The APC was funded by the Erasmus + Programme of the European Union (Framework Agreement No. 2013-0040).

Institutional Review Board Statement: This study was conducted in accordance with the Declaration of Helsinki and approved by the Institutional Review Board of the *Hospital Clinic of Barcelona* (HCB/2017/0642) approved in December 2017, and *Hospital Universitario del Valle, "Evaristo García"* E.S.E. (008-2019) approved in March 2019.

Informed Consent Statement: Informed consent was obtained from all subjects involved in the study.

Data Availability Statement: The data presented in this study are available on request from the corresponding author. The data are not publicly available due to restrictions according to patient privacy regulations.

Acknowledgments: We would like to thank all the Fetal Lung Texture Team members from the previous multicenter study for acquisition of part of the sample included in this study.

Conflicts of Interest: X.P.B.-A. has served and D.C.-G. serves as a Transmural Biotech SL. employee. M.P. has served and E.G. serves as a scientific advisor to Transmural Biotech SL. The other authors declare no competing interests. The funders had no role in the design of the study; in the collection, analyses, or interpretation of data; in the writing of the manuscript; or in the decision to publish the results.

References

1. Tsuda, H.; Kotani, T.; Sumigama, S.; Mano, Y.; Kawabata, I.; Takahashi, Y.; Iwagaki, S.; Hirakawa, A.; Kikkawa, F. Amniotic lamellar body count: Predicting and distinguishing neonatal respiratory complications in twin pregnancies. *Clin. Chim. Acta* **2015**, *441*, 75–78. [CrossRef] [PubMed]
2. Bricelj, K.; Tul, N.; Lasic, M.; Bregar, A.T.; Verdenik, I.; Lucovnik, M.; Blickstein, I. Respiratory morbidity in twins by birth order, gestational age and mode of delivery. *J. Perinat. Med.* **2016**, *44*, 899–902. [CrossRef] [PubMed]
3. Cheong-See, F.; Schuit, E.; Arroyo-Manzano, D.; Khalil, A.; Barrett, J.; Joseph, K.S.; Asztalos, E.; Hack, K.; Lewi, L.; Lim, A.; et al. Prospective risk of stillbirth and neonatal complications in twin pregnancies: Systematic review and meta-analysis. *BMJ* **2016**, *354*, i4353. [CrossRef] [PubMed]
4. Stevenson, D.K.; Tyson, J.E. Beware of the weaker sex: Don't get too close to your twin brother. *Pediatrics* **2007**, *120*, 638–639. [CrossRef]
5. Usta, I.M.; Nassar, A.H.; Awwad, J.T.; Nakad, T.I.; Khalil, A.M.; Karam, K.S. Comparison of the perinatal morbidity and mortality of the presenting twin and its co-twin. *J. Perinatol.* **2002**, *22*, 391–396. [CrossRef]
6. Canpolat, F.E.; Yurdakök, M.; Korkmaz, A.; Yigit, S.; Tekinalp, G. Birthweight discordance in twins and the risk of being heavier for respiratory distress syndrome. *Twin Res. Hum. Genet.* **2006**, *9*, 659–663. [CrossRef]
7. Di Mascio, D.; Acharya, G.; Khalil, A.; Odibo, A.; Prefumo, F.; Liberati, M.; Buca, D.; Manzoli, L.; Flacco, M.E.; Brunelli, R.; et al. Birthweight discordance and neonatal morbidity in twin pregnancies: A systematic review and meta-analysis. *Acta Obstet. Gynecol. Scand.* **2019**, *98*, 1245–1257. [CrossRef]
8. Moreno-Espinosa, A.L.; Hawkins-Villarreal, A.; Burgos-Artizzu, X.P.; Coronado-Gutierrez, D.; Castelazo, S.; Lip-Sosa, D.L.; Fuenzalida, J.; Gallo, D.M.; Peña-Ramirez, T.; Zuazagoitia, P.; et al. Concordance of the risk of neonatal respiratory morbidity assessed by quantitative ultrasound lung texture analysis in fetuses of twin pregnancies. *Sci. Rep.* **2022**, *12*, 9016. [CrossRef]
9. Cobo, T.; Bonet-Carne, E.; Martínez-Terrón, M.; Perez-Moreno, A.; Elías, N.; Luque, J.; Amat-Roldan, I.; Palacio, M. Feasibility and reproducibility of fetal lung texture analysis by automatic quantitative ultrasound analysis and correlation with gestational age. *Fetal Diagn. Ther.* **2012**, *31*, 230–236. [CrossRef]
10. Palacio, M.; Cobo, T.; Martínez-Terrón, M.; Rattá, G.A.; Bonet-Carné, E.; Amat-Roldán, I.; Gratacós, E. Performance of an automatic quantitative ultrasound analysis of the fetal lung to predict fetal lung maturity. *Am. J. Obstet. Gynecol.* **2012**, *207*, 504.e1–504.e5. [CrossRef]
11. Bonet-Carne, E.; Palacio, M.; Cobo, T.; Perez-Moreno, A.; Lopez, M.; Piraquive, J.P.; Ramirez, J.C.; Botet, F.; Marques, F.; Gratacos, E. Quantitative ultrasound texture analysis of fetal lungs to predict neonatal respiratory morbidity. *Ultrasound Obstet. Gynecol.* **2015**, *45*, 427–433. [CrossRef] [PubMed]
12. Palacio, M.; Bonet-Carne, E.; Cobo, T.; Perez-Moreno, A.; Sabrià, J.; Richter, J.; Kacerovsky, M.; Jacobsson, B.; García-Posada, R.A.; Bugatto, F.; et al. Prediction of neonatal respiratory morbidity by quantitative ultrasound lung texture analysis: A multicenter study. *Am. J. Obstet. Gynecol.* **2017**, *217*, 196.e1–196.e14. [CrossRef] [PubMed]
13. Li, S.; Gao, J.; Liu, J.; Hu, J.; Chen, X.; He, J.; Tang, Y.; Liu, X.; Cao, Y. Perinatal Outcomes and Risk Factors for Preterm Birth in Twin Pregnancies in a Chinese Population: A Multi-center Retrospective Study. *Front. Med.* **2021**, *8*, 657862. [CrossRef] [PubMed]
14. Makrydimas, G.; Sotiriadis, A. Prediction of preterm birth in twins. *Best Pract. Res. Clin. Obstet. Gynaecol.* **2014**, *28*, 265–272. [CrossRef] [PubMed]
15. Chauhan, S.P.; Scardo, J.A.; Hayes, E.; Abuhamad, A.Z.; Berghella, V. Twins: Prevalence, problems, and preterm births. *Am. J. Obstet. Gynecol.* **2010**, *203*, 305–315. [CrossRef] [PubMed]
16. Rissanen, A.R.S.; Jernman, R.M.; Gissler, M.; Nupponen, I.K.; Nuutila, M.E. Perinatal outcomes in Finnish twins: A retrospective study. *BMC Pregnancy Childbirth* **2019**, *20*, 2. [CrossRef]
17. Goldenberg, R.L.; Iams, J.D.; Miodovnik, M.; Van Dorsten, J.P.; Thurnau, G.; Bottoms, S.; Mercer, B.M.; Meis, P.J.; Moawad, A.H.; Das, A.; et al. The preterm prediction study: Risk factors in twin gestations. National Institute of Child Health and Human Development Maternal-Fetal Medicine Units Network. *Am. J. Obstet. Gynecol.* **1996**, *175*, 1047–1053. [CrossRef]
18. Whitworth, N.S.; Magann, E.F.; Morrison, J.C. Evaluation of fetal lung maturity in diamniotic twins. *Am. J. Obstet. Gynecol.* **1999**, *180*, 1438–1441. [CrossRef]
19. Leveno, K.J.; Quirk, J.G.; Whalley, P.J.; Herbert, W.N.P.; Trubey, R. Fetal lung maturation in twin gestation. *Am. J. Obstet. Gynecol.* **1984**, *148*, 405–411. [CrossRef]
20. Mackenzie, M.W. Predicting concordance of biochemical lung maturity in the preterm twin gestation. *J. Matern. Neonatal Med.* **2002**, *12*, 50–58. [CrossRef]
21. Burgos-Artizzu, X.P.; Perez-Moreno, Á.; Coronado-Gutierrez, D.; Gratacos, E.; Palacio, M. Evaluation of an improved tool for non-invasive prediction of neonatal respiratory morbidity based on fully automated fetal lung ultrasound analysis. *Sci. Rep.* **2019**, *9*, 1950. [CrossRef] [PubMed]

22. Tsuda, H.; Kotani, T.; Nakano, T.; Imai, K.; Ushida, T.; Hirakawa, A.; Kinoshita, F.; Takahashi, Y.; Iwagaki, S.; Kikkawa, F. The impact of fertility treatment on the neonatal respiratory outcomes and amniotic lamellar body counts in twin pregnancies. *Clin. Chim. Acta* **2018**, *484*, 192–196. [CrossRef] [PubMed]
23. Tsuda, H.; Hirakawa, A.; Kotani, T.; Sumigama, S.; Mano, Y.; Nakano, T.; Imai, K.; Kawabata, I.; Takahashi, Y.; Iwagaki, S.; et al. Risk assessment for neonatal RDS/TTN using gestational age and the amniotic lamellar body count in twin pregnancies. *Clin. Chim. Acta* **2015**, *451*, 301–304. [CrossRef]
24. Viteri, O.A.; Blackwell, S.C.; Chauhan, S.P.; Refuerzo, J.S.; Pedroza, C.; Salazar, X.C.; Sibai, B.M. Antenatal Corticosteroids for the Prevention of Respiratory Distress Syndrome in Premature Twins. *Obstet. Gynecol.* **2016**, *128*, 583–591. [CrossRef] [PubMed]
25. Ben-David, A.; Zlatkin, R.; Bookstein-Peretz, S.; Meyer, R.; Mazaki-Tovi, S.; Yinon, Y. Does antenatal steroids treatment in twin pregnancies prior to late preterm birth reduce neonatal morbidity? Evidence from a retrospective cohort study. *Arch. Gynecol. Obstet.* **2020**, *302*, 1121–1126. [CrossRef]
26. Braun, T.; Weichert, A.; Gil, H.C.; Sloboda, D.M.; Tutschek, B.; Harder, T.; Dudenhausen, J.W.; Plagemann, A.; Henrich, W. Fetal and neonatal outcomes after term and preterm delivery following betamethasone administration in twin pregnancies. *Int. J. Gynecol. Obstet.* **2016**, *134*, 329–335. [CrossRef]
27. Rottenstreich, A.; Levin, G.; Kleinstern, G.; Haj Yahya, R.; Rottenstreich, M.; Yagel, S.; Elchalal, U. Patterns of use and optimal timing of antenatal corticosteroids in twin compared with singleton pregnancies. *Acta Obstet. Gynecol. Scand.* **2018**, *97*, 1508–1514. [CrossRef]
28. Räikkönen, K.; Gissler, M.; Kajantie, E. Associations between Maternal Antenatal Corticosteroid Treatment and Mental and Behavioral Disorders in Children. *JAMA—J. Am. Med. Assoc.* **2020**, *323*, 1924–1933. [CrossRef]
29. Ninan, K.; Liyanage, S.K.; Murphy, K.E.; Asztalos, E.V.; McDonald, S.D. Evaluation of Long-term Outcomes Associated with Preterm Exposure to Antenatal Corticosteroids: A Systematic Review and Meta-analysis. *JAMA Pediatr.* **2022**, *176*, e220483. [CrossRef]

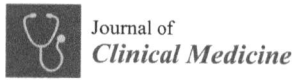

Systematic Review

Evolving the Era of 5D Ultrasound? A Systematic Literature Review on the Applications for Artificial Intelligence Ultrasound Imaging in Obstetrics and Gynecology

Elena Jost [1], Philipp Kosian [1], Jorge Jimenez Cruz [1], Shadi Albarqouni [2,3], Ulrich Gembruch [1], Brigitte Strizek [1] and Florian Recker [1,*]

1. Department of Obstetrics and Gynecology, University Hospital Bonn, Venusberg Campus 1, 53127 Bonn, Germany
2. Department of Diagnostic and Interventional Radiology, University Hospital Bonn, Venusberg Campus 1, 53127 Bonn, Germany
3. Helmholtz AI, Helmholtz Munich, Ingolstädter Landstraße 1, 85764 Neuherberg, Germany
* Correspondence: florian.recker@ukbonn.de; Tel.: +49-228287-37116

Abstract: Artificial intelligence (AI) has gained prominence in medical imaging, particularly in obstetrics and gynecology (OB/GYN), where ultrasound (US) is the preferred method. It is considered cost effective and easily accessible but is time consuming and hindered by the need for specialized training. To overcome these limitations, AI models have been proposed for automated plane acquisition, anatomical measurements, and pathology detection. This study aims to overview recent literature on AI applications in OB/GYN US imaging, highlighting their benefits and limitations. For the methodology, a systematic literature search was performed in the PubMed and Cochrane Library databases. Matching abstracts were screened based on the PICOS (Participants, Intervention or Exposure, Comparison, Outcome, Study type) scheme. Articles with full text copies were distributed to the sections of OB/GYN and their research topics. As a result, this review includes 189 articles published from 1994 to 2023. Among these, 148 focus on obstetrics and 41 on gynecology. AI-assisted US applications span fetal biometry, echocardiography, or neurosonography, as well as the identification of adnexal and breast masses, and assessment of the endometrium and pelvic floor. To conclude, the applications for AI-assisted US in OB/GYN are abundant, especially in the subspecialty of obstetrics. However, while most studies focus on common application fields such as fetal biometry, this review outlines emerging and still experimental fields to promote further research.

Keywords: systematic review; ultrasound imaging; artificial intelligence; deep learning; obstetrics; gynecology; fetal echocardiography; application

Citation: Jost, E.; Kosian, P.; Jimenez Cruz, J.; Albarqouni, S.; Gembruch, U.; Strizek, B.; Recker, F. Evolving the Era of 5D Ultrasound? A Systematic Literature Review on the Applications for Artificial Intelligence Ultrasound Imaging in Obstetrics and Gynecology. *J. Clin. Med.* **2023**, *12*, 6833. https://doi.org/10.3390/jcm12216833

Academic Editor: Michal Kovo

Received: 21 September 2023
Revised: 17 October 2023
Accepted: 25 October 2023
Published: 29 October 2023

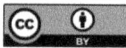

Copyright: © 2023 by the authors. Licensee MDPI, Basel, Switzerland. This article is an open access article distributed under the terms and conditions of the Creative Commons Attribution (CC BY) license (https://creativecommons.org/licenses/by/4.0/).

1. Introduction

Artificial intelligence (AI) is known to be present in everyday life, and over the past years it has gained considerable significance in medical imaging. The term AI refers to various types of computer science technologies, which enable machines to perform tasks simulating human intelligence. AI systems are typically dependent on the input of vast amounts of data, e.g., for pattern recognition, in order to learn to create predictions, classifications, recommendations, or decisions either supervised by humans or without supervision. Terms like machine learning or deep learning represent two of the numerous subcategories of AI [1].

Widely described advantages of AI usage include improved productivity, efficiency, and reduction in human error. These benefits are what make AI exceptionally attractive for application in health care and, particularly, in medical imaging [1]. To comply with the growing demand for AI software in health care, the U.S. Food and Drug Administration has currently certified a list of 178 AI-enabled medical devices, which is continuously growing [2].

The field of obstetrics and gynecology (OB/GYN) is known to be one of the most applied imaging specialties using the diagnostic tools of ultrasound (US), magnetic resonance imaging (MRI), computed tomography (CT), positron emission tomography (PET), laparoscopy, and others. In particular, the subspecialty of obstetrics is profoundly dependent on the diagnostic imaging tool of US because of its non-invasive, cost-effective, real-time, and low-radiation characteristics for fetal scanning [3,4].

However, US imaging has limitations regarding its comparability and reproducibility. Reasons for the high image variability can be low image quality, the need for real-time interpretation, differences in US devices, and the dependence on the sonographer's experience [4]. The limitations increase when US is performed during pregnancy, facing obstacles such as imaging artefacts by maternal (e.g., thickened abdominal wall in obese patient) or fetal (e.g., fetal position or movements) factors, reduced tissue contrast (e.g., with reduced amniotic fluid), and characteristics of increasing gestational age (GA) (e.g., growing fetal volume and increasing ossification of bones) [4]. In clinical settings, US is known to be time consuming and can require a substantial amount of training and experience for specific indications, such as fetal echocardiography or neurosonography [5–7].

To overcome these restrictions, the application of AI assistance in US imaging has been shown to reduce examination time, clinician workload, and inter- and intra-observer variability [8]. US imaging in OB/GYN represents a promising field of application for AI models due to the wide range of indications and generation of high-volume data sets. Various operators with different skill levels and different US devices are challenging aspects influencing AI model performance.

However, the use of AI models is not without discussion about its ethical context [3]. Despite all efforts to automatize US imaging, existing literature still emphasizes the fact that AI is not meant to replace human work and input, but should assist them and reduce the increasing workload [3,6]. As stated in the state-of-the-art review by Drukker et al. [3], to date, no AI method exists that can be generalized to different tasks compared with an OB/GYN specialist capable of performing US scans of different organs and the fetus in various GA periods. Therefore, the variety of AI models in the subspecialties of OB/GYN is tremendous and is worth reviewing within the specific tasks.

So far, most original research articles and literature reviews in OB/GYN have focused on the common fields of AI application in medical imaging, such as the identification of breast or adnexal masses, automated fetal biometry, or fetal echocardiography. To the best of our knowledge, this review is the first to systematically display the variety of fields of applications among the subspecialties of OB/GYN.

The term '5D ultrasound' is derived from the idea to expand the technological US world with a further dimension. While 4D technology extends the 3D view of the scanned object with a time frame, enabling motion visualization, or so-called 'real-time 3D' [9], the term 5D is uncommonly used to describe AI-assisted US imaging including image enhancement processing or automated calculations [10,11]. As there is no clear definition for 5D US, we use the expression of the '5D ultrasound' in this literature review to illustrate the extend of AI models that can create a new dimension in US imaging in OB/GYN by improving work efficacy, accuracy, and visibility in clinical settings.

This study aims at providing an overview of the recent literature on applications for AI in US imaging in the medical field of OB/GYN by working out the benefits and limitations of AI US support systems. Special focus is given to the distribution of research attention among the subspecialties of OB/GYN and researching the emerging and still experimental fields to promote further research for clinical applicability. Assessing the effectiveness of applied AI models is not aim of this study; therefore, all AI technologies are summarized by the term 'AI'. By describing the current research emphasis, possible missing scopes of application may be enlightened.

2. Materials and Methods

This systematic literature review was developed in accordance to the updated Preferred Reporting Items for Systematic Reviews and Meta-Analyses (PRISMA) statement [12,13]. The study was prospectively registered at the International prospective register of systematic reviews (PROSPERO) with registration number CRD42023434218.

For the literature research, the PubMed Database was searched on 14 May 2023 for records using the following search query and using the text availability filter 'abstracts':

((artificial intelligence) OR (deep learning) OR (machine learning) OR (artificial neural networks)) AND (ultrasound) AND ((obstetrics) OR (gynecology) OR (pregnancy)). Additionally, the Cochrane Library was searched on 14 May 2023 with the following query:

(Artificial intelligence OR deep learning OR machine learning OR artificial neural networks) AND ultrasound AND (obstetrics OR gynecology OR pregnancy) [Title Abstract Keyword]

No restriction for year of publication was applied. Relevant records in English or German were independently screened based on the title and abstract by two authors for their accordance with the eligibility criteria. Cases of incongruence were discussed in a consensus meeting. For adequate comprehensiveness of the search process, the PICOS search tool (Participants, Intervention or Exposure, Comparison, Outcome, Study type) was applied and used for judgement [12,13]. Table 1 shows the relevant literature characteristics presented as PICOS search tool headings. Records without the use of AI or US and studies focusing on AI applications in specialties other than OB/GYN were excluded in the screening process. Records describing AI calculations using data obtained from US measures but not the image itself (e.g., crown-rump-length (CRL) or cervical length) were excluded.

Table 1. PICOS search tool headings for literature evaluation [12].

PICOS Search Tool Headings for Literature Evaluation	
Participants	Examiner: Healthcare professionals in OB/GYN or radiology, AI specialists Patients: Healthy pregnant and non-pregnant women or women with any gynecological or obstetric disease/complication, OB/GYN training models
Intervention or Exposure	AI-assisted US applications
Comparison	Comparison of AI US algorithms to human US examiners or another AI algorithm
Outcome	Fields of AI applications in OB/GYN US imaging, benefits and limitations of AI usage, future aspects for emerging fields of applications
Study type	Published literature of any design, excluding trial protocols and reviews

After the initial screening process, full text copies were retrieved for further analysis of the inclusion criteria. By extracting fields of applications, articles were distributed to the sections of either obstetrics or gynecology. By reading all full text copies, the topic of AI application (e.g., fetal neurosonography or identification of breast masses) and the specific benefits and limitations of the AI application in the presented field were extracted. The proportion of research topics for the included literature are illustrated in two figures for the subspecialties of OB/GYN.

3. Results

3.1. Included Literature

Figure 1 depicts the PRISMA flow diagram for the screening process of reports included in this review. A total of 737 records were identified from the searched databases, resulting in 189 records considered adequate for inclusion in this review. Here, 148 records described the application of AI in US imaging in the field of obstetrics compared with 41 records in the field of gynecology (Figure 1). The included articles are displayed in Table S1 of the Supplementary Material for obstetric and Table S2 of the Supplementary Material for gynecological applications. In the following Results section, included articles are evaluated separately for both specialties.

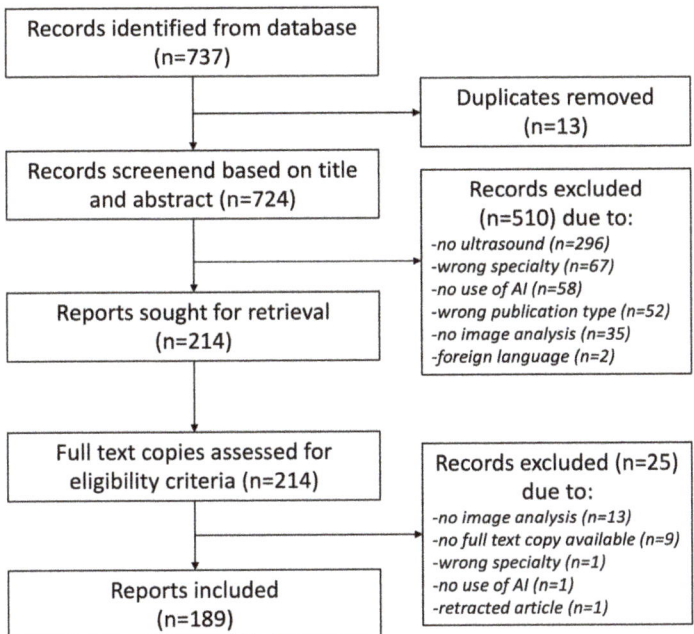

Figure 1. PRISMA flow diagram for the screening process of reports included in this review.

3.2. Applications in Obstetrics

Related to the subspecialty of obstetrics, 148 research articles form part of this systematic literature review. In Figure 2, an overview of the various research topics presented in the included literature is depicted.

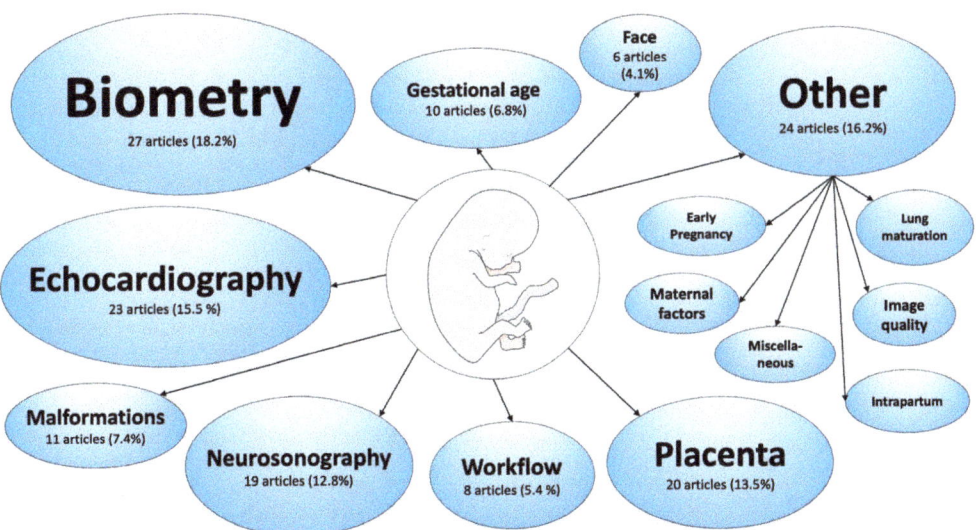

Figure 2. Overview of the distribution of research topics in the analyzed literature (a total of 148 articles) for AI applications in US imaging in the subspecialty of obstetrics. Figure adapted from Servier Medical Art.

3.2.1. Fetal Biometry

The most common application of obstetric US examination remains the assessment of fetal growth, followed by the sonographic examination maternal−fetal perfusion parameters, fetal malformations, placental morphology, or uterine abnormalities. Fetal growth assessment represents a repeated standardized examination throughout pregnancy to monitor fetal development and predict birth weight, and consequently may influence decision making for the timing of delivery. Biometric calculations are based on the acquisition of standard planes for measurements of fetal head circumference (HC), abdominal circumference (AC), and femur length [14]. The accuracy of these measurements is often reduced as a result of operator-, equipment-, patient-, and fetus-related factors.

- Operator-related factors: US in general and obstetric US in particular, are known to require substantial experience and to be extremely training dependent [15]. US examinations are known to inherit high intra- and inter-operator variability [16].
- Equipment-related factors: Especially in hospital settings, repeated examinations may be performed with different US machines, resulting in heterogenous data. Furthermore, image quality depends on resource availability and access to high-end US devices [17], or the use of point-of-care devices [18].
- Patient-related factors: Maternal obesity is known to have an impact on image quality and visualization of the fetus, and thus limits the accuracy of obstetric US examinations [19].
- Fetus-related factors: Fetal size, movements, and position, as well as multiple pregnancies or reduced amniotic fluid resulting in low contrast to surroundings may decrease the accuracy of measurements [20,21].

To minimize operator- and/or equipment-related influences, recently, there have been attempts to automate measurements in obstetric US using AI algorithms. However, these attempts are characterized by their complexity and limitations due to the inevitable patient- and fetus-related constraints.

This review encompasses 27 research articles on the use of AI in the detection, measurement, and assessment of standard planes in obstetric US, with years of publication ranging from 2007 to 2023. Only three of the included studies investigated the use of AI algorithms in 3D US images [22–24], while 24 focused on 2D images. Most studies reported the combined analysis of various standard planes (13 studies, [15,17,23–33]) or exclusively presented an algorithm for the analysis of HC (9 studies, [18,22,34–40]), AC (4 studies, [21,41–43]) or femur length (1 study, [44]). Five studies used the freely available 'HC18' data set [45] for training and testing the algorithms, which contained 1334 2D images from 551 women of the standard fetal head plane [18,34,37,38,40].

AI algorithms for the automated detection of various standard planes in US video scans have been reported by Płotka et al. [25], Chen et al. [28], and Baumgartner et al. [15]. The unique study of Sendra-Balcells et al. presented a deep-learning model to identify standard planes in 2D images showing the transferability of the AI method to six low-income African countries [17]. In comparison with the analysis of 2D US videos, Sridar et al. [26], Burgos-Artizzu et al. [27], Rahman et al. [30], and Carneiro et al. [31,32] reported AI systems for the automated detection or measurement of various standard planes in 2D US images. Zhang et al. proposed an image quality assessment method for evaluating whether US images of standard planes fully show the anatomical structures with clear boundaries [29]. To improve clinical workflow efficiency, Luo et al. evaluated the intelligent Smart Fetus technique for its 'one-touch' approach to search and automatically measure the cine loop for standard planes once the sonographers press the freeze button [33]. Pluym et al. and Yang et al. analyzed 3D US volumes for the localization and measurement of various intracranial standard planes, such as the transventricular, transthalamic, or transcerebellar plane [23,24].

The automated detection and measurement of HC in 2D images was investigated by the research groups Zeng et al. [18,34], Li et al. [36,40], Yang et al. [37], and Zhang et al. [38]. Likewise, Van de Heuvel et al. and Arroyo et al. presented a system for automated analysis of HC, particularity the use of a standardized sweep protocol for data collection to eliminate the need for sonography experts and enable applicability in underserved areas [35,39]. The only study to identify the HC and biparietal diameter from 3D US volumes using the commercially available Smartplanes® software was presented by Ambroise Grandjean et al. [22].

The acquisition and measurement of AC were considered in the studies of Jang et al. and Kim et al. analyzing 2D images [21,41], as well as by Ni et al. and Chen et al. analyzing 2D videos acquired by graduate students [42,43].

Remarkably, only one study, from Zhu et al., reported the automated assessment of femur lengths in 2D US images addressing the difficulties regarding femur lengths acquisition due to the complex background in femur US images [44].

In conclusion, the automated acquisition and measurement of standard planes is an increasingly investigated area, but still faces problems when it comes to clinical applicability and generalization. The benefits of AI usage in standard plane acquisition were found to be the possibility of real-time applicability [15,25,32,33]; the incorporation of clinical aspects into image interpretation [21,23,26]; the feasibility of biometric assessment by non-experts [35,39,43]; the application of a lightweight algorithm in point-of-care devices [18,34,37]; and, as a consequence of the latter two aspects, applicability for medically underserved areas [17,35].

The limitations of AI applications for fetal biometry were found to be reduced algorithm accuracy in poor quality images due to high maternal BMI [22,23], low contrast of anatomical structures [36], and higher GA with large fetuses [21]. Other reported limitations were slow processing times [35,43] and the lack of training for algorithms with pathological cases [28,35].

3.2.2. Fetal Echocardiography

For the detection of the most common congenital malformations, which are known to be congenital heart diseases (CHDs), with an incidence of 6–12/1000 livebirths [46], fetal sonographic examination is usually performed in the second trimester [47,48]. The prenatal diagnosis of CHD is of substantial significance, resulting in improved neonatal outcomes compared with postnatal diagnosis. It allows for appropriate counseling for parents, as well as delivery and treatment planning, and, in some cases, even in utero therapy [49].

Fetal echocardiography is a highly challenging technique, even for experts, and is primarily based on the acquisition of standard views, such as the four-chamber view (4CV), three-vessel view, three-vessel trachea view, and left and right ventricular outflow tract view. The combination of standard views allows for the detection of up to 90% of CHD; however, in clinical practice, the detection rate is only about 30% [48,50]. Reasons for low detection rates were described as insufficient sonographer interpretation and inadequate acquisition of standard views, which were often due to fetus-related factors such as fetal position, movements, and the small size of the fetal heart and its possible defects [50].

This review includes a total of 23 articles from 2007 to 2023 related to fetal echocardiography. Four of the included studies investigated the application of fetal intelligent navigation echocardiography (FINE) as a reliable technique that enabled the automated acquisition of nine standard echocardiographic views from specific 4D volumes of a single cardiac cycle in motion [51–54]. It enabled operator-independent examination and contributed to the standardization of fetal echocardiography [52]. While Yeo et al. reported the time-saving benefits of workflows using FINE in 51 normal fetal cardiac anatomy and 4 different CHD cases [51], Ma et al. confirmed the application of FINE in abnormal anatomical hearts through the successful generation of three standard views in 30 fetuses with double-outlet right ventricles [53]. In a case report, Veronese et al. reported the successful detection of four atrioventricular septum defects using the FINE system [54].

Five of the included studies investigated the performance of AI models that can detect structural abnormalities in cardiac anatomy. Dozen et al. presented a method specific to the interventricular septum [55]; Han et al. focused on the assessment of the left ventricle and left atrium [56]; and Xu et al. aimed at identifying seven anatomical structures, namely right and left atrium and ventricle, thorax, descending aorta, and epicardium [57]. The automated detection of standard views was investigated by Wu et al., Yang et al., and Nurmaini et al. [58–60], while CHD was effectively detected by AI models generated by the research groups of Gong et al. and Nurmaini et al. [61,62], and selectively for the diagnosis of total anomalous pulmonary venous connection by Wang et al. [63].

Three recent studies assessed fetal cardiac function. Yu et al. automatically measured left ventricular volume in 2D US images [64], Herling et al. analyzed the automated measurement of fetal atrioventricular plane displacement in US videos of cardiac cycles using color tissue Doppler [65], and Scharf et al. evaluated the automated assessment of the myocardial performance index as a tool to analyze fetal cardiac function [66]. Lastly, two included studies developed AI models for model improvement itself by synthesizing high-quality 4CV images for model training [67] and by providing existing models with new input data and supporting learning process [68].

The complexity of fetal echocardiography itself is derived from the skill needed to detect even the smallest anatomical abnormalities in a beating organ, which makes it an interesting and challenging research area for AI applications. Advantages are the facilitation of standard view acquisition [58,60] and CHD detection [53,61,62], as well as a significant reduction in examination time [52,55]. Furthermore, Arnaout et al. outlined the benefits of their AI model for telehealth approaches and diagnoses of rare diseases [50]. In case of the study of Emery et al., an AI-based navigation system for needle tracking in fetal aortic valvuloplasty promised increased safety, reduced intervention time, and transferability for other fetal interventions such as amniocentesis [69].

As a result of AI models acquiring US images, the need for quality control mechanisms has arisen to ensure image quality. This issue was addressed by Dong et al. and Pietrolucci et al., who developed quality assessment AI models, of which one is already commercially available, known as 'Heartassist™' [70,71]. Furthermore, to address the 'black box problem', which describes the complexity of algorithms impossible for human understanding, Sakai et al. proposed a method to support fetal echocardiography through 'explainable AI' [7]. This technique aims at promoting the trustworthy use of AI methods for clinicians through the development of specific AI modules for the explanation of the algorithm behavior.

AI assistance in fetal echocardiography showed several limitations. First, most of the studies only used 4CV images as the input for their algorithms [55,57,61–63,67,70], although the detection rate of CHD could be increased by analyzing different standard views [55]. These studies predominantly used apical 4CV, which resulted in AI model limitations when analyzing 4CV from different scanning angles, such as the fetal dorso-anterior position. This issue of the need for the correct identification of the region of interest (ROI) for optimized AI model performance was addressed by the study of Xu et al. [57]. Second, analyzed images have often been obtained only from healthy fetuses with normal cardiac anatomy and AI models lacked training with pathologic findings [52,55,57,64]. Furthermore, even with the assistance of AI methods, experienced sonographers were required for rechecking and the interpretation of results [7,51]. Lastly, the recognition of small CHD or small anatomical structures such as the trachea was limited in some models [55,58].

In summary, fetal echocardiography extensively profits from AI assistance, but shows limitations that need to be addressed in further research. Beside the aforementioned need for the automated detection of ROI, which has been recently proposed in the literature [72,73], other fields of application are of emerging interest. Not only the detection of structural abnormalities in case of CHD, but also cardiac function analysis, is a future topic of AI applications in fetal echocardiography using tissue Doppler US, which can be relevant, e.g., for fetuses diagnosed with hypoplastic left heart syndrome [74–76].

3.2.3. Fetal Neurosonography

Fetal neurosonography focuses on the assessment of fetal brain development and the identification of abnormalities [77]. For sonographic assessment, standard head planes should be acquired following the international guideline of the International Society of Ultrasound in Obstetrics and Gynecology (ISUOG) [77], which enables the detection of key anatomical structures such as lateral ventricles, cavum septum pellucidum, cerebellum, and cisterna magna. Sonographers performing neurosonography require an accurate understanding of fetal neuroanatomy, the skill to interpret 2D planes in a complex 3D structure, and, consequently, substantial clinical experience and training [78].

On the topic of neurosonography, 19 studies were included in this review, ranging from 2017 to 2022 in years of publication. Almost half of the included studies investigated AI applications in US using 3D volumes. Three of the included studies [78–80] used data collected in the Fetal Growth Longitudinal Study of the INTERGROWTH-21st Project, which aimed at developing international standards in fetal growth and size [81].

The research topics in this field are heterogenous, presenting a wide variety of applications for AI-assisted methods. The establishment of a plane localization system as a 3D reference space for locating 2D planes was proposed by Yeung et al., Namburete et al., Yu et al., and Di Vece et al. for improving the acquisition of standard planes and facilitating anatomical orientation for sonographers [78,80,82,83]. In particular, the method by Di Vece et al. used a 23-week synthetic fetal phantom for system development and was the only study to estimate the 6D poses of US planes combining common 3D planes with rotation around the brain center [82]. Xu et al. presented an AI method for authentically simulating third-trimester images from second-trimester images for deep-learning researchers with restricted access to third-trimester images [84]. The automated detection of brain structures and malformations was described by Lin et al. [85,86], Alansary et al. [87], and Gofer et al. [88] in 2D images and videos, and in 3D volumes by Hesse et al. and Huang et al. [79,89]. The image quality assessment of whether a standard plane was correctly acquired, either by human operators or by automated extraction from 3D images, was effectively performed by models developed by the research groups of Lin et al. [90], Yaqub et al. [91], and Skelton et al. [92]. Researchers Xie et al. [6,93] and Sahli et al. [94] reported a method for classifying US images into a binary system of 'normal' and 'abnormal' cases, in which Xie et al. additionally localized the structural lesions, which lead the algorithm to declare it 'abnormal' and thus recommend the clinician to recheck the labeled area. Lastly, the studies of Burgos-Artizzu et al. and Sreelakshmy et al. portrayed AI methods for the estimation of GA through an analysis of transthalamic axial planes or cerebellum measurements [95,96].

The benefits of the usage of AI algorithms in fetal neurosonography were, beside a reduced workload for sonographers due to faster acquisition and measurements [86], the development of guiding methods for skill training [78,83], the measurement of small anatomical structures such as the fetal cortex in first trimester [88], and the accurate estimation of GA in a pregnancy without a valid first trimester scan [95].

The primary limitation of AI US imaging in this topic was described to be the rapid anatomical development of fetal brain structures due to brain maturation, increasing head size and degree of ossification with rising GA [78,80,84]. Ossification of the fetal skull provoked an increase in the shadowing of US images and thus reduced image quality and visibility [80]. To address the heterogeneity in brain images from different GA, studies described the need for matching GA of US images in algorithms [82,94]. Other study limitations were the missing training of AI algorithms with images of pathologies [79,86,95] and the problem of miscalculations when US images were not in accordance with the guidelines for standard planes [6,80].

3.2.4. Fetal Face

With advances in obstetric US and the possibility of 3D and 4D US, the analysis of the fetal face has become feasible and of rising interest. This section encompasses five articles from 2018 to 2023, with heterogenous research topics.

Fetal facial malformations, such as cleft lip and palate, can be assessed by acquiring standard planes such as the ocular axial, median sagittal, and nasolabial coronal plane [97]. Wang et al. and Yu et al. presented AI algorithms to automatically identify standard planes in 2D images [97,98]. However, as facial malformations can be a phenotype of an underlying genetic disorder, Tang et al. used 3D images of fetal faces to develop a novel approach for the early, non-invasive identification of genetic disorders by analyzing key facial regions, such as the jaw, frontal bone, and nasal bone [99].

Additionally, fetal movements and facial expressions were found to be correlated with fetal brain activity and development state [100]. Facial expressions such as eye blinking, mouthing, smiling, and yawning have been described to indicate fetal brain maturation, in utero stress may result in scowling, while the meaning of tongue expulsion and neutral expression remain unclear [101,102]. Miyagi et al. proposed an AI classifier analyzing 4D US volumes to assess fetal facial expressions and classify them into different categories [102,103], and showed that the identification of dense and sparse states of brain activity is possible [104].

3.2.5. Placenta and Umbilical Cord

The placenta is known to play an important role in the pathogenesis of obstetric complications such as placenta previa, abnormally invasive placenta, fetal growth restriction, and hypertensive disorders of pregnancy [105]. Little evidence exists on the neglected role of the placental characteristics and the prediction of these complications [106]. For example, research has shown a correlation between early placental sonographic echogenicity and the prediction of intrauterine growth restriction [107]. To date, sonographic placental assessment is mainly restricted to the identification of placental location, adhesion, or insertion site of umbilical cord [108], and further assessment is limited due to the impossibility to detect minimal change in texture by routine scan and time-consuming examinations. The use of AI imaging algorithms has recently enabled automated assessment of the placental volume, tissue texture, and vascularization, and is thus of rising research interest.

In this review, 20 articles were included that were published from 1994 to 2023, whereby the three studies from 1994–1996 investigated umbilical cord Doppler analysis and studies from 2014–2023 focused on placental analysis. While part of the included studies focused on the automated assessment of placental localization and volume, others reported efforts to identify or predict the presence of placenta-related obstetric complications by analyzing echogenic tissue texture.

Andreasen et al. and Schilpzand et al. presented an effective AI algorithm for placental localization, including heterogenous data through differences in sonographers' expertise [109], or using a previous established sweep protocol in low-resource settings [110]. It is known that early reduced placental volume is associated with small-for-gestational-age fetuses [111]. Schwartz et al. and Looney et al. presented an effective model to automatically assess placenta volumes from 2D and 3D images in first trimester [112,113]. Hu et al. performed an echotexture analysis in 2D placental images [108], while Qi et al. reported successful automated localization of the placental lacunae in 2D images as a potential tool for screening abnormally invasive placenta [114,115]. The automated classification of placental maturity was proposed by Lei et al. and Li et al. [116,117]. Early and small changes in placental tissue texture were detected by Gupta et al. and Sun et al. through using AI-assisted US and microvascular Doppler imaging in women with hypertensive disorders of pregnancy [118,119] and gestational diabetes [120].

Further examples of adverse pregnancy events with an often disastrous maternal and fetal outcome are placental abruption and pernicious placenta previa. Yang et al., therefore, investigated the predictive role of a scoring system for the occurrence of pernicious placenta previa [121], while the research group of Asadpour et al. reported a method for identifying placental abruption [122].

In addition to placental characteristics, research exists on the role of umbilical cord anatomy and blood flow. Pradipta et al. investigated the use of machine learning methods to classify 2D color Doppler US images of umbilical cords along the umbilical coiling index and its possible impact on fetal growth [123]. In the earliest studies included in this review, Beksaç et al. and Baykal et al. presented an automated diagnostic, interpretation, and classification method to analyze umbilical artery blood flow Doppler US images [124–126].

The importance of pre-operative planning for surgical interventions such as laser-therapy in twin-to-twin-transfusion syndrome was addressed by the research group of Torrents-Barrena et al. [127,128]. They proposed a new AI algorithm for the simulation and planning of fetoscopic surgery through the detection and mapping of the maternal soft tissue, uterus, placenta, and umbilical cord via MRI in combination with the detection of the placenta and its vascular tree in 3D US. This model fully simulates the intraabdominal environment and enables the correct entry point planning and surgeon's training [127,128].

In summary, placental AI-based US diagnostic may propose a promising non-invasive, predictive tool to improve patient counseling and management to prevent adverse pregnancy outcomes. Reported limitations in applications arose from the difficulty of identifying the interface between the placenta and myometrium, especially in first trimester scans [113], and low accuracy rates in the assessment of posterior wall placentas [109]. Further research is necessary to identify the link between placental health and obstetric complications.

3.2.6. Fetal Malformations

First Trimester Scan

The timing of the first trimester scan is standardized to 11 + 0 and 13 + 6 weeks of gestation and its performance of image acquisition is defined by a protocol of the Fetal Medicine Foundation [129] and the ISUOG [130]. The purpose of this US examination includes confirmation of viability; assessment of GA; screening for preeclampsia; and detecting chromosomal anomalies such as trisomy 13, 18, or 21 or other malformations. Combining clinical information (maternal age and serum parameters) with sonographic assessment of fetal characteristics, predominantly the assessment of nuchal translucency (NT), is recommended practice [131].

Seven studies included in this review focused on the AI application for first trimester scans, ranging from 2012 to 2022. The research groups Walker et al. [132], Zhang et al. [133], Sciortino et al. [134], and Deng et al. [135] addressed the time consuming process of NT measurement by introducing AI models for its automated detection and measurement, in particular for the diagnosis of trisomy 21 [133] or cystic hygroma [132]. Tsai et al. aimed at facilitating the preliminary step for NT measurement, which was the automated detection of the correct mid-sagittal plane in 3D volumes [136], and Ryou et al. and Yang et al. proposed a model for the assessment of the whole fetus in 3D volumes [137,138]. The potential benefits of these models were the highly accurate non-invasive method for anomaly screening [134] and reduced workload [133,135–137]. Limitations could be uncovered when assessing fetal limbs due to its small anatomy and close surroundings [136–138], small data sets in rare anomalies [132,133], and missing real-time application for clinical applicability [133,134,138].

Second Trimester Scan

The timing of the second trimester scan is standardized to 18 + 0 to 23 + 6 weeks of gestation and is intended for the evaluation of fetal growth and detection of fetal malformations [139].

Four studies included in this review focussed on the detection of fetal malformations in mid-trimester US scans. Matthew et al. prospectively evaluated a model for automated image acquisition, measurements, and report production [140]. Cengizler et al. proposed an algorithm for the identification of the fetal spine and proofed the model's performance in cases of fetuses with spina bifida [141]. Furthermore, Meenakshi et al. focused on the identification of fetal kidneys [142] and Shozu et al. presented an AI model for the identification of the thoracic wall, which enabled plane detection for 4CV, but also allowed for the detection of thoracic malformations [143]. All of the studies showed a reduction in examination time, which helps sonographers concentrate on interpretation instead of repetitive tasks [140].

3.2.7. Prediction of Gestational Age

The estimation of GA is one of the important indications for obstetric US in early pregnancy that helps to adjust maternity care and identify complications such as prematurity or fetal growth disorders [144]. It is usually calculated using the last menstrual period and is confirmed with fetal CRL and biometry. In low-resource countries, access to medical care is constrained and ultrasonography and their operators are rare. In these areas especially, pregnancy complications play an important role and improvement in diagnostic resources for correct GA measurement as a prerequisite for adequate maternity care is thus necessary [145].

This literature review includes 10 studies on the assessment of GA, starting in 1996 with a pioneering study of Beksaç et al. on the estimation of GA via the calculation of the fetal biparietal diameter and HC [146]. In addition to this, the studies of Namburete et al. and Alzubaidi et al. similarly used the anatomy and growth of the fetal head for GA estimation [147,148]. Dan et al. developed a DeepGA model that used the three main factors of fetal head, abdomen, and femur [149], while Lee et al. proposed a machine learning method to accurately estimate GA with standard US planes [150]. The recent topic of point-of-care-US was addressed in the research of Maraci et al., who successfully showed automated head plane detection and GA estimation with point-of-care devices [151]. Lastly, four studies used data from the Fetal Age Machine Learning Initiative (FAMLI), which is an obstetrical US development project in low-income settings. The purpose of these studies, which were based on US data from the US and Zambia, was the successful establishment of an AI algorithm for GA estimation from simplified blind US sweeps of US novices in low-resource countries [144,145,152,153]. The benefits of the GA AI models were the possibility for application in low-resource countries [144,145,148,149,152], even without internet connectivity [145], and in portable devices [148], promising high accuracy with an error of 3.9 to 5 days in GA estimation [149,152]. An important limitation of the AI models was described to be application in very early [144,147] or very late stages of pregnancy [146,147,152], the latter of which was due to the thickened texture of the fetal skull.

3.2.8. Workflow Analysis of Obstetric Ultrasound Scans

Over the past decades, obstetrics US has gained immense advances in US technology and computational power, including AI processes, but the procedure of acquiring the image itself by a bedside-acting clinician has remained unchanged. As it is known that acquiring obstetric US skills is a long-lasting and highly demanding task, efforts have been made to analyze the workflow of experienced sonographers and draw conclusions about the interaction between the sonographer, probe, and image [154].

All eight included studies investigating this topic arose from the same working group of the University of Oxford, UK. The PULSE (Perception Ultrasound by Learning Sonographer Experience) project, presented by Drukker et al., was designed to enable insights into experts' sonography workflow and to transform the learning process of obstetric US using deep-learning algorithms [154]. Its data set was within the framework of all of the included studies. While Drukker et al. analyzed eye and transducer movements, actions during scanning, and audio recordings to generate automated image captioning of the sonographer's explanation, Sharma et al. added the pupillometric data to objectify not only the localization of the sonographer's gaze on the screen, but also the intensity of concentration in this focus [155]. Completeness, precision, and speed of sonographic performance were assessed by Wang et al. to quantify operator skill level [156]. Zhao et al. presented a method for virtual-assisted probe movement guidance along a virtual 3D fetus model with automatic labeling of the captured images [157]. Sharma et al. and Drukker et al. analyzed full-length scanning videos to assess workflow by building timeline models illustrating the scanning sequence of anatomical regions over time [155,158]. Lastly, Alsharid et al. developed a novel video captioning model for the description of second-trimester US scans by training an AI model with speech recordings and gaze-tracking information of sonographers while performing US scans [159].

To sum up, the included studies on this topic showed clinical benefits of AI in scan workflow through automating image labeling [154,157], enabling transfer learning for US novices [160], reducing clinician's mental workload, and optimizing workflow [155]. Limitations in application were reported to be the impossibility of the generalization of workflow sequences due to maternal–fetal factors and different skill levels of sonographers for different anatomical regions during a full routine scan [155,158].

3.2.9. Other Applications in Obstetrics

Fetal Lung Maturation

The maturation process of the fetal lung is an important aspect in clinical practice as it implies the leading cause for neonatal morbidity and mortality [161]. The GA of the fetal lung does not always correlate with the actual GA and can be influenced by pregnancy complications disrupting lung maturation.

Five included studies analyzed fetal lung US images for the prediction of neonatal outcomes. Du et al. proposed an AI model to classify the lung textures in pregnancies affected by gestational diabetes or preeclampsia [162], while Xia et al. and Chen et al. developed a lung maturation grading model that can be implemented for identifying abnormal development and evaluating the effectiveness of antenatal corticosteroid therapy [161,163]. The study of Bonet-Carne et al. and a further study of Du et al. showed that automated fetal lung ultrasound was able to accurately predict neonatal respiratory morbidity [164,165]. While Du et al. analyzed lung images from healthy and affected pregnant women, the studies of Xia et al. and Chen et al. were limited by the analysis of only healthy fetuses [161,163].

Maternal Factors

US in OB/GYN usually focusses on the examination of the fetus; however, there are several indications to evaluate maternal structures.

Four included studies were summarized in this section. The early study of Wu et al. proposed a tool for preterm labor prediction by using computer-assisted measurement of the cervix on transvaginal US images to overcome the issues of poor reproducibility and sonographer dependency on manual cervical length measurements [166]. The model of He et al. addressed the challenge of the identification and classification of intrauterine pregnancy residues that had the potential to reduce associated complications and improve surgical outcomes of curettages [167]. Wang et al. presented an algorithm to assess the color Doppler US images of fetal and maternal vessels as an approach to facilitate the diagnosis of severe preeclampsia linked to the medical outcome [168]. Lastly, Liu et al. proposed a Doppler US model for the prediction of fetal distress in women with pregnancy-induced hypertension [169]. These algorithms may improve medical diagnosis and potentially reduce clinical workload by replacing the sonographer's manual tracing [168].

Early Pregnancy

Three studies included in this review focused on the US examination in early pregnancy, which is often performed to confirm intrauterine localization and vitality of pregnancy, to estimate GA via measuring CRL, or to diagnose adverse pregnancy outcomes such as miscarriages.

While Wang et al. prospectively analyzed an automated assessment of the gestational sac as a predictor for early miscarriages in 2D images in pregnancies of 6–8 weeks of gestation [170], the research groups Sur et al. and Looney et al. proposed an 3D AI model to provide volumetric measurements of the embryo, placenta, gestational sac, yolk sac, and amniotic fluid [113,171]. The potential benefits of these models were the development of fetal volume nomograms for precise fetal growth assessment [171] and the establishment of an early screening method for the prediction of adverse pregnancy outcomes [113], which facilitates adequate consultancy and recommendation for follow-up US examinations [170]. However, validation of the results is difficult in this field of application, which limits clinical applicability.

Intrapartum Sonography

The application of US during the second stage of labor to assess the progression of childbirth is a recent development to improve obstetric management. Transperineal US is, therefore, used to objectivate vaginal digital examination when estimating fetal head descent.

In a prospective, multicenter study, Ghi et al. established an AI model for automatically classifying fetal head position and distinguishing between occiput anterior and non-occiput anterior position of the fetal head, because the latter may result in protracted labor and increased risk of a poor obstetric outcome [172]. In addition to this, Lu et al. and Bai et al. proposed a method for the automated measurement of the angle of progression, which allowed for the estimation of fetal head descent by identifying the symphysis and fetal head contour [173,174]. All three studies showed promising results but lacked clinical applicability for their missing real-time application.

Image Quality

In terms of the quality control of US images, four studies were included in this review that applied their algorithms to different aspects.

Wu et al. proposed a computerized quality assessment scheme for quality control of US images by identifying the ROI in fetal abdominal images [175]. Meng et al. established a model for the classification of shadow-rich and shadow-free regions in various US images [176] and Gupta et al. presented an algorithm for a better separation between the fetus and surrounding information in fetal US, such as maternal tissue, placenta, or amniotic fluid [177]. Lastly, Yin et al. showed improved image quality when using an AI algorithm for image processing in US images of the pelvic floor [178]. Beside improved US image quality [176–178], the benefits of automated quality control algorithms are the facilitation of image acquisition by novices and experts, reduced workload, and the development of toolkits for education [175].

Miscellaneous

Five studies investigating various areas are summarized in this section.

The study of Cho et al. proposed a model for the automated estimation of amniotic fluid, as it is known to be a particular observer-dependent factor and, therefore, benefits from automation [179]. Compagnone et al. presented a clinical case report of a successful AI-image-guided placement of an epidural catheter in an extremely obese patient for delivery [180]. The research group Maraci et al. developed an AI model to detect the fetal position and heart beat from predefined US sweeps. Further, Rueda et al. aimed at investigating the fetal nutritional status using AI-assisted assessment of the adipose and fat-free tissue of the fetal arm in US images [181]. Lastly, an AI model for the automated classification of fetal sex in 2D US images of the genital area was established by Kaplan et al. that helped reduce misclassification and facilitate screening [182].

3.3. Applications in Gynecology

Focusing on the specialty of gynecology, 41 research articles were included in this review. Figure 3 provides an overview of research topics on AI applications in gynecological US.

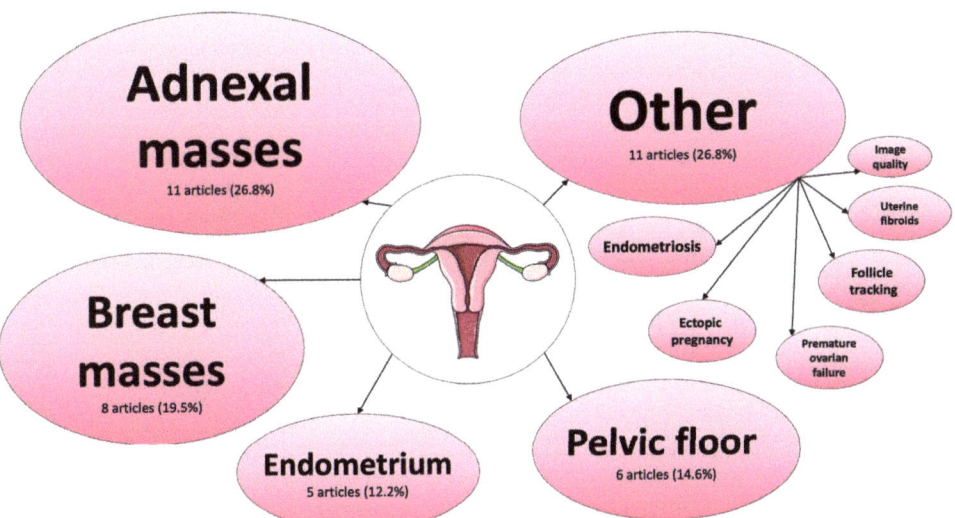

Figure 3. Overview of the distribution of research topics in the analyzed literature (a total of 41 articles) for AI applications in US imaging in the subspecialty of gynecology. Figure adapted from Servier Medical Art.

3.3.1. Adnexal Masses

Adnexal masses are among the common reasons for US examination in gynecology due to the importance of ovarian cancer detection. The assessment of adnexal findings is crucial for further diagnostic steps and therapy planning, which differ significantly between benign and malignant tumors. In the clinical setting, the examination of adnexal masses is primarily performed via transvaginal US, combining grayscale 2D images with color Doppler imaging to assess vascularization. The identification and especially classification of adnexal findings represents a challenging task even for experienced examiners and thus the International Ovarian Tumor Analysis (IOTA) group has established US-based rules for classification of adnexal tumors [183]. In recent years, the automated analysis of US images of adnexal masses has gained attention due to its advantage in supporting unexperienced examiners and assisting experienced examiners in diagnostic decision making.

Of the 11 extracted articles, only two were designed as prospective studies [184,185]. Included studies were published from 2009–2023, whereby the research group Amor et al. was the first to describe AI application in sonographic assessment using a non-specified pattern recognition analysis to classify adnexal masses in a new reporting system [184]. All but one of the studies analyzed 2D images, with only three of them including color Doppler images.

Enabling an automated discrimination between benign and malignant tumors was a predominant focus of the current research, represented in six studies included [185–190]. Three studies assessed the performance of automated tumor classification [184,191,192], one study developed a population-based screening method for BRCA mutations [193], and one study focused on the automated elimination of artefacts and objects in US images to increase the accuracy of the AI model [194]. Aramendía-Vidaurreta et al. was the only group to investigate the automated discrimination of benign and malignant masses in 3D US images [187] and Hsu et al. distinguished between transabdominal and transvaginal US images [185].

All of the included studies showed a high accuracy and sensitivity of AI performance. The study by Gao et al. used a large, multicenter, and heterogenous data set, which disclosed that AI-enabled US outperformed an average trained radiologist in discriminating malignant and benign ovarian masses and improved the examiner's accuracy [189]. These findings were consistent with other studies [185,186], but there were also studies with smaller sample sizes that showed a level of performance reaching those of human experts [188,191,192].

Nevertheless, a described limiting aspect was the fact that clinicians using AI image analyzing algorithms must still take clinical aspects into account [188,189]. Furthermore, metastases or secondary ovarian cancer in pelvic images may be misinterpreted because of their different clinical presentation and their low representation in the data set [189]. Frequent described limitations of studies on AI applications in US imaging were homogeneity of data due to a single examiner or single center study [188,192], a single investigated ethnicity [189], absent external validation [192,193], poor image quality [186,190], and, most importantly, small sample sizes not sufficient enough to train the algorithm [184,185,187,188,192,193].

3.3.2. Breast Masses

Breast cancer represents the most common malignancy in women worldwide and its incidence still shows a rising tendency [195]. To address this health issue, screening programs and early diagnosis are of the utmost importance. While primary screening is often performed and recommend through mammography, the advantages of breast US are numerous. Especially in women with dense breast tissue, e.g., predominantly in young women or in Asian ethnicity, and for underserved areas, US diagnostics and screening are crucial [196].

This review includes eight articles on AI application in US imaging of the breast, all of which were published in the past three years and focused on 2D images.

All of the included studies worked on either the detection of breast lesions, classification, or both. Two studies used AI algorithms in combination with handheld US devices [197,198]. Berg et al. pointed out the importance of training for sonographers to obtain a reasonable image quality for AI analysis [197], while Huang et al. compared handheld US to robotically performed AI-assisted US and showed reduced costs, shorter examination times, and a higher detection rate in the latter [198]. The possibility of avoiding unnecessary breast biopsies was the result of two further studies, of which one used an AI-assisted multi-modal shear wave elastography model [199,200]. In a retrospective study, Dong et al. promoted the importance of an increased confidence in AI assistance in health care, which can be addressed by understanding the algorithm of the black box and encouraging the concept of 'explainable AI' [201]. Limitations to AI usage in breast US were the missing clinical context in unimodal approaches only focusing on image analysis [202], small data sets for algorithm training, and a lower accuracy in borderline findings [201].

3.3.3. Endometrium

In gynecologic US examinations, evaluation of the endometrium is part of normal routine and obtains its significance due to the frequency of endometrial abnormalities, e.g., endometrial fibroids, polyps, endometrial hyperplasia or atrophy, and carcinoma [203]. In particular, endometrial thickness is known to show dynamics in premenopausal women throughout the menstrual cycle, while an increase in thickness in postmenopausal women represents a risk factor for the presence of malignancy [204]. However, the identification of the endometrial–myometrial junction represents a challenging task due to heterogenous textures, irregular boundaries, and different sizes of the endometrium in the menstrual phases, which is why the application of AI in US is a field of research interest.

For this topic, five articles were extracted from the current literature. Publication years ranged from 2019 to 2023. Wang et al. and Zhao et al. conducted their studies based on 3D US images [205,206]. All but one study investigated the AI performance for the assessment of endometrial thickness, texture, or uterine adhesions [205–208]. Moro et al. aimed at establishing an AI model for risk stratification in endometrial cancer, but could not prove increased performance [209].

The application of AI US to assess endometrial characteristics showed a high accuracy and similar level of performance compared with human examiners [205,208], which could be further increased by setting human-selected key points in the images as a demarcation of the ROI for the AI algorithm [207]. The only two studies using 3D imaging outlined the superiority of this data to 2D imaging for its improved capability in identifying the endometrial–myometrial junction [205,206]. Extracted limiting aspects for AI application were reduced accuracy in assessing endometria smaller than 3 mm [208], operator-dependence, limited data for algorithm training [205,206], and the need for human experts selecting images before analysis [205,207,209].

3.3.4. Pelvic Floor

The assessment of pelvic floor dysfunction is a highly essential and sensitive topic in gynecological examination due to its consequences on women's health-related quality of life. Transvaginal US is the preferred diagnostic method, enabling the assessment of pelvic organ integrity, dynamic of pelvic floor function during Valsalva maneuver, and diagnosis of pelvic organ prolapse.

This review includes six articles on the introduced topic, with only one being designed as a prospective, randomized-controlled clinical trial [210]. Publication years ranged from 2019 to 2023. Two studies used 3D US images [211,212], two 2D [213–215], two of them derived 2D images from a 3D/4D data set [214,215], and one did not specify the type of image [210].

The assessment of the pelvic floor muscles and measurement of pelvic anatomical landmarks were addressed in all studies, while two focused on the diagnosis of pelvic organ prolapse [212,213]. Reliable automated plane detection and measurements were obtained results in all of the studies. Three studies were able to show the significantly reduced time between manual and automatic image evaluation, from up to 15 minutes to 1.27 seconds [211–213], concluding in saved clinician's time for better bedside patient care. Limiting aspects encompassed high operator dependency [211,212], homogeneity of data when exclusively using cases of affected women [212,213], and the need for manual selection of ROI before AI image processing [211,213,214].

3.3.5. Other Applications in Gynecology

Further fields of applications were found in the process of this literature review. In total, 11 articles were summarized in this section, including the topics of endometriosis [216,217], premature ovarian failure [218,219], uterine fibroids [220,221], follicle tracking [222,223], and ectopic pregnancies [224,225]. Another study addressed the issue of poor image quality in 3D US images due to data processing and showed that AI image enhancement methods could produce increased 3D image quality with user-preferential flexibility in both gynecological and obstetric US images [226]. The retrospective study of Huo et al. showed that AI-assisted US improved the accuracy of uterine fibroid assessment of young sonographers, but, summarized that AI applications rather assist than replace human observers [50].

Endometriosis

Two included articles discussed the sensitive topic of endometriosis, which can be problematic for both physician and patient due to complex clinical management and impaired quality of life in affected women [216,217]. Both studies had the usage of transvaginal 2D US videos and the missing histopathological or surgical confirmation in common, but focused on two different manifestations of endometriosis. Maicas et al. developed a highly accurate AI model for the classification of the pouch of Douglas obliteration as a cause of pelvic inflammation often seen in endometriosis via detection of the so-called 'sliding sign' [216]. In comparison, the results of Raimondo et al. showed a low sensitivity of the AI model to detect adenomyosis, but a high specificity, interpreted as a useful tool to rather exclude than detect adenomyosis [217].

Uterine Fibroids

In two of the included studies, the automated detection of uterine fibroids was analyzed. The retrospective study of Huo et al. showed that AI-assisted US improved the accuracy of uterine fibroid assessment of young sonographers, but, summarized that AI applications rather assist than replace human observers [220]. Yang et al. proposed an AI algorithm for the detection of fibroids, which facilitated pre-operative guidance and interventional therapy [221].

Premature Ovarian Failure

Premature ovarian failure or insufficiency is defined by the interruption of ovarian function before the onset of menopause, affects around 1% in women aged 40, and can cause amenorrhea or infertility [227]. Beside anamnesis and laboratory results on the hormone level, transvaginal US is the primary diagnostic tool to assess ovarian characteristics. This review lists two studies on this topic, evidencing that ovarian artery flow parameters obtained by AI analyzed color Doppler imaging can be used as a predictive factor, and both AI models showed reliability for disease prediction [210,218].

Follicle Tracking

In reproductive medicine, the evaluation of follicles after ovarian stimulation or the functional ovarian reserve in patients suffering from infertility is an important diagnostic component performed via US. Two included studies, of which one had a prospective, randomized-controlled design, showed increased accuracy of follicle evaluation and reduced examination time by using AI-assisted 2D and 3D US [222,223]. The mentioned limitations included cost-intensified AI-assisted machines and possible reduced image quality in obese patients [223].

Ectopic Pregnancy

In comparison with the use of AI in US for image analysis, two studies published an approach to use US images of ectopic pregnancies to build an ontology with a reference image collection for specific diagnostic signs (e.g., 'ring of fire'). The prognosis of ectopic pregnancy is known to be dependent on the correctness and timing of diagnosis, for which the research groups Maurice et al. and Dhombres et al. showed that a knowledge base for US image annotations as a clinical decision support system based on this ontology significantly improved the timing of diagnosis [224,225].

4. Discussion

This systematic literature review presents an overview on applications for AI in US imaging in the medical field of OB/GYN. Relatively more publications were found to be suitable for inclusion that focused on applications in the field of obstetrics (148 versus 41 studies), possibly due to the predominance of US indications in this field. US is the preferred imaging method during pregnancy for fetal and maternal disorders for its low radiation exposure and possibility of real-time examination. In contrast with that, gynecological disorders such as different cancer entities and pelvis-related diseases benefit from other imaging methods such as MRI or CT. In the current literature, not only US, but also MRI applications profit from AI assistance, for example in fetal lung texture analysis [228,229] or cervical cancer diagnosis [230]. In the following, the benefits and limitations of AI application in OB/GYN US imaging are summarized.

4.1. Benefits

In general, AI in US imaging has the potential to reduce inter- and intra-observer variability by automating processes of image acquisition and interpretation [8]. AI-assisted US is able to significantly reduce examination time, showing decreased image acquisition times from minutes to seconds [211,212], thus, minimizing clinician's workload [33] and enabling the sonographer to focus on the interpretation of the obtained images [140].

These advantages are of the utmost importance, especially in the clinical setting and in times of shortage of experienced health care personnel. In addition to this, AI models have been designed for image acquisition and classification, but also for facilitating or omitting repetitive work-intense tasks such as scan report production or captioning of US videos [140,159].

Not only clinicians profit from AI usage in US, but also patients, as AI helps to improve diagnostic accuracy and provides diagnostic safety. For example, the use of AI-assisted US has been shown to reduce the amount of unnecessary hospital admissions due to misdiagnosis and unnecessary breast biopsies [197,199,200]. This fact may reduce not only heath care costs, but, more importantly, diminish psychological burden for patients with unsecure diagnosis fearing the need for further diagnostic and intervention in inconclusive imaging results. In this context, AI in clinical settings can positively impact an individual patients' life. Another example of direct patient benefit is the finding that in high-risk patients with ectopic pregnancies, reduced timing of diagnosis may result in an improved outcome [224]. AI models can also help to increase diagnostic accuracy, for example when US image quality is impeded by a thickened abdominal wall in obese patients [180]. Moreover, the advantages in pre-operative risk stratification or intraoperative assistance are described in both subspecialties of OB/GYN, e.g., in pre-operative endometrial cancer staging [209] and for fetoscopic surgical interventions [69,127]. Because of its reduction in examination time, AI-assisted US also has the potential to allow for cost-effective, population-based screening methods, e.g., for breast US [193,198,199]. Remarkably, when contextual clinical information is additionally incorporated in the AI model, the level of misclassification and misdiagnosis has been shown to be reduced [23,26]. To sum up, AI is not only a technical advantage when focusing on the imaging quality and accuracy, but, even more importantly, there is a clear benefit for an individual patient's health care.

Nevertheless, AI-assisted US also helps to improve clinical education, which is well known to be neglected by a shortage of experienced clinicians and increased workload, especially in the recent pandemic times. It can support US novices in skill training and enables non-experts the acquisition of US images [160], e.g., for telehealth approaches in times of shortage of expert sonographers [50]. It, therefore, is of public health relevance, by reducing costs and the need for sonography experts [35,39]. In this framework, AI models are additionally able to enhance image acquisition and diagnostic accuracy in point-of-care US devices, which is of particular significance for application in low-resource settings and medically underserved areas [34,145,148,199].

4.2. Limitations

The main limitation of AI models in US imaging described in the summarized literature was the fact that most AI models still need experts for image acquisition, image or ROI selection to obtain an adequate image quality for accurate model performance [6,205,209,216], and for interpretation of the results [51,220]. In applications of tissue analysis such as assessment of the endometrium in gynecology [207,209] and fetal lung texture [162], or identification of the cervix [166] in obstetrics, manual selection of the ROI is still a limiting aspect in AI performance. These findings are in accordance with the often noted statement that AI models are primarily intended to assist the clinician, not to replace them [6,231]. This limitation is of major importance to discuss as it underlines the requirement for humans in performing, analyzing, supervising, interpreting, and taking clinical consequences of AI produced results.

The irreplaceable need for experts will be understandable when working out other limitations of AI usage. In pattern recognition tasks, some AI models can fail when subtle differences are diagnosis-relevant, e.g., in borderline findings or in small regions of interest such as endometrial thickness or fetal brain structures [95,201,208]. A change in US probe or modality may also lead to misclassification, e.g., when comparing abdominal or vaginal US images [185]. Furthermore, AI model performance in 2D and 3D US imaging can be limited due to imaging artefacts and noise, especially when automated tissue analysis is intended, for example, for fetal lung assessment, whereas the method of MRI for this specific application seems future-oriented and promising [127,163]. In the clinical setting, the assessment of fetal lungs in terms of texture and volume can be relevant for prenatal diagnosis, risk classification, prediction of prognosis, and therapy planning in fetal congenital diaphragmatic hernia, profiting from the combination of the imaging modalities of US and MRI [228,232].

In obstetric US, AI models designed for automatic biometric measurements are usually restraint to a specific range of GA and can fail in images of different GA [34,40,78]. Small structures such as the fetal limbs are prone to failing AI recognition [26,138,140], as well as the differentiation of structures within similar tissue textures [113]. Furthermore, real-time application is of particular importance in obstetric US and some authors noted the missing possibility for real-time application of various AI models, interestingly affecting especially those that are designed for intrapartum application [42,127,172–174]. This limitation may be due to the great use of computational power and memory of AI algorithms. One leading limitation of AI algorithms in obstetric US is the dependence on fetal position and movement. In fetal echocardiography in particular, most presented AI models have been trained with apical 4CV, ignoring the reality of heterogenous US images obtained from different scanning angles in clinical routine [57]. As a solution to this issue and an emerging research focus, the detection of the fetal heart as a ROI in US images can be performed by AI models [72,73].

However, not only the AI models itself, but also the study designs for model development and analysis summarized in this review bear some limitations that have an influence on model development and performance. As AI algorithms are usually dependent on large data sets for training, the detection of rare pathologies is limited due to missing training of pattern recognition models [132,133]. As most of the studies are performed with data obtained from healthy subjects or healthy fetuses, miscalculation or misdiagnosis may occur in case of pathologies [35,95,145]. Other factors based on study design that influence model performance are single study center, single observer or sonographer, single US device, small sample sizes, missing long-term data, and missing clinical validation.

Nevertheless, as perfectly outlined in the state-of-the-art review by Drukker et al., the clinical applicability of AI algorithms is still limited due to fears and concerns of clinicians regarding the safety or stability of the algorithms, trustworthiness, ethical background, privacy, and professional liability [3]. Where there is research about AI, it is also indispensable to mention ethical aspects of its application. The World Health Organization guidance for the ethics and governance of artificial intelligence for health states that it "recognizes that AI holds great promise for the practice of public health and medicine" [233], but also stresses the important aspect of ethical challenges, which must be addressed due to the fast-developing technologies. Drukker et al. stressed the importance of a better interdisciplinary research on AI applications of technicians and clinicians to reduce the difficulties and insecurities of clinicians when facing the complex methods of AI systems resulting in missing trust in these systems [3]. This aspect is particularly addressed by the concept of 'explainable AI', which is used in the studies of Sakai et al. and Dong et al. [7,201]. To sum up, limitations in the applications of AI algorithms are abundant, especially because most study settings seem inadequate for the evaluation of clinical applicability. Considering the fact that the technique of AI and its emerging systems is relatively new in the medical field, it is comprehensible that clinical approved results are missing.

4.3. Strengths and Limitations of This Review

One important advantage of this review is the inclusion of a reasonable number of publications over an extensive period of time, with no restrictions regarding year of publication. The included literature is categorized among their subspecialty and research topics, allowing for a visualized overview of the current research interest on the one hand, as well as an idea of still underrepresented tasks for AI applications in further research on the other hand.

Regarding the distribution of literature among the subspecialties of OB/GYN, one limiting aspect of this study may be the search query containing the extra keyword 'pregnancy', which is likely to have influenced a discrepancy in the obtained records in favor of obstetric studies. Another important limiting aspect might be the fact that this review includes research articles from engineering literature, which are known to have a technical viewpoint and fail to assess clinical applicability. Most applications of AI US imaging in these technical articles are still experimental and preliminary work and have not been sufficiently assessed for clinical applicability, which was also stated in the review of Dhombres et al. [234]. As these technical studies are developed by engineers, they are difficult to understand for clinicians, bringing up the discussion about the urgent need for an improved interface between AI specialists and clinicians applying AI technology in real-life scenarios [231]. Lastly, a classification of the presented AI applications in the technologic subcategories of regression modeling, population classification, and image segmentation would be of further interest and should be considered for further research. In the realm of regression modeling, AI algorithms can predict crucial parameters, such as fetal growth, aiding clinicians in identifying potential complications early on. Moreover, AI-driven classification systems can enhance the accuracy of diagnoses, ensuring a higher level of precision in identifying abnormalities or diseases. The segmentation applications of AI can assess the way organs and structures are delineated in ultrasound images, offering accuracy in complex anatomical analyses.

5. Conclusions

Applications for AI-assisted US widely range from fetal biometry, echocardiography, neurosonography, or the estimation of gestational age in obstetrics, to the identification of adnexal or breast masses and the assessment of endometrium or pelvic floor in gynecology. The applications for AI-assisted US in OB/GYN are especially numerous in the subspecialty of obstetrics, where the imaging method of US is of particular significance. However, while most studies are of technical nature and studies are designed by AI engineers, most of presented literature lack clinical applicability. This systematic literature review displays the variety of research topics on AI applications in US imaging in OB/GYN, including sparsely represented and potentially emerging topics for further research.

In conclusion, with abundant evidence, we can pronounce to live and evolve the era of 5D ultrasound, as AI algorithms add and will add a momentous further dimension to the existing US imaging methods in OB/GYN.

Supplementary Materials: The following supporting information can be downloaded at: https://www.mdpi.com/article/10.3390/jcm12216833/s1, Table S1: Overview of included literature on artificial intelligence applications in ultrasound for the subspecialty of obstetrics; Table S2: Overview of included literature on artificial intelligence applications in ultrasound for the subspecialty of gynecology.

Author Contributions: Conceptualization, F.R. and E.J.; methodology, E.J.; validation, F.R., E.J.; formal analysis, F.R. and E.J.; investigation, E.J.; resources, S.A. and J.J.C.; data curation, E.J. and P.K.; writing—original draft preparation, E.J.; writing—review and editing, F.R, U.G., B.S., and S.A.; visualization, E.J.; supervision, F.R.; project administration, F.R. All authors have read and agreed to the published version of the manuscript.

Funding: This work was supported by the Open Access Publication Fund of the University of Bonn.

Institutional Review Board Statement: Not applicable.

Informed Consent Statement: Not applicable.

Data Availability Statement: The data presented in this study are available in the article or Supplementary Material here.

Conflicts of Interest: The authors declare no conflict of interest.

Abbreviations

2/3/4/5D	Two/three/four/five-dimensional
4CV	Four-chamber view
AC	Abdominal circumference
AI	Artificial intelligence
CHD	Congenital heart disease
CRL	Crown-rump-length
CT	Computed tomography
FINE	Fetal intelligent navigation echocardiography
GA	Gestational age
HC	Head circumference
ISUOG	International Society of Ultrasound in Obstetrics & Gynecology
MRI	Magnetic resonance imaging
NT	Nuchal translucency
OB/GYN	Obstetrics and gynecology
ROI	Region of interest
US	Ultrasound

References

1. Shen, Y.T.; Chen, L.; Yue, W.W.; Xu, H.X. Artificial intelligence in ultrasound. *Eur. J. Radiol.* **2021**, *139*, 109717. [CrossRef] [PubMed]
2. U.S. Food and Drug Administration. Artificial Intelligence and Machine Learning (AI/ML)-Enabled Medical Devices. Available online: https://www.fda.gov/medical-devices/software-medical-device-samd/artificial-intelligence-and-machine-learning-aiml-enabled-medical-devices (accessed on 21 August 2023).
3. Drukker, L.; Noble, J.A.; Papageorghiou, A.T. Introduction to artificial intelligence in ultrasound imaging in obstetrics and gynecology. *Ultrasound Obstet. Gynecol.* **2020**, *56*, 498–505. [CrossRef] [PubMed]
4. Diniz, P.H.B.; Yin, Y.; Collins, S. Deep Learning Strategies for Ultrasound in Pregnancy. *EMJ Reprod. Health* **2020**, *6*, 73–80. [CrossRef]
5. Reddy, C.D.; van den Eynde, J.; Kutty, S. Artificial intelligence in perinatal diagnosis and management of congenital heart disease. *Semin. Perinatol.* **2022**, *46*, 151588. [CrossRef] [PubMed]
6. Xie, H.N.; Wang, N.; He, M.; Zhang, L.H.; Cai, H.M.; Xian, J.B.; Lin, M.F.; Zheng, J.; Yang, Y.Z. Using deep-learning algorithms to classify fetal brain ultrasound images as normal or abnormal. *Ultrasound Obstet. Gynecol.* **2020**, *56*, 579–587. [CrossRef] [PubMed]
7. Sakai, A.; Komatsu, M.; Komatsu, R.; Matsuoka, R.; Yasutomi, S.; Dozen, A.; Shozu, K.; Arakaki, T.; Machino, H.; Asada, K.; et al. Medical Professional Enhancement Using Explainable Artificial Intelligence in Fetal Cardiac Ultrasound Screening. *Biomedicines* **2022**, *10*, 551. [CrossRef] [PubMed]
8. Sarno, L.; Neola, D.; Carbone, L.; Saccone, G.; Carlea, A.; Miceli, M.; Iorio, G.G.; Mappa, I.; Rizzo, G.; Di Girolamo, R.; et al. Use of artificial intelligence in obstetrics: Not quite ready for prime time. *Am. J. Obstet. Gynecol. MFM* **2023**, *5*, 100792. [CrossRef]
9. Leung, K.-Y. Applications of Advanced Ultrasound Technology in Obstetrics. *Diagnostics* **2021**, *11*, 1217. Available online: https://pubmed.ncbi.nlm.nih.gov/34359300/ (accessed on 21 August 2023). [CrossRef]
10. Rizzo, G.; Aiello, E.; Elena Pietrolucci, M.; Arduini, D. The feasibility of using 5D CNS software in obtaining standard fetal head measurements from volumes acquired by three-dimensional ultrasonography: Comparison with two-dimensional ultrasound. *J. Matern.-Fetal Neonatal Med.* **2016**, *29*, 2217–2222. [CrossRef]
11. Deshmukh, N.P.; Caban, J.J.; Taylor, R.H.; Hager, G.D.; Boctor, E.M. Five-dimensional ultrasound system for soft tissue visualization. *Int. J. Comput. Assist. Radiol. Surg.* **2015**, *10*, 1927–1939. [CrossRef]
12. Page, M.J.; McKenzie, J.E.; Bossuyt, P.M.; Boutron, I.; Hoffmann, T.C.; Mulrow, C.D.; Shamseer, L.; Tetzlaff, J.M.; Moher, D. The PRISMA 2020 statement: An updated guideline for reporting systematic reviews. *BMJ* **2021**, *29*, n71. [CrossRef] [PubMed]
13. Liberati, A.; Altman, D.G.; Tetzlaff, J.; Mulrow, C.; Gotzsche, P.C.; Ioannidis, J.P.A.; Clarke, M.; Devereaux, P.J.; Kleijnen, J.; Moher, D. The PRISMA Statement for Reporting Systematic Reviews and Meta-Analyses of Studies That Evaluate Healthcare Interventions: Explanation and Elaboration. *BMJ* **2009**, *339*, b2700. [CrossRef] [PubMed]
14. Hadlock, F.P.; Harrist, R.B.; Sharman, R.S.; Deter, R.L.; Park, S.K. Estimation of fetal weight with the use of head, body, and femur measurements—A prospective study. *Am. J. Obstet. Gynecol.* **1985**, *151*, 333–337. [CrossRef] [PubMed]
15. Baumgartner, C.F.; Kamnitsas, K.; Matthew, J.; Fletcher, T.P.; Smith, S.; Koch, L.M.; Kainz, B.; Rueckert, D. SonoNet: Real-Time Detection and Localisation of Fetal Standard Scan Planes in Freehand Ultrasound. *IEEE Trans. Med. Imaging* **2017**, *36*, 2204–2215. [CrossRef] [PubMed]
16. Sarris, I.; Ioannou, C.; Chamberlain, P.; Ohuma, E.; Roseman, F.; Hoch, L.; Altman, D.G.; Papageorghiou, A.T.; International Fetal and Newborn Growth Consortium for the 21st Century (INTERGROWTH-21st). Intra- and interobserver variability in fetal ultrasound measurements. *Ultrasound Obstet. Gynecol.* **2012**, *39*, 266–273. [CrossRef] [PubMed]

17. Sendra-Balcells, C.; Campello, V.M.; Torrents-Barrena, J.; Ahmed, Y.A.; Elattar, M.; Ohene-Botwe, B.; Nyangulu, P.; Stones, W.; Ammar, M.; Benamer, L.N.; et al. Generalisability of fetal ultrasound deep learning models to low-resource imaging settings in five African countries. *Sci. Rep.* **2023**, *13*, 2728. [CrossRef] [PubMed]
18. Zeng, W.; Luo, J.; Cheng, J.; Lu, Y. Efficient fetal ultrasound image segmentation for automatic head circumference measurement using a lightweight deep convolutional neural network. *Med. Phys.* **2022**, *49*, 5081–5092. [CrossRef] [PubMed]
19. Dashe, J.S.; McIntire, D.D.; Twickler, D.M. Effect of Maternal Obesity on the Ultrasound Detection of Anomalous Fetuses. *Obstet. Gynecol.* **2009**, *113*, 1001–1007. [CrossRef]
20. Song, J.; Liu, J.; Liu, L.; Jiang, Y.; Zheng, H.; Ke, H.; Yang, L.; Zhang, Z. The birth weight of macrosomia influence the accuracy of ultrasound estimation of fetal weight at term. *J. Clin. Ultrasound* **2022**, *50*, 967–973. [CrossRef]
21. Jang, J.; Park, Y.; Kim, B.; Lee, S.M.; Kwon, J.-Y.; Seo, J.K. Automatic Estimation of Fetal Abdominal Circumference from Ultrasound Images. *IEEE J. Biomed. Health Inform.* **2018**, *22*, 1512–1520. [CrossRef]
22. Grandjean, G.A.; Hossu, G.; Bertholdt, C.; Noble, P.; Morel, O.; Grangé, G. Artificial intelligence assistance for fetal head biometry: Assessment of automated measurement software. *Diagn. Interv. Imaging* **2018**, *99*, 709–716. [CrossRef] [PubMed]
23. Pluym, I.D.; Afshar, Y.; Holliman, K.; Kwan, L.; Bolagani, A.; Mok, T.; Silver, B.; Ramirez, E.; Han, C.S.; Platt, L.D. Accuracy of automated three-dimensional ultrasound imaging technique for fetal head biometry. *Ultrasound Obstet. Gynecol.* **2021**, *57*, 798–803. [CrossRef] [PubMed]
24. Yang, X.; Dou, H.; Huang, R.; Xue, W.; Huang, Y.; Qian, J.; Zhang, Y.; Luo, H.; Guo, H.; Wang, T.; et al. Agent with Warm Start and Adaptive Dynamic Termination for Plane Localization in 3D Ultrasound. *IEEE Trans. Med. Imaging* **2021**, *40*, 1950–1961. [CrossRef] [PubMed]
25. Płotka, S.; Klasa, A.; Lisowska, A.; Seliga-Siwecka, J.; Lipa, M.; Trzciński, T.; Sitek, A. Deep learning fetal ultrasound video model match human observers in biometric measurements. *Phys. Med. Biol.* **2022**, *67*, 045013. [CrossRef] [PubMed]
26. Sridar, P.; Kumar, A.; Quinton, A.; Nanan, R.; Kim, J.; Krishnakumar, R. Decision Fusion-Based Fetal Ultrasound Image Plane Classification Using Convolutional Neural Networks. *Ultrasound Med. Biol.* **2019**, *45*, 1259–1273. [CrossRef]
27. Burgos-Artizzu, X.P.; Coronado-Gutiérrez, D.; Valenzuela-Alcaraz, B.; Bonet-Carne, E.; Eixarch, E.; Crispi, F.; Gratacos, E. Evaluation of deep convolutional neural networks for automatic classification of common maternal fetal ultrasound planes. *Sci. Rep.* **2020**, *10*, 10200. [CrossRef]
28. Chen, H.; Wu, L.; Dou, Q.; Qin, J.; Li, S.; Cheng, J.-Z.; Ni, D.; Heng, P.-A. Ultrasound Standard Plane Detection Using a Composite Neural Network Framework. *IEEE Trans. Cybern.* **2017**, *47*, 1576–1586. [CrossRef]
29. Zhang, B.; Liu, H.; Luo, H.; Li, K. Automatic quality assessment for 2D fetal sonographic standard plane based on multitask learning. *Medicine* **2021**, *100*, e24427. [CrossRef]
30. Rahman, R.; Alam, M.d.G.R.; Reza, M.d.T.; Huq, A.; Jeon, G.; Uddin, M.d.Z.; Hassan, M.M. Demystifying evidential Dempster Shafer-based CNN architecture for fetal plane detection from 2D ultrasound images leveraging fuzzy-contrast enhancement and explainable AI. *Ultrasonics* **2023**, *132*, 107017. [CrossRef]
31. Carneiro, G.; Georgescu, B.; Good, S.; Comaniciu, D. Automatic Fetal Measurements in Ultrasound Using Constrained Probabilistic Boosting Tree. In *Medical Image Computing and Computer-Assisted Intervention—MICCAI 2007, Proceedings of the 10th International Conference, Brisbane, Australia, 29 October–2 November 2007*; Ayache, N., Ourselin, S., Maeder, A., Eds.; Lecture Notes in Computer Science; Springer: Berlin/Heidelberg, Germany, 2007; Volume 4792, pp. 571–579. Available online: http://link.springer.com/10.1007/978-3-540-75759-7_69 (accessed on 9 June 2023).
32. Carneiro, G.; Georgescu, B.; Good, S.; Comaniciu, D. Detection and Measurement of Fetal Anatomies from Ultrasound Images using a Constrained Probabilistic Boosting Tree. *IEEE Trans. Med. Imaging* **2008**, *27*, 1342–1355. [CrossRef]
33. Luo, D.; Wen, H.; Peng, G.; Lin, Y.; Liang, M.; Liao, Y.; Qin, Y.; Zeng, Q.; Dang, J.; Li, S. A Prenatal Ultrasound Scanning Approach: One-Touch Technique in Second and Third Trimesters. *Ultrasound Med. Biol.* **2021**, *47*, 2258–2265. [CrossRef] [PubMed]
34. Zeng, Y.; Tsui, P.-H.; Wu, W.; Zhou, Z.; Wu, S. Fetal Ultrasound Image Segmentation for Automatic Head Circumference Biometry Using Deeply Supervised Attention-Gated V-Net. *J. Digit. Imaging* **2021**, *34*, 134–148. [CrossRef] [PubMed]
35. Heuvel, T.L.v.d.; Petros, H.; Santini, S.; de Korte, C.L.; van Ginneken, B. Automated Fetal Head Detection and Circumference Estimation from Free-Hand Ultrasound Sweeps Using Deep Learning in Resource-Limited Countries. *Ultrasound Med. Biol.* **2019**, *45*, 773–785. [CrossRef] [PubMed]
36. Li, J.; Wang, Y.; Lei, B.; Cheng, J.-Z.; Qin, J.; Wang, T.; Li, S.; Ni, D. Automatic Fetal Head Circumference Measurement in Ultrasound Using Random Forest and Fast Ellipse Fitting. *IEEE J. Biomed. Health Inform.* **2018**, *22*, 215–223. [CrossRef] [PubMed]
37. Yang, C.; Yang, Z.; Liao, S.; Guo, J.; Yin, S.; Liu, C.; Kang, Y. A new approach to automatic measure fetal head circumference in ultrasound images using convolutional neural networks. *Comput. Biol. Med.* **2022**, *147*, 105801. [CrossRef] [PubMed]
38. Zhang, J.; Petitjean, C.; Ainouz, S. Segmentation-Based vs. Regression-Based Biomarker Estimation: A Case Study of Fetus Head Circumference Assessment from Ultrasound Images. *J. Imaging* **2022**, *8*, 23. [CrossRef] [PubMed]
39. Arroyo, J.; Marini, T.J.; Saavedra, A.C.; Toscano, M.; Baran, T.M.; Drennan, K.; Dozier, A.; Zhao, Y.T.; Egoavil, M.; Tamayo, L.; et al. No sonographer, no radiologist: New system for automatic prenatal detection of fetal biometry, fetal presentation, and placental location. *PLoS ONE* **2022**, *17*, e0262107. [CrossRef]
40. Li, P.; Zhao, H.; Liu, P.; Cao, F. Automated measurement network for accurate segmentation and parameter modification in fetal head ultrasound images. *Med. Biol. Eng. Comput.* **2020**, *58*, 2879–2892. [CrossRef]

41. Kim, B.; Kim, K.C.; Park, Y.; Kwon, J.-Y.; Jang, J.; Seo, J.K. Machine-learning-based automatic identification of fetal abdominal circumference from ultrasound images. *Physiol. Meas.* **2018**, *39*, 105007. [CrossRef]
42. Ni, D.; Yang, X.; Chen, X.; Chin, C.-T.; Chen, S.; Heng, P.A.; Li, S.; Qin, J.; Wang, T. Standard Plane Localization in Ultrasound by Radial Component Model and Selective Search. *Ultrasound Med. Biol.* **2014**, *40*, 2728–2742. [CrossRef]
43. Chen, H.; Ni, D.; Qin, J.; Li, S.; Yang, X.; Wang, T.; Heng, P.A. Standard Plane Localization in Fetal Ultrasound via Domain Transferred Deep Neural Networks. *IEEE J. Biomed. Health Inform.* **2015**, *19*, 1627–1636. [CrossRef] [PubMed]
44. Zhu, F.; Liu, M.; Wang, F.; Qiu, D.; Li, R.; Dai, C. Automatic measurement of fetal femur length in ultrasound images: A comparison of random forest regression model and SegNet. *Math. Biosci. Eng.* **2021**, *18*, 7790–7805. [CrossRef] [PubMed]
45. Van Den Heuvel, T.L.A.; De Bruijn, D.; De Korte, C.L.; Ginneken, B.V. Automated measurement of fetal head circumference using 2D ultrasound images. *PLoS ONE* **2018**, *13*, e0200412. [CrossRef] [PubMed]
46. Donofrio, M.T.; Moon-Grady, A.J.; Hornberger, L.K.; Copel, J.A.; Sklansky, M.S.; Abuhamad, A.; Cuneao, B.F.; Huhta, J.C.; Jonas, R.A.; Krishnan, A.; et al. Diagnosis and Treatment of Fetal Cardiac Disease: A Scientific Statement from the American Heart Association. *Circulation* **2014**, *129*, 2183–2242. [CrossRef] [PubMed]
47. Gembruch, U. Prenatal diagnosis of congenital heart disease. *Prenat. Diagn.* **1997**, *17*, 1283–1298. [CrossRef]
48. Carvalho, J.; Allan, L.; Chaoui, R.; Copel, J.; DeVore, G.; Hecher, K.; Lee, W.; Munoz, H.; Paladini, D.; Tutschek, B.; et al. ISUOG Practice Guidelines (updated): Sonographic screening examination of the fetal heart. *Ultrasound Obstet. Gynecol.* **2013**, *41*, 348–359. [CrossRef] [PubMed]
49. Bensemlali, M.; Bajolle, F.; Laux, D.; Parisot, P.; Ladouceur, M.; Fermont, L.; Levy, M.; Le Bidois, J.; Raimondi, F.; Ville, Y.; et al. Neonatal management and outcomes of prenatally diagnosed CHDs. *Cardiol. Young* **2017**, *27*, 344–353. [CrossRef] [PubMed]
50. Arnaout, R.; Curran, L.; Zhao, Y.; Levine, J.C.; Chinn, E.; Moon-Grady, A.J. An ensemble of neural networks provides expert-level prenatal detection of complex congenital heart disease. *Nat. Med.* **2021**, *27*, 882–891. [CrossRef]
51. Yeo, L.; Romero, R. Fetal Intelligent Navigation Echocardiography (FINE): A novel method for rapid, simple, and automatic examination of the fetal heart: Fetal intelligent navigation echocardiography (FINE). *Ultrasound Obstet. Gynecol.* **2013**, *42*, 268–284. [CrossRef]
52. Gembicki, M.; Hartge, D.R.; Dracopoulos, C.; Weichert, J. Semiautomatic Fetal Intelligent Navigation Echocardiography Has the Potential to Aid Cardiac Evaluations Even in Less Experienced Hands. *J. Ultrasound Med.* **2020**, *39*, 301–309. [CrossRef]
53. Ma, M.; Li, Y.; Chen, R.; Huang, C.; Mao, Y.; Zhao, B. Diagnostic performance of fetal intelligent navigation echocardiography (FINE) in fetuses with double-outlet right ventricle (DORV). *Int. J. Cardiovasc. Imaging* **2020**, *36*, 2165–2172. [CrossRef] [PubMed]
54. Veronese, P.; Guariento, A.; Cattapan, C.; Fedrigo, M.; Gervasi, M.T.; Angelini, A.; Riva, A.; Vida, V. Prenatal Diagnosis and Fetopsy Validation of Complete Atrioventricular Septal Defects Using the Fetal Intelligent Navigation Echocardiography Method. *Diagnostics* **2023**, *13*, 456. [CrossRef] [PubMed]
55. Dozen, A.; Komatsu, M.; Sakai, A.; Komatsu, R.; Shozu, K.; Machino, H.; Yasutomi, S.; Arakaki, T.; Asada, K.; Kaneko, S.; et al. Image Segmentation of the Ventricular Septum in Fetal Cardiac Ultrasound Videos Based on Deep Learning Using Time-Series Information. *Biomolecules* **2020**, *10*, 1526. [CrossRef] [PubMed]
56. Han, G.; Jin, T.; Zhang, L.; Guo, C.; Gui, H.; Na, R.; Wang, X.; Bai, H. Adoption of Compound Echocardiography under Artificial Intelligence Algorithm in Fetal Congenital Heart Disease Screening during Gestation. *Appl. Bionics Biomech.* **2022**, *2022*, 6410103. [CrossRef] [PubMed]
57. Xu, L.; Liu, M.; Shen, Z.; Wang, H.; Liu, X.; Wang, X.; Wang, S.; Li, T.; Yu, S.; Hou, M.; et al. DW-Net: A cascaded convolutional neural network for apical four-chamber view segmentation in fetal echocardiography. *Comput. Med. Imaging Graph.* **2020**, *80*, 101690. [CrossRef]
58. Wu, H.; Wu, B.; Lai, F.; Liu, P.; Lyu, G.; He, S.; Dai, J. Application of Artificial Intelligence in Anatomical Structure Recognition of Standard Section of Fetal Heart. *Comput. Math. Methods Med.* **2023**, *2023*, 5650378. [CrossRef]
59. Yang, Y.; Wu, B.; Wu, H.; Xu, W.; Lyu, G.; Liu, P.; He, S. Classification of normal and abnormal fetal heart ultrasound images and identification of ventricular septal defects based on deep learning. *J. Perinat. Med.* **2023**, *51*, 1052–1058. [CrossRef] [PubMed]
60. Nurmaini, S.; Rachmatullah, M.N.; Sapitri, A.I.; Darmawahyuni, A.; Tutuko, B.; Firdaus, F.; Partan, R.U.; Bernolian, N. Deep Learning-Based Computer-Aided Fetal Echocardiography: Application to Heart Standard View Segmentation for Congenital Heart Defects Detection. *Sensors* **2021**, *21*, 8007. [CrossRef]
61. Gong, Y.; Zhang, Y.; Zhu, H.; Lv, J.; Cheng, Q.; Zhang, H.; He, Y.; Wang, S. Fetal Congenital Heart Disease Echocardiogram Screening Based on DGACNN: Adversarial One-Class Classification Combined with Video Transfer Learning. *IEEE Trans. Med. Imaging* **2020**, *39*, 1206–1222. [CrossRef]
62. Nurmaini, S.; Partan, R.U.; Bernolian, N.; Sapitri, A.I.; Tutuko, B.; Rachmatullah, M.N.; Darmawahyuni, A.; Firdaus, F.; Mose, J.C. Deep Learning for Improving the Effectiveness of Routine Prenatal Screening for Major Congenital Heart Diseases. *J. Clin. Med.* **2022**, *11*, 6454. [CrossRef]
63. Wang, X.; Yang, T.; Zhang, Y.; Liu, X.; Zhang, Y.; Sun, L.; Gu, X.; Chen, Z.; Guo, Y.; Xue, C.; et al. Diagnosis of fetal total anomalous pulmonary venous connection based on the post-left atrium space ratio using artificial intelligence. *Prenat. Diagn.* **2022**, *42*, 1323–1331. [CrossRef]
64. Yu, L.; Guo, Y.; Wang, Y.; Yu, J.; Chen, P. Determination of Fetal Left Ventricular Volume Based on Two-Dimensional Echocardiography. *J. Healthc. Eng.* **2017**, *2017*, 4797315. [CrossRef] [PubMed]

65. Herling, L.; Johnson, J.; Ferm-Widlund, K.; Zamprakou, A.; Westgren, M.; Acharya, G. Automated quantitative evaluation of fetal atrioventricular annular plane systolic excursion. *Ultrasound Obstet. Gynecol.* **2021**, *58*, 853–863. [CrossRef] [PubMed]
66. Scharf, J.L.; Dracopoulos, C.; Gembicki, M.; Welp, A.; Weichert, J. How Automated Techniques Ease Functional Assessment of the Fetal Heart: Applicability of MPI+^{TM} for Direct Quantification of the Modified Myocardial Performance Index. *Diagnostics* **2023**, *13*, 1705. [CrossRef] [PubMed]
67. Qiao, S.; Pan, S.; Luo, G.; Pang, S.; Chen, T.; Singh, A.K.; Lv, Z. A Pseudo-Siamese Feature Fusion Generative Adversarial Network for Synthesizing High-Quality Fetal Four-Chamber Views. *IEEE J. Biomed. Health Informatics* **2023**, *27*, 1193–1204. [CrossRef] [PubMed]
68. Patra, A.; Noble, J.A. Hierarchical Class Incremental Learning of Anatomical Structures in Fetal Echocardiography Videos. *IEEE J. Biomed. Health Informatics* **2020**, *24*, 1046–1058. [CrossRef] [PubMed]
69. Emery, S.P.; Kreutzer, J.; Sherman, F.R.; Fujimoto, K.L.; Jaramaz, B.; Nikou, C.; Tobita, K.; Keller, B.B. Computer-assisted navigation applied to fetal cardiac intervention. *Int. J. Med. Robot. Comput. Assist. Surg.* **2007**, *3*, 187–198. [CrossRef]
70. Dong, J.; Liu, S.; Liao, Y.; Wen, H.; Lei, B.; Li, S.; Wang, T. A Generic Quality Control Framework for Fetal Ultrasound Cardiac Four-Chamber Planes. *IEEE J. Biomed. Health Inform.* **2020**, *24*, 931–942. [CrossRef] [PubMed]
71. Pietrolucci, M.E.; Maqina, P.; Mappa, I.; Marra, M.C.; D' Antonio, F.; Rizzo, G. Evaluation of an artificial intelligent algorithm (Heartassist^{TM}) to automatically assess the quality of second trimester cardiac views: A prospective study. *J. Perinat. Med.* **2023**, *51*, 920–924. [CrossRef]
72. Vijayalakshmi, S.; Sriraam, N.; Suresh, S.; Muttan, S. Automated region mask for four-chamber fetal heart biometry. *J. Clin. Monit. Comput.* **2013**, *27*, 205–209. [CrossRef]
73. Sriraam, N.; Punyaprabha, V.; Sushma Tv Suresh, S. Performance evaluation of computer-aided automated master frame selection techniques for fetal echocardiography. *Med. Biol. Eng. Comput.* **2023**, *61*, 1723–1744. [CrossRef] [PubMed]
74. Graupner, O.; Enzensberger, C.; Wieg, L.; Willruth, A.; Steinhard, J.; Gembruch, U.; Doelle, A.; Bahlmann, F.; Kawecki, A.; Degenhardt, J.; et al. Evaluation of right ventricular function in fetal hypoplastic left heart syndrome by color tissue Doppler imaging: Right ventricular function in fetal HLHS. *Ultrasound Obstet. Gynecol.* **2016**, *47*, 732–738. [CrossRef] [PubMed]
75. Sun, L.; Wang, J.; Su, X.; Chen, X.; Zhou, Y.; Zhang, X.; Lu, H.; Niu, J.; Yu, L.; Sun, C.; et al. Reference ranges of fetal heart function using a Modified Myocardial Performance Index: A prospective multicentre, cross-sectional study. *BMJ Open* **2021**, *11*, e049640. [CrossRef] [PubMed]
76. Lane, E.S.; Jevsikov, J.; Shun-Shin, M.J.; Dhutia, N.; Matoorian, N.; Cole, G.D.; Francis, D.P.; Zolgharni, M. Automated multi-beat tissue Doppler echocardiography analysis using deep neural networks. *Med. Biol. Eng. Comput.* **2023**, *61*, 911–926. [CrossRef] [PubMed]
77. Sonographic examination of the fetal central nervous system: Guidelines for performing the 'basic examination' and the 'fetal neurosonogram'. *Ultrasound Obstet. Gynecol.* **2007**, *29*, 109–116. [CrossRef] [PubMed]
78. Yeung, P.-H.; Aliasi, M.; Papageorghiou, A.T.; Haak, M.; Xie, W.; Namburete, A.I. Learning to map 2D ultrasound images into 3D space with minimal human annotation. *Med. Image Anal.* **2021**, *70*, 101998. [CrossRef] [PubMed]
79. Hesse, L.S.; Aliasi, M.; Moser, F.; INTERGROWTH-21(st) Consortium; Haak, M.C.; Xie, W.; Jenkinson, M.; Namburete, A.I. Subcortical segmentation of the fetal brain in 3D ultrasound using deep learning. *NeuroImage* **2022**, *254*, 119117. [CrossRef] [PubMed]
80. Namburete, A.I.; Xie, W.; Yaqub, M.; Zisserman, A.; Noble, J.A. Fully-automated alignment of 3D fetal brain ultrasound to a canonical reference space using multi-task learning. *Med. Image Anal.* **2018**, *46*, 1–14. [CrossRef]
81. Papageorghiou, A.T.; Ohuma, E.O.; Altman, D.G.; Todros, T.; Ismail, L.C.; Lambert, A.; Jaffer, Y.A.; Bertino, E.; Gravett, M.G.; Purwar, M.; et al. International standards for fetal growth based on serial ultrasound measurements: The Fetal Growth Longitudinal Study of the INTERGROWTH-21st Project. *Lancet* **2014**, *384*, 869–879. [CrossRef]
82. Di Vece, C.; Dromey, B.; Vasconcelos, F.; David, A.L.; Peebles, D.; Stoyanov, D. Deep learning-based plane pose regression in obstetric ultrasound. *Int. J. Comput. Assist. Radiol. Surg.* **2022**, *17*, 833–839. [CrossRef]
83. Yu, Y.; Chen, Z.; Zhuang, Y.; Yi, H.; Han, L.; Chen, K.; Lin, J. A guiding approach of Ultrasound scan for accurately obtaining standard diagnostic planes of fetal brain malformation. *J. X-ray Sci. Technol.* **2022**, *30*, 1243–1260. [CrossRef]
84. Xu, Y.; Lee, L.H.; Drukker, L.; Yaqub, M.; Papageorghiou, A.T.; Noble, A.J. Simulating realistic fetal neurosonography images with appearance and growth change using cycle-consistent adversarial networks and an evaluation. *J. Med. Imaging* **2020**, *7*, 057001. [CrossRef] [PubMed]
85. Lin, Q.; Zhou, Y.; Shi, S.; Zhang, Y.; Yin, S.; Liu, X.; Peng, Q.; Huang, S.; Jiang, Y.; Cui, C.; et al. How much can AI see in early pregnancy: A multi-center study of fetus head characterization in week 10–14 in ultrasound using deep learning. *Comput. Methods Programs Biomed.* **2022**, *226*, 107170. [CrossRef]
86. Lin, M.; He, X.; Guo, H.; He, M.; Zhang, L.; Xian, J.; Lei, T.; Xu, Q.; Zheng, J.; Feng, J.; et al. Use of real-time artificial intelligence in detection of abnormal image patterns in standard sonographic reference planes in screening for fetal intracranial malformations. *Ultrasound Obstet. Gynecol.* **2022**, *59*, 304–316. [CrossRef] [PubMed]
87. Alansary, A.; Oktay, O.; Li, Y.; Le Folgoc, L.; Hou, B.; Vaillant, G.; Kamnitsas, K.; Vlontzos, A.; Glocker, B.; Kainz, B.; et al. Evaluating reinforcement learning agents for anatomical landmark detection. *Med. Image Anal.* **2019**, *53*, 156–164. [CrossRef]
88. Gofer, S.; Haik, O.; Bardin, R.; Gilboa, Y.; Perlman, S. Machine Learning Algorithms for Classification of First-Trimester Fetal Brain Ultrasound Images. *J. Ultrasound Med.* **2022**, *41*, 1773–1779. [CrossRef] [PubMed]

89. Huang, R.; Xie, W.; Noble, J.A. VP-Nets: Efficient automatic localization of key brain structures in 3D fetal neurosonography. *Med. Image Anal.* **2018**, *47*, 127–139. [CrossRef]
90. Lin, Z.; Li, S.; Ni, D.; Liao, Y.; Wen, H.; Du, J.; Chen, S.; Wang, T.; Lei, B. Multi-task learning for quality assessment of fetal head ultrasound images. *Med. Image Anal.* **2019**, *58*, 101548. [CrossRef]
91. Yaqub, M.; Kelly, B.; Papageorghiou, A.T.; Noble, J.A. A Deep Learning Solution for Automatic Fetal Neurosonographic Diagnostic Plane Verification Using Clinical Standard Constraints. *Ultrasound Med. Biol.* **2017**, *43*, 2925–2933. [CrossRef]
92. Skelton, E.; Matthew, J.; Li, Y.; Khanal, B.; Martinez, J.C.; Toussaint, N.; Gupta, C.; Knight, C.; Kainz, B.; Hajnal, J.; et al. Towards automated extraction of 2D standard fetal head planes from 3D ultrasound acquisitions: A clinical evaluation and quality assessment comparison. *Radiography* **2021**, *27*, 519–526. [CrossRef]
93. Xie, B.; Lei, T.; Wang, N.; Cai, H.; Xian, J.; He, M.; Zhang, L.; Xie, H. Computer-aided diagnosis for fetal brain ultrasound images using deep convolutional neural networks. *Int. J. Comput. Assist. Radiol. Surg.* **2020**, *15*, 1303–1312. [CrossRef] [PubMed]
94. Sahli, H.; Mouelhi, A.; Ben Slama, A.; Sayadi, M.; Rachdi, R. Supervised classification approach of biometric measures for automatic fetal defect screening in head ultrasound images. *J. Med. Eng. Technol.* **2019**, *43*, 279–286. [CrossRef] [PubMed]
95. Burgos-Artizzu, X.P.; Coronado-Gutiérrez, D.; Valenzuela-Alcaraz, B.; Vellvé, K.; Eixarch, E.; Crispi, F.; Bonet-Carne, E.; Bennasar, M.; Gratacos, E. Analysis of maturation features in fetal brain ultrasound via artificial intelligence for the estimation of gestational age. *Am. J. Obstet. Gynecol. MFM* **2021**, *3*, 100462. [CrossRef] [PubMed]
96. Sreelakshmy, R.; Titus, A.; Sasirekha, N.; Logashanmugam, E.; Begam, R.B.; Ramkumar, G.; Raju, R. An Automated Deep Learning Model for the Cerebellum Segmentation from Fetal Brain Images. *BioMed Res. Int.* **2022**, *2022*, 8342767. [CrossRef] [PubMed]
97. Wang, X.; Liu, Z.; Du, Y.; Diao, Y.; Liu, P.; Lv, G.; Zhang, H. Recognition of Fetal Facial Ultrasound Standard Plane Based on Texture Feature Fusion. *Comput. Math. Methods Med.* **2021**, *2021*, 656942. [CrossRef] [PubMed]
98. Yu, Z.; Tan, E.-L.; Ni, D.; Qin, J.; Chen, S.; Li, S.; Lei, B.; Wang, T. A Deep Convolutional Neural Network-Based Framework for Automatic Fetal Facial Standard Plane Recognition. *IEEE J. Biomed. Health Inform.* **2018**, *22*, 874–885. [CrossRef] [PubMed]
99. Tang, J.; Han, J.; Xie, B.; Xue, J.; Zhou, H.; Jiang, Y.; Hu, L.; Chen, C.; Zhang, K.; Zhu, F.; et al. The Two-Stage Ensemble Learning Model Based on Aggregated Facial Features in Screening for Fetal Genetic Diseases. *Int. J. Environ. Res. Public Health* **2023**, *20*, 2377. [CrossRef]
100. Hata, T. Current status of fetal neurodevelopmental assessment: Four-dimensional ultrasound study: Fetal neurodevelopmental assessment. *J. Obstet. Gynaecol. Res.* **2016**, *42*, 1211–1221. [CrossRef]
101. AboEllail, M.A.M.; Hata, T. Fetal face as important indicator of fetal brain function. *J. Perinat. Med.* **2017**, *45*, 729–736. [CrossRef]
102. Miyagi, Y.; Hata, T.; Bouno, S.; Koyanagi, A.; Miyake, T. Artificial intelligence to understand fluctuation of fetal brain activity by recognizing facial expressions. *Int. J. Gynecol. Obstet.* **2023**, *161*, 877–885. [CrossRef]
103. Miyagi, Y.; Hata, T.; Bouno, S.; Koyanagi, A.; Miyake, T. Recognition of facial expression of fetuses by artificial intelligence (AI). *J. Perinat. Med.* **2021**, *49*, 596–603. [CrossRef] [PubMed]
104. Miyagi, Y.; Hata, T.; Miyake, T. Fetal brain activity and the free energy principle. *J. Perinat. Med.* **2023**, *51*, 925–931. [CrossRef] [PubMed]
105. Sun, C.; Groom, K.M.; Oyston, C.; Chamley, L.W.; Clark, A.R.; James, J.L. The placenta in fetal growth restriction: What is going wrong? *Placenta* **2020**, *96*, 10–18. [CrossRef] [PubMed]
106. Maltepe, E.; Fisher, S.J. Placenta: The Forgotten Organ. *Annu. Rev. Cell Dev. Biol.* **2015**, *31*, 523–552. [CrossRef] [PubMed]
107. Walter, A.; Böckenhoff, P.; Geipel, A.; Gembruch, U.; Engels, A.C. Early sonographic evaluation of the placenta in cases with IUGR: A pilot study. *Arch. Gynecol. Obstet.* **2020**, *302*, 337–343. [CrossRef] [PubMed]
108. Hu, R.; Singla, R.; Yan, R.; Mayer, C.; Rohling, R.N. Automated Placenta Segmentation with a Convolutional Neural Network Weighted by Acoustic Shadow Detection. In Proceedings of the 41st Annual International Conference of the IEEE Engineering in Medicine and Biology Society (EMBC), Berlin, Germany, 23–27 July 2019; IEEE: New York, NY, USA, 2019; pp. 6718–6723. Available online: https://ieeexplore.ieee.org/document/8857448/ (accessed on 9 July 2023).
109. Andreasen, L.A.; Feragen, A.; Christensen, A.N.; Thybo, J.K.; Svendsen, M.B.S.; Zepf, K.; Lekadir, K.; Tolsgaard, M.G. Multi-centre deep learning for placenta segmentation in obstetric ultrasound with multi-observer and cross-country generalization. *Sci. Rep.* **2023**, *13*, 2221. [CrossRef] [PubMed]
110. Schilpzand, M.; Neff, C.; van Dillen, J.; van Ginneken, B.; Heskes, T.; de Korte, C.; Heuvel, T.v.D. Automatic Placenta Localization from Ultrasound Imaging in a Resource-Limited Setting Using a Predefined Ultrasound Acquisition Protocol and Deep Learning. *Ultrasound Med. Biol.* **2022**, *48*, 663–674. [CrossRef]
111. Plasencia, W.; Akolekar, R.; Dagklis, T.; Veduta, A.; Nicolaides, K.H. Placental Volume at 11–13 Weeks' Gestation in the Prediction of Birth Weight Percentile. *Fetal Diagn. Ther.* **2011**, *30*, 23–28. [CrossRef]
112. Schwartz, N.; Oguz, I.; Wang, J.; Pouch, A.; Yushkevich, N.; Parameshwaran, S.; Gee, J.; Yushkevich, P.; Oguz, B. Fully Automated Placental Volume Quantification From 3D Ultrasound for Prediction of Small-for-Gestational-Age Infants. *J. Ultrasound Med.* **2022**, *41*, 1509–1524. [CrossRef]
113. Looney, P.; Yin, Y.; Collins, S.L.; Nicolaides, K.H.; Plasencia, W.; Molloholli, M.; Natsis, S.; Stevenson, G.N. Fully Automated 3-D Ultrasound Segmentation of the Placenta, Amniotic Fluid, and Fetus for Early Pregnancy Assessment. *IEEE Trans. Ultrason. Ferroelectr. Freq. Control* **2021**, *68*, 2038–2047. [CrossRef]

114. Qi, H.; Collins, S.; Noble, J.A. Automatic Lacunae Localization in Placental Ultrasound Images via Layer Aggregation. In *Medical Image Computing and Computer Assisted Intervention—MICCAI 2018, Proceedings of the 1st International Conference, Granada, Spain, 16–20 September 2018*; Frangi, A.F., Schnabel, J.A., Davatzikos, C., Alberola-López, C., Fichtinger, G., Eds.; Lecture Notes in Computer Science; Springer International Publishing: Cham, Switzerland, 2018; Volume 11071, pp. 921–929. Available online: http://link.springer.com/10.1007/978-3-030-00934-2_102 (accessed on 9 June 2023).
115. Qi, H.; Collins, S.; Noble, A. Weakly Supervised Learning of Placental Ultrasound Images with Residual Networks. In *Medical Image Understanding and Analysis*; Valdés Hernández, M., González-Castro, V., Eds.; Communications in Computer and Information Science; Springer International Publishing: Cham, Switzerland, 2017; Volume 723, pp. 98–108. Available online: http://link.springer.com/10.1007/978-3-319-60964-5_9 (accessed on 9 June 2023).
116. Lei, B.; Yao, Y.; Chen, S.; Li, S.; Li, W.; Ni, D.; Wang, T. Discriminative Learning for Automatic Staging of Placental Maturity via Multi-layer Fisher Vector. *Sci. Rep.* **2015**, *5*, 12818. [CrossRef] [PubMed]
117. Li, X.; Yao, Y.; Ni, D.; Chen, S.; Li, S.; Lei, B.; Wang, T. Automatic staging of placental maturity based on dense descriptor. *Bio-Med. Mater. Eng.* **2014**, *24*, 2821–2829. [CrossRef] [PubMed]
118. Gupta, K.; Balyan, K.; Lamba, B.; Puri, M.; Sengupta, D.; Kumar, M. Ultrasound placental image texture analysis using artificial intelligence to predict hypertension in pregnancy. *J. Matern. Neonatal Med.* **2022**, *35*, 5587–5594. [CrossRef] [PubMed]
119. Sun, H.; Jiao, J.; Ren, Y.; Guo, Y.; Wang, Y. Multimodal fusion model for classifying placenta ultrasound imaging in pregnancies with hypertension disorders. *Pregnancy Hypertens.* **2023**, *31*, 46–53. [CrossRef] [PubMed]
120. Sun, H.; Jiao, J.; Ren, Y.; Guo, Y.; Wang, Y. Model application to quantitatively evaluate placental features from ultrasound images with gestational diabetes. *J. Clin. Ultrasound* **2022**, *50*, 976–983. [CrossRef] [PubMed]
121. Yang, X.; Chen, Z.; Jia, X. Deep Learning Algorithm-Based Ultrasound Image Information in Diagnosis and Treatment of Pernicious Placenta Previa. *Comput. Math. Methods Med.* **2022**, *2022*, 3452176. [CrossRef] [PubMed]
122. Asadpour, V.; Puttock, E.J.; Getahun, D.; Fassett, M.J.; Xie, F. Automated placental abruption identification using semantic segmentation, quantitative features, SVM, ensemble and multi-path CNN. *Heliyon* **2023**, *9*, e13577. [CrossRef]
123. Pradipta, G.A.; Wardoyo, R.; Musdholifah, A.; Sanjaya, I.N.H. Machine learning model for umbilical cord classification using combination coiling index and texture feature based on 2-D Doppler ultrasound images. *Health Inform. J.* **2022**, *28*, 146045822210842. [CrossRef]
124. Beksaç, M.; Egemen, A.; Izzetoğlu, K.; Ergün, G.; Erkmen, A.M. An automated intelligent diagnostic system for the interpretation of umbilical artery Doppler velocimetry. *Eur. J. Radiol.* **1996**, *23*, 162–167. [CrossRef]
125. Beksaç, M.; Başaran, F.; Eskiizmirliler, S.; Erkmen, A.M.; Yörükan, S. A computerized diagnostic system for the interpretation of umbilical artery blood flow velocity waveforms. *Eur. J. Obstet. Gynecol. Reprod. Biol.* **1996**, *64*, 37–42. [CrossRef]
126. Baykal, N.; A Reggia, J.; Yalabik, N.; Erkmen, A.; Beksac, M.S. Interpretation of Doppler blood flow velocity waveforms using neural networks. *Proc. Annu. Symp. Comput. Appl. Med. Care* **1994**, 865–869.
127. Torrents-Barrena, J.; Monill, N.; Piella, G.; Gratacós, E.; Eixarch, E.; Ceresa, M.; Ballester, M.A.G. Assessment of Radiomics and Deep Learning for the Segmentation of Fetal and Maternal Anatomy in Magnetic Resonance Imaging and Ultrasound. *Acad. Radiol.* **2021**, *28*, 173–188. [CrossRef] [PubMed]
128. Torrents-Barrena, J.; López-Velazco, R.; Piella, G.; Masoller, N.; Valenzuela-Alcaraz, B.; Gratacós, E.; Eixarch, E.; Ceresa, M.; Ballester, M.G. TTTS-GPS: Patient-specific preoperative planning and simulation platform for twin-to-twin transfusion syndrome fetal surgery. *Comput. Methods Programs Biomed.* **2019**, *179*, 104993. [CrossRef] [PubMed]
129. Nicolaides, K.H. *The 11–13+6 Weeks Scan*; Fetal Medicine Foundation: London, UK, 2004.
130. Salomon, L.J.; Alfirevic, Z.; Bilardo, C.M.; Chalouhi, G.E.; Ghi, T.; Kagan, K.O.; Lau, T.K.; Papageorghiou, A.T.; Raine-Fenning, N.J.; Stirnemann, J.; et al. ISUOG Practice Guidelines: Performance of first-trimester fetal ultrasound scan. *Ultrasound Obstet. Gynecol.* **2013**, *41*, 102–113. [PubMed]
131. Snijders, R.; Noble, P.; Sebire, N.; Souka, A.; Nicolaides, K. UK multicentre project on assessment of risk of trisomy 21 by maternal age and fetal nuchal-translucency thickness at 10–14 weeks of gestation. *Lancet* **1998**, *352*, 343–346. [CrossRef] [PubMed]
132. Walker, M.C.; Willner, I.; Miguel, O.X.; Murphy, M.S.Q.; El-Chaâr, D.; Moretti, F.; Harvey, A.L.J.D.; White, R.R.; Muldoon, K.A.; Carrington, A.M.; et al. Using deep-learning in fetal ultrasound analysis for diagnosis of cystic hygroma in the first trimester. *PLoS ONE* **2022**, *17*, e0269323. [CrossRef] [PubMed]
133. Zhang, L.; Dong, D.; Sun, Y.; Hu, C.; Sun, C.; Wu, Q.; Tian, J. Development and Validation of a Deep Learning Model to Screen for Trisomy 21 During the First Trimester from Nuchal Ultrasonographic Images. *JAMA Netw. Open* **2022**, *5*, e2217854. [CrossRef]
134. Sciortino, G.; Tegolo, D.; Valenti, C. Automatic detection and measurement of nuchal translucency. *Comput. Biol. Med.* **2017**, *82*, 12–20. [CrossRef]
135. Deng, Y.; Wang, Y.; Chen, P.; Yu, J. A hierarchical model for automatic nuchal translucency detection from ultrasound images. *Comput. Biol. Med.* **2012**, *42*, 706–713. [CrossRef]
136. Tsai, P.-Y.; Hung, C.-H.; Chen, C.-Y.; Sun, Y.-N. Automatic Fetal Middle Sagittal Plane Detection in Ultrasound Using Generative Adversarial Network. *Diagnostics* **2020**, *11*, 21. [CrossRef]
137. Ryou, H.; Yaqub, M.; Cavallaro, A.; Papageorghiou, A.T.; Noble, J.A. Automated 3D ultrasound image analysis for first trimester assessment of fetal health. *Phys. Med. Biol.* **2019**, *64*, 185010. [CrossRef] [PubMed]
138. Yang, X.; Yu, L.; Li, S.; Wen, H.; Luo, D.; Bian, C.; Qin, J.; Ni, D.; Heng, P.-A. Towards Automated Semantic Segmentation in Prenatal Volumetric Ultrasound. *IEEE Trans. Med Imaging* **2019**, *38*, 180–193. [CrossRef] [PubMed]

139. Salomon, L.J.; Alfirevic, Z.; Berghella, V.; Bilardo, C.; Hernandez-Andrade, E.; Johnsen, S.L.; Kalache, K.; Leung, K.; Malinger, G.; Munoz, H.; et al. Practice guidelines for performance of the routine mid-trimester fetal ultrasound scan. *Ultrasound Obstet. Gynecol.* **2010**, *37*, 116–126. [CrossRef] [PubMed]
140. Matthew, J.; Skelton, E.; Day, T.G.; Zimmer, V.A.; Gomez, A.; Wheeler, G.; Toussaint, N.; Liu, T.; Budd, S.; Lloyd, K.; et al. Exploring a new paradigm for the fetal anomaly ultrasound scan: Artificial intelligence in real time. *Prenat. Diagn.* **2022**, *42*, 49–59. [CrossRef] [PubMed]
141. Cengizler, Ç.; Ün, M.K.; Büyükkurt, S. A Nature-Inspired Search Space Reduction Technique for Spine Identification on Ultrasound Samples of Spina Bifida Cases. *Sci. Rep.* **2020**, *10*, 9280. [CrossRef] [PubMed]
142. Meenakshi, S.; Suganthi, M.; Sureshkumar, P. Segmentation and Boundary Detection of Fetal Kidney Images in Second and Third Trimesters Using Kernel-Based Fuzzy Clustering. *J. Med Syst.* **2019**, *43*, 203. [CrossRef] [PubMed]
143. Shozu, K.; Komatsu, M.; Sakai, A.; Komatsu, R.; Dozen, A.; Machino, H.; Yasutomi, S.; Arakaki, T.; Asada, K.; Kaneko, S.; et al. Model-Agnostic Method for Thoracic Wall Segmentation in Fetal Ultrasound Videos. *Biomolecules* **2020**, *10*, 1691. [CrossRef] [PubMed]
144. Lee, C.; Willis, A.; Chen, C.; Sieniek, M.; Watters, A.; Stetson, B.; Uddin, A.; Wong, J.; Pilgrim, R.; Chou, K.; et al. Development of a Machine Learning Model for Sonographic Assessment of Gestational Age. *JAMA Netw. Open* **2023**, *6*, e2248685. [CrossRef]
145. Gomes, R.G.; Vwalika, B.; Lee, C.; Willis, A.; Sieniek, M.; Price, J.T.; Chen, C.; Kasaro, M.P.; Taylor, J.A.; Stringer, E.M.; et al. A mobile-optimized artificial intelligence system for gestational age and fetal malpresentation assessment. *Commun. Med.* **2022**, *2*, 128. [CrossRef]
146. Beksaç, M.S.; Odçikin, Z.; Egemen, A.; Karakaş, U. An intelligent diagnostic system for the assessment of gestational age based on ultrasonic fetal head measurements. *Technol. Health Care* **1996**, *4*, 223–231. [CrossRef]
147. Namburete, A.I.; Stebbing, R.V.; Kemp, B.; Yaqub, M.; Papageorghiou, A.T.; Noble, J.A. Learning-based prediction of gestational age from ultrasound images of the fetal brain. *Med. Image Anal.* **2015**, *21*, 72–86. [CrossRef] [PubMed]
148. Alzubaidi, M.; Agus, M.; Shah, U.; Makhlouf, M.; Alyafei, K.; Househ, M. Ensemble Transfer Learning for Fetal Head Analysis: From Segmentation to Gestational Age and Weight Prediction. *Diagnostics* **2022**, *12*, 2229. [CrossRef] [PubMed]
149. Dan, T.; Chen, X.; He, M.; Guo, H.; He, X.; Chen, J.; Xian, J.; Hu, Y.; Zhang, B.; Wang, N.; et al. DeepGA for automatically estimating fetal gestational age through ultrasound imaging. *Artif. Intell. Med.* **2023**, *135*, 102453. [CrossRef] [PubMed]
150. Lee, L.H.; Bradburn, E.; Craik, R.; Yaqub, M.; Norris, S.A.; Ismail, L.C.; Ohuma, E.O.; Barros, F.C.; Lambert, A.; Carvalho, M.; et al. Machine learning for accurate estimation of fetal gestational age based on ultrasound images. *NPJ Digit. Med.* **2023**, *6*, 36. [CrossRef] [PubMed]
151. Maraci, M.A.; Yaqub, M.; Craik, R.; Beriwal, S.; Self, A.; Von Dadelszen, P.; Papageorghiou, A.; Noble, J.A. Toward point-of-care ultrasound estimation of fetal gestational age from the trans-cerebellar diameter using CNN-based ultrasound image analysis. *J. Med. Imaging* **2020**, *7*, 1. [CrossRef] [PubMed]
152. Pokaprakarn, T.; Prieto, J.C.; Price, J.T.; Kasaro, M.P.; Sindano, N.; Shah, H.R.; Peterson, M.; Akapelwa, M.M.; Kapilya, F.M.; Sebastião, Y.V.; et al. AI Estimation of Gestational Age from Blind Ultrasound Sweeps in Low-Resource Settings. *NEJM Évid.* **2022**, *1*, EVIDoa2100058. [CrossRef] [PubMed]
153. Prieto, J.C.; Shah, H.; Rosenbaum, A.; Jiang, X.; Musonda, P.; Price, J.; Stringer, E.M.; Vwalika, B.; Stamilio, D.M.; Stringer, J.S.A. An automated framework for image classification and segmentation of fetal ultrasound images for gestational age estimation. In *Medical Imaging 2021: Image Processing*; Landman, B.A., Išgum, I., Eds.; SPIE: Bellingham, WA, USA, 2021; p. 55. Available online: https://www.spiedigitallibrary.org/conference-proceedings-of-spie/11596/2582243/An-automated-framework-for-image-classification-and-segmentation-of-fetal/10.1117/12.2582243.full (accessed on 16 October 2023).
154. Drukker, L.; Sharma, H.; Droste, R.; Alsharid, M.; Chatelain, P.; Noble, J.A.; Papageorghiou, A.T. Transforming obstetric ultrasound into data science using eye tracking, voice recording, transducer motion and ultrasound video. *Sci. Rep.* **2021**, *11*, 14109. [CrossRef]
155. Sharma, H.; Drukker, L.; Chatelain, P.; Droste, R.; Papageorghiou, A.T.; Noble, J.A. Knowledge representation and learning of operator clinical workflow from full-length routine fetal ultrasound scan videos. *Med. Image Anal.* **2021**, *69*, 101973. [CrossRef]
156. Wang, Y.; Yang, Q.; Drukker, L.; Papageorghiou, A.; Hu, Y.; Noble, J.A. Task model-specific operator skill assessment in routine fetal ultrasound scanning. *Int. J. CARS* **2022**, *17*, 1437–1444. [CrossRef]
157. Zhao, C.; Droste, R.; Drukker, L.; Papageorghiou, A.T.; Noble, J.A. Visual-Assisted Probe Movement Guidance for Obstetric Ultrasound Scanning Using Landmark Retrieval. In *Medical Image Computing and Computer Assisted Intervention—MICCAI 2021, Proceedings of the 24th International Conference, Strasbourg, France, 27 September–1 October 2021*; De Bruijne, M., Cattin, P.C., Cotin, S., Padoy, N., Speidel, S., Zheng, Y., Eds.; Lecture Notes in Computer Science; Springer International Publishing: Cham, Switzerland, 2021; Volume 12908, pp. 670–679. Available online: https://link.springer.com/10.1007/978-3-030-87237-3_64 (accessed on 9 June 2023).
158. Drukker, L.; Sharma, H.; Karim, J.N.; Droste, R.; Noble, J.A.; Papageorghiou, A.T. Clinical workflow of sonographers performing fetal anomaly ultrasound scans: Deep-learning-based analysis. *Ultrasound Obstet. Gynecol.* **2022**, *60*, 759–765. [CrossRef]
159. Alsharid, M.; Cai, Y.; Sharma, H.; Drukker, L.; Papageorghiou, A.T.; Noble, J.A. Gaze-assisted automatic captioning of fetal ultrasound videos using three-way multi-modal deep neural networks. *Med. Image Anal.* **2022**, *82*, 102630. [CrossRef] [PubMed]

160. Sharma, H.; Drukker, L.; Papageorghiou, A.T.; Noble, J.A. Multi-Modal Learning from Video, Eye Tracking, and Pupillometry for Operator Skill Characterization in Clinical Fetal Ultrasound. In Proceedings of the 2021 IEEE 18th International Symposium on Biomedical Imaging (ISBI), Nice, France, 13–16 April 2021; pp. 1646–1649. Available online: https://ieeexplore.ieee.org/document/9433863/ (accessed on 9 June 2023).
161. Xia, T.-H.; Tan, M.; Li, J.-H.; Wang, J.-J.; Wu, Q.-Q.; Kong, D.-X. Establish a normal fetal lung gestational age grading model and explore the potential value of deep learning algorithms in fetal lung maturity evaluation. *Chin. Med. J.* **2021**, *134*, 1828–1837. [CrossRef] [PubMed]
162. Du, Y.; Fang, Z.; Jiao, J.; Xi, G.; Zhu, C.; Ren, Y.; Guo, Y.; Wang, Y. Application of ultrasound-based radiomics technology in fetal-lung-texture analysis in pregnancies complicated by gestational diabetes and/or pre-eclampsia. *Ultrasound Obstet. Gynecol.* **2021**, *57*, 804–812. [CrossRef] [PubMed]
163. Chen, P.; Chen, Y.; Deng, Y.; Wang, Y.; He, P.; Lv, X.; Yu, J. A preliminary study to quantitatively evaluate the development of maturation degree for fetal lung based on transfer learning deep model from ultrasound images. *Int. J. Comput. Assist. Radiol. Surg.* **2020**, *15*, 1407–1415. [CrossRef] [PubMed]
164. Du, Y.; Jiao, J.; Ji, C.; Li, M.; Guo, Y.; Wang, Y.; Zhou, J.; Ren, Y. Ultrasound-based radiomics technology in fetal lung texture analysis prediction of neonatal respiratory morbidity. *Sci. Rep.* **2022**, *12*, 12747. [CrossRef] [PubMed]
165. Bonet-Carne, E.; Palacio, M.; Cobo, T.; Perez-Moreno, A.; Lopez, M.; Piraquive, J.P.; Ramirez, J.C.; Botet, F.; Marques, F.; Gratacos, E. Quantitative ultrasound texture analysis of fetal lungs to predict neonatal respiratory morbidity. *Ultrasound Obstet. Gynecol.* **2015**, *45*, 427–433. [CrossRef] [PubMed]
166. Wu, M.; Fraser, R.F.; Chen, C.W. A Novel Algorithm for Computer-Assisted Measurement of Cervical Length from Transvaginal Ultrasound Images. *IEEE Trans. Inform. Technol. Biomed.* **2004**, *8*, 333–342. [CrossRef]
167. He, H.; Liu, R.; Zhou, X.; Zhang, Y.; Yu, B.; Xu, Z.; Huang, H. B-Ultrasound Image Analysis of Intrauterine Pregnancy Residues after Mid-Term Pregnancy Based on Smart Medical Big Data. *J. Healthc. Eng.* **2022**, *2022*, 9937051. [CrossRef]
168. Wang, Q.; Liu, D.; Liu, G. Value of Ultrasonic Image Features in Diagnosis of Perinatal Outcomes of Severe Preeclampsia on account of Deep Learning Algorithm. *Comput. Math. Methods Med.* **2022**, *2022*, 4010339. [CrossRef]
169. Liu, S.; Sun, Y.; Luo, N. Doppler Ultrasound Imaging Combined with Fetal Heart Detection in Predicting Fetal Distress in Pregnancy-Induced Hypertension under the Guidance of Artificial Intelligence Algorithm. *J. Healthc. Eng.* **2021**, *2021*, 4405189. [CrossRef]
170. Wang, Y.; Zhang, Q.; Yin, C.; Chen, L.; Yang, Z.; Jia, S.; Sun, X.; Bai, Y.; Han, F.; Yuan, Z. Automated prediction of early spontaneous miscarriage based on the analyzing ultrasonographic gestational sac imaging by the convolutional neural network: A case-control and cohort study. *BMC Pregnancy Childbirth* **2022**, *22*, 621. [CrossRef] [PubMed]
171. Sur, S.D.; Jayaprakasan, K.; Jones, N.W.; Clewes, J.; Winter, B.; Cash, N.; Campbell, B.; Raine-Fenning, N.J. A Novel Technique for the Semi-Automated Measurement of Embryo Volume: An Intraobserver Reliability Study. *Ultrasound Med. Biol.* **2010**, *36*, 719–725. [CrossRef] [PubMed]
172. Ghi, T.; Conversano, F.; Zegarra, R.R.; Pisani, P.; Dall'Asta, A.; Lanzone, A.; Lau, W.; Vimercati, A.; Iliescu, D.G.; Mappa, I.; et al. Novel artificial intelligence approach for automatic differentiation of fetal occiput anterior and non-occiput anterior positions during labor. *Ultrasound Obstet. Gynecol.* **2021**, *59*, 93–99. [CrossRef] [PubMed]
173. Lu, Y.; Zhi, D.; Zhou, M.; Lai, F.; Chen, G.; Ou, Z.; Zeng, R.; Long, S.; Qiu, R.; Zhou, M.; et al. Multitask Deep Neural Network for the Fully Automatic Measurement of the Angle of Progression. *Comput. Math. Methods Med.* **2022**, *2022*, 5192338. [CrossRef] [PubMed]
174. Bai, J.; Sun, Z.; Yu, S.; Lu, Y.; Long, S.; Wang, H.; Qiu, R.; Ou, Z.; Zhou, M.; Zhi, D.; et al. A framework for computing angle of progression from transperineal ultrasound images for evaluating fetal head descent using a novel double branch network. *Front. Physiol.* **2022**, *13*, 940150. [CrossRef] [PubMed]
175. Wu, L.; Cheng, J.-Z.; Li, S.; Lei, B.; Wang, T.; Ni, D. FUIQA: Fetal Ultrasound Image Quality Assessment with Deep Convolutional Networks. *IEEE Trans. Cybern.* **2017**, *47*, 1336–1349. [CrossRef] [PubMed]
176. Meng, Q.; Housden, J.; Matthew, J.; Rueckert, D.; Schnabel, J.A.; Kainz, B.; Sinclair, M.; Zimmer, V.; Hou, B.; Rajchl, M.; et al. Weakly Supervised Estimation of Shadow Confidence Maps in Fetal Ultrasound Imaging. *IEEE Trans. Med. Imaging* **2019**, *38*, 2755–2767. [CrossRef]
177. Gupta, L.; Sisodia, R.S.; Pallavi, V.; Firtion, C.; Ramachandran, G. Segmentation of 2D fetal ultrasound images by exploiting context information using conditional random fields. In Proceedings of the 2011 Annual International Conference of the IEEE Engineering in Medicine and Biology Society, Boston, MA, USA, 30 August–3 September 2011; IEEE: New York, NY, USA, 2011; pp. 7219–7222.
178. Yin, P.; Wang, H. Evaluation of Nursing Effect of Pelvic Floor Rehabilitation Training on Pelvic Organ Prolapse in Postpartum Pregnant Women under Ultrasound Imaging with Artificial Intelligence Algorithm. *Comput. Math. Methods Med.* **2022**, *2022*, 1786994. [CrossRef]
179. Cho, H.C.; Sun, S.; Hyun, C.M.; Kwon, J.-Y.; Kim, B.; Park, Y.; Seo, J.K. Automated ultrasound assessment of amniotic fluid index using deep learning. *Med. Image Anal.* **2021**, *69*, 101951. [CrossRef]
180. Compagnone, C.; Borrini, G.; Calabrese, A.; Taddei, M.; Bellini, V.; Bignami, E. Artificial intelligence enhanced ultrasound (AI-US) in a severe obese parturient: A case report. *Ultrasound J.* **2022**, *14*, 34. [CrossRef]

181. Rueda, S.; Knight, C.L.; Papageorghiou, A.T.; Noble, J.A. Feature-based fuzzy connectedness segmentation of ultrasound images with an object completion step. *Med. Image Anal.* **2015**, *26*, 30–46. [CrossRef]
182. Kaplan, E.; Ekinci, T.; Kaplan, S.; Barua, P.D.; Dogan, S.; Tuncer, T.; Tan, R.S.; Arunkumar, N.; Acharya, U.R. PFP-LHCINCA: Pyramidal Fixed-Size Patch-Based Feature Extraction and Chi-Square Iterative Neighborhood Component Analysis for Automated Fetal Sex Classification on Ultrasound Images. *Contrast Media Mol. Imaging* **2022**, *2022*, 6034971. [CrossRef] [PubMed]
183. Timmerman, D.; Testa, A.C.; Bourne, T.; Ameye, L.; Jurkovic, D.; Van Holsbeke, C.; Paladini, D.; Van Calster, B.; Vergote, I.; Van Huffel, S.; et al. Simple ultrasound-based rules for the diagnosis of ovarian cancer. *Ultrasound Obstet. Gynecol.* **2008**, *31*, 681–690. [CrossRef] [PubMed]
184. Amor, F.; Vaccaro, H.; Alcázar, J.L.; León, M.; Craig, J.M.; Martinez, J. Gynecologic Imaging Reporting and Data System: A New Proposal for Classifying Adnexal Masses on the Basis of Sonographic Findings. *J. Ultrasound Med.* **2009**, *28*, 285–291. [CrossRef] [PubMed]
185. Hsu, S.-T.; Su, Y.-J.; Hung, C.-H.; Chen, M.-J.; Lu, C.-H.; Kuo, C.-E. Automatic ovarian tumors recognition system based on ensemble convolutional neural network with ultrasound imaging. *BMC Med. Inform. Decis. Mak.* **2022**, *22*, 298. [CrossRef] [PubMed]
186. Al-Karawi, D.; Al-Assam, H.; Du, H.; Sayasneh, A.; Landolfo, C.; Timmerman, D.; Bourne, T.; Jassim, S. An Evaluation of the Effectiveness of Image-based Texture Features Extracted from Static B-mode Ultrasound Images in Distinguishing between Benign and Malignant Ovarian Masses. *Ultrason. Imaging* **2021**, *43*, 124–138. [CrossRef] [PubMed]
187. Aramendía-Vidaurreta, V.; Cabeza, R.; Villanueva, A.; Navallas, J.; Alcázar, J.L. Ultrasound Image Discrimination between Benign and Malignant Adnexal Masses Based on a Neural Network Approach. *Ultrasound Med. Biol.* **2016**, *42*, 742–752. [CrossRef]
188. Christiansen, F.; Epstein, E.L.; Smedberg, E.; Åkerlund, M.; Smith, K. Ultrasound image analysis using deep neural networks for discriminating between benign and malignant ovarian tumors: Comparison with expert subjective assessment. *Ultrasound Obstet. Gynecol.* **2021**, *57*, 155–163. [CrossRef]
189. Gao, Y.; Zeng, S.; Xu, X.; Li, H.; Yao, S.; Song, K.; Li, X.; Chen, L.; Tang, J.; Xing, H.; et al. Deep learning-enabled pelvic ultrasound images for accurate diagnosis of ovarian cancer in China: A retrospective, multicentre, diagnostic study. *Lancet Digit. Health* **2022**, *4*, e179–e187. [CrossRef]
190. Jung, Y.; Kim, T.; Han, M.R.; Kim, S.; Kim, G.; Lee, S.; Choi, Y.J. Ovarian tumor diagnosis using deep convolutional neural networks and a denoising convolutional autoencoder. *Sci Rep.* **2022**, *12*, 17024. [CrossRef]
191. Martínez-Más, J.; Bueno-Crespo, A.; Khazendar, S.; Remezal-Solano, M.; Martínez-Cendán, J.-P.; Jassim, S.; Du, H.; Al Assam, H.; Bourne, T.; Timmerman, D. Evaluation of machine learning methods with Fourier Transform features for classifying ovarian tumors based on ultrasound images. *PLoS ONE* **2019**, *14*, e0219388. [CrossRef] [PubMed]
192. Chen, H.; Yang, B.-W.; Qian, L.; Meng, Y.-S.; Bai, X.-H.; Hong, X.-W.; He, X.; Jiang, M.-J.; Yuan, F.; Du, Q.-W.; et al. Deep Learning Prediction of Ovarian Malignancy at US Compared with O-RADS and Expert Assessment. *Radiology* **2022**, *304*, 106–113. [CrossRef] [PubMed]
193. Nero, C.; Ciccarone, F.; Boldrini, L.; Lenkowicz, J.; Paris, I.; Capoluongo, E.D.; Testa, A.C.; Fagotti, A.; Valentini, V.; Scambia, G. Germline BRCA 1-2 status prediction through ovarian ultrasound images radiogenomics: A hypothesis generating study (PROBE study). *Sci. Rep.* **2020**, *10*, 16511. [CrossRef] [PubMed]
194. Chen, L.; Qiao, C.; Wu, M.; Cai, L.; Yin, C.; Yang, M.; Sang, X.; Bai, W. Improving the Segmentation Accuracy of Ovarian-Tumor Ultrasound Images Using Image Inpainting. *Bioengineering* **2023**, *10*, 184. [CrossRef] [PubMed]
195. Sung, H.; Ferlay, J.; Siegel, R.L.; Laversanne, M.; Soerjomataram, I.; Jemal, A.; Bray, F. Global Cancer Statistics 2020: GLOBOCAN Estimates of Incidence and Mortality Worldwide for 36 Cancers in 185 Countries. *CA Cancer J. Clin.* **2021**, *71*, 209–249. [CrossRef] [PubMed]
196. Ren, W.; Chen, M.; Qiao, Y.; Zhao, F. Global guidelines for breast cancer screening: A systematic review. *Breast* **2022**, *64*, 85–99. [CrossRef] [PubMed]
197. Berg, W.A.; Aldrete, A.-L.L.; Jairaj, A.; Parea, J.C.L.; García, C.Y.; McClennan, R.C.; Cen, S.Y.; Larsen, L.H.; de Lara, M.T.S.; Love, S. Toward AI-supported US Triage of Women with Palpable Breast Lumps in a Low-Resource Setting. *Radiology* **2023**, *307*, e223351. [CrossRef]
198. Huang, X.; Qiu, Y.; Bao, F.; Wang, J.; Lin, C.; Lin, Y.; Wu, J.; Yang, H. Artificial intelligence breast ultrasound and handheld ultrasound in the BI-RADS categorization of breast lesions: A pilot head to head comparison study in screening program. *Front. Public Health* **2023**, *10*, 1098639. [CrossRef]
199. Browne, J.L.; Pascual, M.Á.; Perez, J.; Salazar, S.; Valero, B.; Rodriguez, I.; Cassina, D.; Alcazar, J.L.; Guerriero, S.; Graupera, B. AI: Can It Make a Difference to the Predictive Value of Ultrasound Breast Biopsy? *Diagnostics* **2023**, *13*, 811. [CrossRef]
200. Pfob, A.; Sidey-Gibbons, C.; Barr, R.G.; Duda, V.; Alwafai, Z.; Balleyguier, C.; Clevert, D.-A.; Fastner, S.; Gomez, C.; Goncalo, M.; et al. Intelligent multi-modal shear wave elastography to reduce unnecessary biopsies in breast cancer diagnosis (INSPiRED 002): A retrospective, international, multicentre analysis. *Eur. J. Cancer* **2022**, *177*, 1–14. [CrossRef]
201. Dong, F.; She, R.; Cui, C.; Shi, S.; Hu, X.; Zeng, J.; Wu, H.; Xu, J.; Zhang, Y. One step further into the blackbox: A pilot study of how to build more confidence around an AI-based decision system of breast nodule assessment in 2D ultrasound. *Eur. Radiol.* **2021**, *31*, 4991–5000. [CrossRef] [PubMed]

202. Pfob, A.; Sidey-Gibbons, C.; Barr, R.G.; Duda, V.; Alwafai, Z.; Balleyguier, C.; Clevert, D.-A.; Fastner, S.; Gomez, C.; Goncalo, M.; et al. The importance of multi-modal imaging and clinical information for humans and AI-based algorithms to classify breast masses (INSPiRED 003): An international, multicenter analysis. *Eur. Radiol.* **2022**, *32*, 4101–4115. [CrossRef] [PubMed]
203. Heremans, R.; Bosch, T.V.D.; Valentin, L.; Wynants, L.; Pascual, M.A.; Fruscio, R.; Testa, A.C.; Buonomo, F.; Guerriero, S.; Epstein, E.; et al. Ultrasound features of endometrial pathology in women without abnormal uterine bleeding: Results from the International Endometrial Tumor Analysis study (IETA3). *Ultrasound Obstet. Gynecol.* **2022**, *60*, 243–255. [CrossRef] [PubMed]
204. Vitale, S.G.; Riemma, G.; Haimovich, S.; Carugno, J.; Pacheco, L.A.; Perez-Medina, T.; Parry, J.P.; Török, P.; Tesarik, J.; Della Corte, L.; et al. Risk of endometrial cancer in asymptomatic postmenopausal women in relation to ultrasonographic endometrial thickness: Systematic review and diagnostic test accuracy meta-analysis. *Am. J. Obstet. Gynecol.* **2022**, *228*, 22–35.e2. [CrossRef] [PubMed]
205. Zhao, X.; Wu, S.; Zhang, B.; Burjoo, A.; Yang, Y.; Xu, D. Artificial intelligence diagnosis of intrauterine adhesion by 3D ultrasound imaging: A prospective study. *Quant. Imaging Med. Surg.* **2023**, *13*, 2314–2327. [CrossRef] [PubMed]
206. Wang, X.; Bao, N.; Xin, X.; Tan, J.; Li, H.; Zhou, S.; Liu, H. Automatic evaluation of endometrial receptivity in three-dimensional transvaginal ultrasound images based on 3D U-Net segmentation. *Quant. Imaging Med. Surg.* **2022**, *12*, 4095–4108. [CrossRef] [PubMed]
207. Park, H.; Lee, H.J.; Kim, H.G.; Ro, Y.M.; Shin, D.; Lee, S.R.; Kim, S.H.; Kong, M. Endometrium segmentation on transvaginal ultrasound image using key-point discriminator. *Med. Phys.* **2019**, *46*, 3974–3984. [CrossRef]
208. Liu, Y.; Zhou, Q.; Peng, B.; Jiang, J.; Fang, L.; Weng, W.; Wang, W.; Wang, S.; Zhu, X. Automatic Measurement of Endometrial Thickness from Transvaginal Ultrasound Images. *Front. Bioeng. Biotechnol.* **2022**, *10*, 853845. [CrossRef]
209. Moro, F.; Albanese, M.; Boldrini, L.; Chiappa, V.; Lenkowicz, J.; Bertolina, F.; Mascilini, F.; Moroni, R.; Gambacorta, M.A.; Raspagliesi, F.; et al. Developing and validating ultrasound-based radiomics models for predicting high-risk endometrial cancer. *Ultrasound Obstet. Gynecol.* **2022**, *60*, 256–268. [CrossRef]
210. Zhu, Y.; Zhang, J.; Ji, Z.; Liu, W.; Li, M.; Xia, E.; Zhang, J.; Wang, J. Ultrasound Evaluation of Pelvic Floor Function after Transumbilical Laparoscopic Single-Site Total Hysterectomy Using Deep Learning Algorithm. *Comput. Math. Methods Med.* **2022**, *2022*, 1116332. [CrossRef]
211. Williams, H.; Cattani, L.; Van Schoubroeck, D.; Yaqub, M.; Sudre, C.; Vercauteren, T.; D'Hooge, J.; Deprest, J. Automatic Extraction of Hiatal Dimensions in 3-D Transperineal Pelvic Ultrasound Recordings. *Ultrasound Med. Biol.* **2021**, *47*, 3470–3479. [CrossRef] [PubMed]
212. Szentimrey, Z.; Ameri, G.; Hong, C.X.; Cheung, R.Y.K.; Ukwatta, E.; Eltahawi, A. Automated segmentation and measurement of the female pelvic floor from the mid-sagittal plane of 3D ultrasound volumes. *Med. Phys.* **2023**, *50*, 6215–6227. [CrossRef] [PubMed]
213. Van Den Noort, F.; Manzini, C.; Van Der Vaart, C.H.; Van Limbeek, M.A.J.; Slump, C.H.; Grob, A.T.M. Automatic identification and segmentation of slice of minimal hiatal dimensions in transperineal ultrasound volumes. *Ultrasound Obstet. Gynecol.* **2022**, *60*, 570–576. [CrossRef] [PubMed]
214. Van den Noort, F.; van der Vaart, C.H.; Grob, A.T.M.; van de Waarsenburg, M.K.; Slump, C.H.; van Stralen, M. Deep learning enables automatic quantitative assessment of puborectalis muscle and urogenital hiatus in plane of minimal hiatal dimensions. *Ultrasound Obstet. Gynecol.* **2019**, *54*, 270–275. [CrossRef] [PubMed]
215. Wu, S.; Ren, Y.; Lin, X.; Huang, Z.; Zheng, Z.; Zhang, X. Development and validation of a composite AI model for the diagnosis of levator ani muscle avulsion. *Eur. Radiol.* **2022**, *32*, 5898–5906. [CrossRef] [PubMed]
216. Maicas, G.; Leonardi, M.; Avery, J.; Panuccio, C.; Carneiro, G.; Hull, M.L.; Condous, G. Deep learning to diagnose pouch of Douglas obliteration with ultrasound sliding sign. *Reprod. Fertil.* **2021**, *2*, 236–243. [CrossRef]
217. Raimondo, D.; Raffone, A.; Aru, A.C.; Giorgi, M.; Giaquinto, I.; Spagnolo, E.; Travaglino, A.; Galatolo, F.A.; Cimino, M.G.C.A.; Lenzi, J.; et al. Application of Deep Learning Model in the Sonographic Diagnosis of Uterine Adenomyosis. *Int. J. Environ. Res. Public Health* **2023**, *20*, 1724. [CrossRef]
218. Zhang, Y.; Hou, J.; Wang, Q.; Hou, A.; Liu, Y. Application of Transfer Learning and Feature Fusion Algorithms to Improve the Identification and Prediction Efficiency of Premature Ovarian Failure. *J. Healthc. Eng.* **2022**, *2022*, 3269692. [CrossRef]
219. Yu, L.; Qing, X. Diagnosis of Idiopathic Premature Ovarian Failure by Color Doppler Ultrasound under the Intelligent Segmentation Algorithm. *Comput. Math. Methods Med.* **2022**, *2022*, 2645607. [CrossRef]
220. Huo, T.; Li, L.; Chen, X.; Wang, Z.; Zhang, X.; Liu, S.; Huang, J.; Zhang, J.; Yang, Q.; Wu, W.; et al. Artificial intelligence-aided method to detect uterine fibroids in ultrasound images: A retrospective study. *Sci. Rep.* **2023**, *13*, 3714. [CrossRef]
221. Yang, T.; Yuan, L.; Li, P.; Liu, P. Real-Time Automatic Assisted Detection of Uterine Fibroid in Ultrasound Images Using a Deep Learning Detector. *Ultrasound Med. Biol.* **2023**, *49*, 1616–1626. [CrossRef] [PubMed]
222. Singh, V.K.; Yousef Kalafi, E.; Cheah, E.; Wang, S.; Wang, J.; Ozturk, A.; Li, Q.; Eldar, Y.C.; Samir, A.E.; Kumar, V. HaTU-Net: Harmonic Attention Network for Automated Ovarian Ultrasound Quantification in Assisted Pregnancy. *Diagnostics* **2022**, *12*, 3213. [CrossRef] [PubMed]

223. Noor, N.; Vignarajan, C.; Malhotra, N.; Vanamail, P. Three-Dimensional Automated Volume Calculation (Sonography-Based Automated Volume Count) versus Two-Dimensional Manual Ultrasonography for Follicular Tracking and Oocyte Retrieval in Women Undergoing in vitro Fertilization-Embryo Transfer: A Randomized Controlled Trial. *J. Hum. Reprod. Sci.* **2020**, *13*, 296. [PubMed]
224. Maurice, P.; Dhombres, F.; Blondiaux, E.; Friszer, S.; Guilbaud, L.; Lelong, N.; Khoshnood, B.; Charlet, J.; Perrot, N.; Jauniaux, E.; et al. Towards ontology-based decision support systems for complex ultrasound diagnosis in obstetrics and gynecology. *J. Gynecol. Obstet. Hum. Reprod.* **2017**, *46*, 423–429. [CrossRef] [PubMed]
225. Dhombres, F.; Maurice, P.; Friszer, S.; Guilbaud, L.; Lelong, N.; Khoshnood, B.; Charlet, J.; Perrot, N.; Jauniaux, E.; Jurkovic, D.; et al. Developing a knowledge base to support the annotation of ultrasound images of ectopic pregnancy. *J. Biomed. Semant.* **2017**, *8*, 4. [CrossRef] [PubMed]
226. Huh, J.; Khan, S.; Choi, S.; Shin, D.; Lee, J.E.; Lee, E.S.; Ye, J.C. Tunable image quality control of 3-D ultrasound using switchable CycleGAN. *Med. Image Anal.* **2023**, *83*, 102651. [CrossRef] [PubMed]
227. Kalantaridou, S.N.; Nelson, L.M. Premature ovarian failure is not premature menopause. *Ann. N. Y. Acad. Sci.* **2006**, *900*, 393–402. [CrossRef]
228. Watzenboeck, M.L.; Heidinger, B.H.; Rainer, J.; Schmidbauer, V.; Ulm, B.; Rubesova, E.; Prayer, D.; Kasprian, G.; Prayer, F. Reproducibility of 2D versus 3D radiomics for quantitative assessment of fetal lung development: A retrospective fetal MRI study. *Insights Imaging* **2023**, *14*, 31. [CrossRef]
229. Prayer, F.; Watzenböck, M.L.; Heidinger, B.H.; Rainer, J.; Schmidbauer, V.; Prosch, H.; Ulm, B.; Rubesova, E.; Prayer, D.; Kasprian, G. Fetal MRI radiomics: Non-invasive and reproducible quantification of human lung maturity. *Eur. Radiol.* **2023**, *33*, 4205–4213. [CrossRef]
230. Liu, Y.; Zhang, Y.; Cheng, R.; Liu, S.; Qu, F.; Yin, X.; Wang, Q.; Xiao, B.; Ye, Z. Radiomics analysis of apparent diffusion coefficient in cervical cancer: A preliminary study on histological grade evaluation: Radiomic Features in Uterine Cervical Cancer. *J. Magn. Reson. Imaging* **2019**, *49*, 280–290. [CrossRef]
231. Drukker, L.; Noble, J.A.; Papageorghiou, A.T. Introduction to Artificial Intelligence in Ultrasound Imaging in Obstetrics and Gynecology. *Obstet. Gynecol. Surv.* **2021**, *76*, 127–129. [CrossRef]
232. Jani, J.; Peralta, C.F.A.; Benachi, A.; Deprest, J.; Nicolaides, K.H. Assessment of lung area in fetuses with congenital diaphragmatic hernia. *Ultrasound Obstet. Gynecol.* **2007**, *30*, 72–76. [CrossRef]
233. World Health Organization. *Ethics and Governance of Artificial Intelligence for Health: WHO Guidance*; Licence: CC BY-NC-SA 3.0 IGO; WHO: Switzerland, Geneva, 2021.
234. Dhombres, F.; Bonnard, J.; Bailly, K.; Maurice, P.; Papageorghiou, A.T.; Jouannic, J.-M. Contributions of Artificial Intelligence Reported in Obstetrics and Gynecology Journals: Systematic Review. *J. Med. Internet Res.* **2022**, *24*, e35465. [CrossRef]

Disclaimer/Publisher's Note: The statements, opinions and data contained in all publications are solely those of the individual author(s) and contributor(s) and not of MDPI and/or the editor(s). MDPI and/or the editor(s) disclaim responsibility for any injury to people or property resulting from any ideas, methods, instructions or products referred to in the content.

Protocol

Study Protocol of a Prospective, Monocentric, Single-Arm Study Investigating the Safety and Efficacy of Local Ablation of Symptomatic Uterine Fibroids with US-Guided High-Intensity Focused Ultrasound (HIFU)

Dieter M. Matlac [1,†], Tolga Tonguc [2,3,†], Nikola Mutschler [1], Florian Recker [4], Olga Ramig [2], Holger M. Strunk [5], Tatjana Dell [2], Claus C. Pieper [2], Martin Coenen [6], Christine Fuhrmann [6], Oregan Vautey [7], Eva-Katharina Egger [1], Jim Küppers [7], Rupert Conrad [8], Markus Essler [7], Alexander Mustea [1] and Milka Marinova [7,*]

1. Department of Gynecology and Gynecological Oncology, University Hospital Bonn, University Bonn, 53127 Bonn, Germany
2. Department of Diagnostic and Interventional Radiology, University Hospital Bonn, University Bonn, 53127 Bonn, Germany
3. Department of Neuroradiology, University Hospital Bonn, University Bonn, 53127 Bonn, Germany
4. Department of Obstetrics and Prenatal Medicine, University Hospital Bonn, University Bonn, 53127 Bonn, Germany
5. Medical Center, University Bonn, 53115 Bonn, Germany
6. Clinical Study Core Unit Bonn, Institute of Clinical Chemistry and Clinical Pharmacology, University Hospital Bonn, University Bonn, 53127 Bonn, Germany; christine.fuhrmann@ukbonn.de (C.F.)
7. Department of Nuclear Medicine, University Hospital Bonn, 53127 Bonn, Germany
8. Department of Psychosomatic Medicine and Psychotherapy, University Hospital Muenster, 48149 Muenster, Germany

* Correspondence: milka.marinova@ukbonn.de
† These authors contributed equally to this work.

Abstract: Uterine fibroids are the most common benign tumors of the uterus. Approximately 20–50% of women with myomas experience a variety of symptoms such as vaginal bleeding, abdominal pain, pelvic pain and pressure, and urological problems, possibly interfering with fertility and pregnancy. Although surgery remains the standard treatment option for fibroids, non-invasive therapeutic options, such as high-intensity focused ultrasound (HIFU), have emerged over the last decade. During HIFU, ultrasound is focused on the target tissue causing coagulation necrosis. HIFU has, meanwhile, become an established method for treating uterine fibroids in many countries. Clinical data have shown that it effectively alleviates fibroid-related symptoms and reduces fibroid size with a very low rate of side effects. However, there is a lack of data on how this treatment affects laboratory parameters and structural features of uterine tissue. As our center is the only one in German-speaking countries where ultrasound-guided HIFU technology is currently established, the aim of this prospective, monocentric, single-arm trial is not only to evaluate the safety and efficacy of local US-guided HIFU in symptomatic uterine fibroid patients according to GCP standards but also to explore its effects on blood parameters and the structural integrity of uterine tissue using elastographic methods.

Keywords: symptomatic uterine fibroids; high-intensity focused ultrasound; structural integrity of uterine tissue; US and MRI elastographic methods

1. Uterine Fibroids

Uterine fibroids are the most common benign tumors of the uterus. As their growth depends on the female sexual hormone estrogen, fibroids mostly occur in women of childbearing age. In a methodologically sound systematic review, the following twelve risk or protective factors were identified: black race, age, premenopausal state, hypertension, family history, time since last birth, and food additive and soybean milk consumption increase fibroid risk; the use of oral contraceptives or the injectable contraceptive depot medroxyprogesterone acetate and smoking in women with low body mass index and parity are protective factors [1]. Other large datasets suggest that a clinical history of obesity, current alcohol use, and chronic psychological stress may increase the risk/prevalence of uterine fibroids [2,3]. Interestingly, an increase in the frequency of fibroids is shown in women with a history of benign breast disease and particularly of breast biopsies [4]. Moreover, the evolution of uterine fibroids during pregnancy and puerperium appears to follow a non-linear trend, with systematic enlargement observed in the first trimester, while changes during the second and third trimesters are supported by inconsistent evidence, and the overall modifications of myomas during this period remain uncertain [5].

Most uterine fibroids do not cause any symptoms, only 25–30% of the patients experience fibroid-associated symptoms [6]. These include abnormal uterine bleeding, pain or pressure in the lower abdomen with potential effects on the bladder or rectum, and even dyspareunia and fertility [7]. Especially submucosal myomas (classified as type 3 according to the FIGO classification) are notably associated with reduced implantation rates, cumulative pregnancy rates, and live birth rates [8]. Moreover, their negative influence on IVF outcomes becomes more pronounced with larger size and an increased number of such myomas. In addition, uterine fibroids can be associated with pregnancy complications [9].

As long as fibroids do not cause any symptoms and there is no evidence of malignancy, no treatment is necessary. For symptomatic fibroids, there are various treatment options, including pharmacological (hormone) therapy, surgical therapies such as myomectomy or hysterectomy, and minimally invasive therapies such as uterine artery embolization (UAE) [7] and local ablation with high-intensity focused ultrasound (HIFU) as a non-invasive procedure [10].

2. Pharmacological Therapy of Uterine Myomas

Several groups of pharmacological agents, such as gonadotropin-releasing hormone agonists, oral combined contraceptives, progesterone receptor modulators, and intrauterine progestogen coils, are available for drug therapy of symptomatic uterine fibroids [11,12]. The progesterone receptor modulator ulipristal acetate (Esmya®) was commonly used in the past for symptom relief and fibroid volume reduction prior to pending surgery. However, the usefulness of this drug has been out of perspective since 2018 due to observed side effects and an unfavorable risk–benefit profile [13].

The most recent change in the pharmacological therapy of fibroids has been the approval of Ryeqo® (Gedeon Richter) in June 2021. Ryeqo® is a combinational drug containing relugolix, a selective GnRH-receptor antagonist, estradiol, and norethisterone acetate. It has been shown to significantly reduce fibroid-associated symptoms in two approval studies. The combination of these three drugs is supposed to reduce fibroid-induced symptoms while keeping symptoms due to estrogen shortage low and preventing a higher risk of endometrial carcinoma [14].

3. Gynecological Surgical Treatment of Uterine Fibroids

Surgical therapy remains the most direct treatment for uterine fibroids as a primary therapeutic option. It can either be performed laparoscopically or through an abdominal incision. Depending on the size, number, location of the fibroids, and the patient's desire for uterus preservation, there are different surgical approaches. For submucosal fibroids, hysteroscopy can be usually performed. For subserosal fibroids, enucleation by laparoscopy may be an option, and if laparoscopy is not feasible, a surgical procedure by laparotomy is necessary. Removal of the uterus is indeed the most effective treatment, although several factors have to be considered. If removal of the uterus is desired, a choice can be made between open and laparoscopic procedures depending on the size of the uterus. Moreover, in rare cases (under 0.03%), malignant sarcoma may be present [15]. Considering aspects of oncological safety, morcellement of the uterus is avoided in our clinic.

4. HIFU for Uterine Fibroids

High-intensity focused ultrasound (HIFU; high-intensity focused ultrasound) represents an innovative and non-invasive therapeutic option for symptomatic uterine fibroids [16]. This technique allows targeted thermal ablation of solid tumors accessible to sonography [17]. The decision on the indication for HIFU treatment is made individually for each patient in an interdisciplinary team of the HIFU center at the University Hospital Bonn. Fibroid ablation with HIFU represents a low-risk intervention compared with other procedures with few and, in the rarest cases, severe side effects [18].

In contrast to diagnostic ultrasound, HIFU generates much higher energies in the target area during ablation. The ultrasound waves are focused by special transducers in the lesion, and the focus measures only a few millimeters. This results in local heating of the target tissue up to more than 60 °C, inducing coagulation necrosis.

In recent years, HIFU has been increasingly used for the local therapy of different benign and malignant solid tumors [19]. The clinical value of HIFU treatment for uterine fibroids has been investigated in numerous studies involving large patient populations over the past decade. All of these studies have described the procedure as safe and effective, with a significant clinical benefit for patients through the reduction in myoma-related symptoms. Symptom reduction and a decrease in fibroid volume have been shown in all types of treated fibroids [20]. Special attention should be given to submucosal fibroids, as they may have potential negative effects on the fertility of patients in their childbearing age [8]. Therefore, a comprehensive and individual evaluation of the prospects and feasibility of HIFU treatment is warranted in this context.

Side effects are rare and less frequent than after surgical procedures like myomectomy and hysterectomy [16]. Moderate pain during the procedure, which is performed under conscious sedation, may last for a few hours in some cases, and cutaneous/subcutaneous edema of the anterior lower abdominal wall in the acoustic pathway are common side effects [21]. However, fever, urinary tract infections, hematuria, bowel lesions, and back pain are possible, but these are very rare nowadays.

The duration of the procedure depends on the size, number, and location of the target fibroids and lasts normally 1–2 h but may take up to 3–4 h. The HIFU treatment can be performed on an outpatient basis; after a rest period of four to six hours, the patient can usually leave the clinic and resume her normal daily routine the next day. HIFU treatment of fibroids requires good coordination between interventionalists, anesthesiologists, and gynecologists, as previously described [22]. In the course of this prospective study, the patients are hospitalized for one night in the local gynecology department in order to accurately evaluate the treatment-associated side effects.

5. Rationale of the Study

The study has a prospective, monocentric, and single-arm design and is intended to evaluate the safety and efficacy of local therapy with ultrasound-guided HIFU in patients with symptomatic uterine fibroids according to GCP standards. To the best of our knowledge, the University Hospital Bonn is currently the only center in German-speaking countries where an ultrasound-guided HIFU system (TTS, tumor therapeutic system, Chongqing Haifu Medical Technology, China) is available and in use as opposed to several other centers that use MRI-guided HIFU. The evaluation of study results is based on clinical gynecological investigation, records, and assessment of side effects; the UFS-QOL questionnaire on disease-related symptoms (symptom severity score) and health-related quality of life (QOL); and changes in fibroid volume over time using MRI [19]. This present study aims to identify patients who would benefit the most from HIFU treatment and collect data to plan a confirmatory phase III trial assessing the efficacy of combining HIFU with other therapies. Additionally, this study investigates the effects of HIFU treatment on laboratory parameters, including its potential to induce an immune response. Another exploratory endpoint is an assessment of elastographic features of uterine fibroid tissue before and after HIFU treatment, utilizing both sonographic share wave elastography and MR imaging techniques.

6. Trial Design

The current investigation is a prospective, monocentric, single-arm, and open-label study (Figures 1 and 2). The entire study duration per patient is 8 months, including screening visits. The HIFU procedure typically lasts for 2–5 h, with a hospital stay for one night. Each patient is monitored for a follow-up period of 6 months. The clinical trial will be conducted in the interdisciplinary HIFU center at the University Hospital Bonn, and all investigators meet the requirements to perform the planned study-specific examinations and therapies.

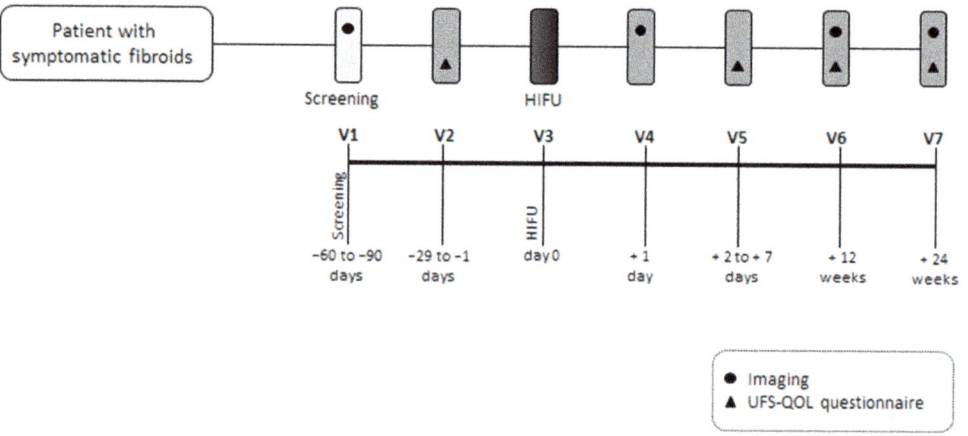

Figure 1. Intervention scheme.

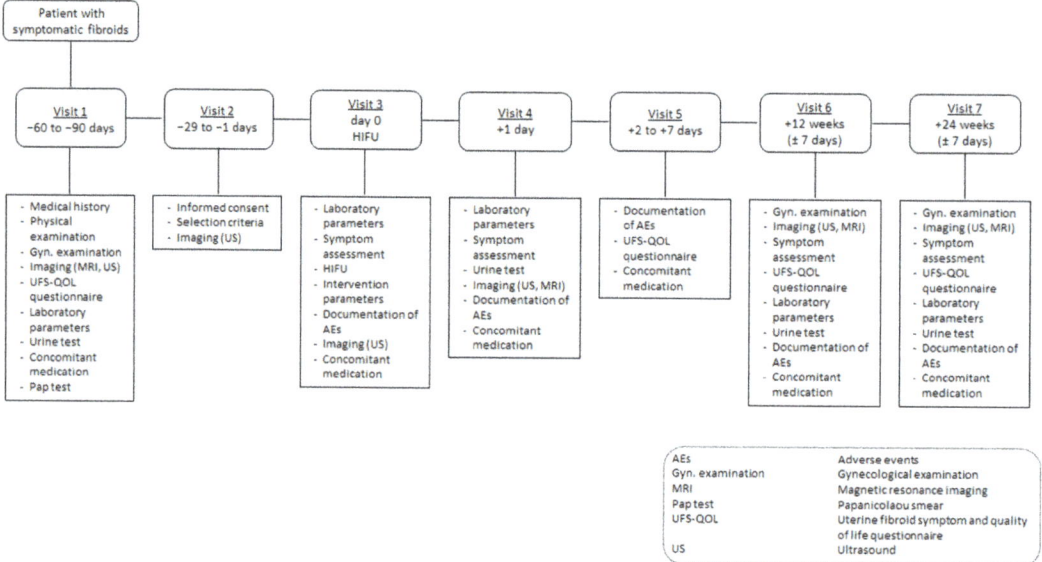

Figure 2. Trial flow.

7. Study Population

Twenty eligible patients will be recruited for this study. Potential participants who present at the gynecology department will be informed about the study and given adequate time to reflect before providing written informed consent to participate. Patients who do not meet the inclusion criteria (outlined in Table 1) will not be included in the study.

Table 1. Selection criteria for HIFU treatment and study participation.

Inclusion Criteria	Exclusion Criteria
− Age ≥ 18 years − Written informed consent − Ability to follow study instructions and participate in required study visits − Fibroid visualization on diagnostic ultrasound − Minimum fibroid diameter of 2 cm − Maximum fibroid diameter ≤ 12 cm − No evidence of malignancy − Safe acoustic access path to the fibroid − Distance between skin surface and deepest fibroid regions of max. 11 cm − Fibroid-related symptoms − Patient's MRI suitability	− Current pregnancy or breastfeeding − Suspected malignancy − Abnormal cervical cancer screening result − Acute cystitis − Acute infection (e.g., pneumonia) − Pedunculated or subserosal fibroids − Thick scar tissue on the skin or in the acoustic pathway − History of ileum conduit − Simultaneous participation in a clinical trial up to 30 days prior to participation in this clinical trial − Non-eligibility for conscious sedation

Fertile study patients will be informed that pregnancy or breastfeeding are contraindications to participating in the study and will be instructed to use reliable contraceptive methods throughout the study period. Reliable contraceptive methods with a Pearl Index below 1 include hormonal methods, barrier methods, and hormonal medication. Patients will be required to abstain from sexual intercourse during the first month after the HIFU procedure, and transvaginal ultrasound should be avoided during this period. Eligible patients will be mainly recruited from the outpatient clinic of the Department of Gyneco-logy, but patients referred by external gynecologists or those who present themselves will be also included.

The interdisciplinary uterine fibroid conference, which convenes weekly, will determine whether HIFU treatment is indicated for each patient on an individual basis. Potentially suitable patients will receive detailed information about their participation in the study and the procedures involved by the investigator. The study has been initiated after professional ethical consultation by the responsible ethics committee at the University Hospital Bonn.

8. Measurements

8.1. Primary Endpoints

The primary objective of this study is to evaluate the safety and tolerability of local HIFU treatment in patients with symptomatic uterine fibroids. This involves evaluating incidents and product defects as well as adverse events after HIFU therapy. Adverse events will be graded according to the Common Terminology Criteria for Adverse Events (CTCAE, Version 5.0), with grades 1–5 indicating increasing severity.

In addition to the frequency and severity of adverse events according to CTCAE, the expected treatment-associated adverse events will be recorded, including pain during and immediately after the HIFU procedure (measured on a pain scale NRS/VAS 0–10, with 0 indicating no pain and 10 indicating the most severe pain), pain within the first day after the procedure, skin edema, skin redness, skin burning, ascites, cystitis, vaginal discharge, and vaginal bleeding.

8.2. Secondary Endpoints

The following objectives are defined as secondary endpoints:

- Evaluation of symptom severity score (SSS) and health-related quality of life score using UFS-QOL questionnaire (baseline scores versus scores 1 week, 3 months, and 6 months after HIFU procedure).
- Evaluation of fibroid volume using MRI measurements (baseline volume versus volume 1 week, 3 months, and 6 months after HIFU procedure).
- Evaluation of the correlation between intervention parameters (sonication time, treatment time, total energy, and energy per milliliter of fibroid volume), achieved non-perfused volume, fibroid type according to Funaki classification, and fibroid shrinkage over time.
- Evaluation of tissue stiffness properties of uterine fibroids using elastography measurements on transabdominal ultrasound and MRI before and after HIFU procedure.
- Effects of HIFU treatment on blood parameters.

9. Data Collection

Several kinds of data will be assessed in this study at each visit (Table 2). Data related to symptoms will be gained through communication with the patients and objectivation via established questionnaires. In addition, blood samples will be taken and analyzed for several parameters with emphasis on immune system-related parameters. Moreover, changes in the physical quality of fibroid tissue before and after HIFU treatment will be monitored through follow-up ultrasound and MRI examinations, including elastography.

Table 2. Schedule of activities at each visit.

	Visit 1 −60 to −90 Days Screening	Visit 2 −29 to −1 Days Baseline	Visit 3 Day 0	Visit 4 +1 Day	Visit 5 +2 to +7 Days	Visit 6 +12 Weeks (±7 Days)	Visit 7 +24 Weeks (± 7 Days)
Selection criteria	(X)	X					
Informed consent	(X)	X					
Medical history	X						
Physical examination	X						
Vital signs	X						
Gynecological examination	X					X	X
Pap test	X						
Laboratory parameters	X	X	X	X		X	X
Urine test	X			X		X	X
MRI	X			X		X	X
Ultrasound inc. elastography	(X)	X	X	X		X	X
Records of concomitant medications	X		X	X	X	X	X
Records of pre-treatments	X						
Bowel preparation		X (day −1)					
Premedication		X					
Urinary catheter			X				
Preparation of abdominal wall			X				
HIFU treatment			X				
Assessment of pain (VAS 0–10)			X	X	X	X	X
Assessment of treatment-related AEs and SAEs			X	X	X	X	X
Assessment of additional AEs and SAEs			X	X	X	X	X

Table 2. Cont.

	Visit 1 −60 to −90 Days Screening	Visit 2 −29 to −1 Days Baseline	Visit 3 Day 0	Visit 4 +1 Day	Visit 5 +2 to +7 Days	Visit 6 +12 Weeks (±7 Days)	Visit 7 +24 Weeks (± 7 Days)
UFS-QOL		X			X	X	X
Imaging assessment		X	(X)	X		X	X
Intervention parameters (J/mL)			X				
NPV (%)					X		

AE: Adverse event; Gyn. Examination: Gynecological examination; HIFU: High-intensity focused ultrasound; MRI: Magnetic resonance imaging; NPV: Non-perfused volume; Pap test: Papanicolaou test, Papanicolaou smear; SAE: Serious adverse event; UFS-QOL: Uterine Fibroid Symptom and Quality of Life questionnaire; US: Ultrasound; VAS: Visual analog scale.

10. Statistical Analysis

Data from this prospective observational longitudinal study will be analyzed using Stata (latest version, StataCorp, StataCorp LP, College Station, TX, USA) and SPSS (latest version, SPSS Inc., Chicago, IL, USA). Evaluation of changes in fibroid volumes, symptom severity, and quality of life scores will be performed by using a longitudinal mixed model considering values at baseline and each follow-up as dependent variables. The influence of various interventional parameters (total energy, sonication time, and power) and assignment to corresponding Funaki types on non-perfused volumes and volume reduction over time will be analyzed using logistic regression and a mixed model, respectively. A p-value of < 0.05 is considered statistically significant.

11. Strengths and Limitations

The present study offers several strengths, including its prospective design and focus on ultrasound-guided HIFU therapy in a German cohort. Notably, the University Hospital Bonn is currently the only center in Germany-speaking countries where US-guided HIFU technology is available and in use. For this reason, the primary endpoint of the study is to investigate the incidence and severity of treatment-related adverse events using the CTCAE classification. In addition to evaluating patients' symptoms and well-being using standardized questionnaires, this study also employs innovative diagnostic modalities such as sonographic and MRI-based technologies to assess fibroid stiffness and provide a more comprehensive understanding of the effects of HIFU treatment beyond just changes in fibroid size. Moreover, the study focuses on early ablation-related laboratory changes and potential inflammatory reactions. While the strength of the study lies in its prospective design and the use of ultrasound-guided HIFU therapy on a German cohort, the limitation is referred to the relatively small sample size and the inability to directly compare the results to other treatment methods due to the single-arm study design.

12. Summary

Previous clinical research has demonstrated that high-intensity focused ultrasound (HIFU) is a non-invasive and low-risk treatment option for symptomatic uterine fibroids, as long as the fibroids are accessible to therapeutic ultrasound. HIFU provides effective symptom control while avoiding the potential risks and drawbacks of surgery, which is currently the standard treatment option. This study assesses the safety, efficacy, and clinical outcomes of US-guided HIFU treatment in 20 patients with symptomatic fibroids. The study aims to identify patients who would benefit most from this innovative treatment compared to other methods and to collect data that will serve as a foundation for future research on diagnostic and therapeutic approaches.

Author Contributions: Conceptualization, F.R., H.M.S., R.C. and M.M.; methodology, D.M.M., T.T., N.M. and M.M.; software, O.R., M.C., C.F. and M.M.; validation, M.C., C.F. and M.M.; formal analysis, M.M.; investigation, D.M.M., N.M., O.R., T.D., and M.M; resources, M.M.; data curation, D.M.M., T.T., O.R. and M.M.; writing—original draft preparation, D.M.M., T.T. and M.M.; writing—review and editing, H.M.S., T.D., C.C.P., E.-K.E., J.K., R.C., M.E., A.M. and M.M.; visualization, O.V., J.K. and M.M.; supervision, H.M.S., M.C., C.F., R.C., M.E. and A.M.; project administration, D.M.M., T.T., N.M., F.R., O.R., M.C., C.F., O.V., E.-K.E. and M.M.; funding acquisition, F.R. and M.M. All authors have read and agreed to the published version of the manuscript.

Funding: This study is an Investigator Initiated Trial (IIT), which is supported by grants from the Clinical Trials Commission at the University Hospital Bonn. Trial registration number: DRKS00017490; German Cllinical Trials Register; Deutsches Register Klinischer Studien.

Institutional Review Board Statement: The study was conducted in accordance with the Declaration of Helsinki, and approved by the Institutional Review Board, Ethics Committee of the University Hospital Bonn (protocol code 055/19, date of approval 12 April 2019).

Informed Consent Statement: Informed consent is obtained from all subjects involved in the study.

Data Availability Statement: This article represents a study protocol. Data will be generated in the course of the study and published later.

Conflicts of Interest: The authors declare no conflict of interest.

References

1. Stewart, E.A.; Cookson, C.L.; Gandolfo, R.A.; Schulze-Rath, R. Epidemiology of uterine fibroids: A systematic review. *BJOG* **2017**, *124*, 1501–1512. [CrossRef] [PubMed]
2. Qin, H.; Lin, Z.; Vásquez, E.; Luan, X.; Guo, F.; Xu, L. Association between obesity and the risk of uterine fibroids: A systematic review and meta-analysis. *J. Epidemiol. Community Health* **2021**, *75*, 197–204. [CrossRef] [PubMed]
3. Salehi, A.M.; Jenabi, E.; Farashi, S.; Aghababaei, S.; Salimi, Z. The environmental risk factors related to uterine leiomyoma: An umbrella review. *J. Gynecol. Obstet. Hum. Reprod.* **2023**, *52*, 102517. [CrossRef] [PubMed]
4. Parazzini, F.; Chiaffarino, F.; Polverino, G.; Chiantera, V.; Surace, M.; La Vecchia, C. Uterine fibroids risk and history of selected medical conditions linked with female hormones. *Eur. J. Epidemiol.* **2004**, *19*, 249–253. [CrossRef] [PubMed]
5. Vitagliano, A.; Noventa, M.; Di Spiezio Sardo, A.; Saccone, G.; Gizzo, S.; Borgato, S.; Vitale, S.G.; Laganà, A.S.; Nardelli, G.B.; Litta, P.S.; et al. Uterine fibroid size modifications during pregnancy and puerperium: Evidence from the first systematic review of literature. *Arch. Gynecol. Obstet.* **2018**, *297*, 823–835. [CrossRef] [PubMed]
6. Yang, Q.; Ciebiera, M.; Bariani, M.V.; Ali, M.; Elkafas, H.; Boyer, T.G.; Al-Hendy, A. Comprehensive Review of Uterine Fibroids: Developmental Origin, Pathogenesis, and Treatment. *Endocr. Rev.* **2022**, *43*, 678–719. [CrossRef] [PubMed]
7. Williams, A.R.W. Uterine fibroids—What's new? *F1000Research* **2017**, *6*, 2109. [CrossRef] [PubMed]
8. Favilli, A.; Etrusco, A.; Chiantera, V.; Laganà, A.S.; Cicinelli, E.; Gerli, S.; Vitagliano, A. Impact of FIGO type 3 uterine fibroids on in vitro fertilization outcomes: A systematic review and meta-analysis. *Int. J. Gynaecol. Obstet.* **2023**. [CrossRef] [PubMed]
9. Parazzini, F.; Tozzi, L.; Bianchi, S. Pregnancy outcome and uterine fibroids. *Best. Pract. Res. Clin. Obstet. Gynaecol.* **2016**, *34*, 74–84. [CrossRef] [PubMed]
10. Liu, L.; Wang, T.; Lei, B. High-intensity focused ultrasound (HIFU) ablation versus surgical interventions for the treatment of symptomatic uterine fibroids: A meta-analysis. *Eur. Radiol.* **2022**, *32*, 1195–1204. [CrossRef] [PubMed]
11. The American College of Obstetricians and Gynecologists. Uterine Fibroids. Available online: https://www.acog.org/womens-health/faqs/uterine-fibroids (accessed on 10 April 2023).
12. Gurusamy, K.S.; Vaughan, J.; Fraser, I.S.; Best, L.M.J.; Richards, T. Medical Therapies for Uterine Fibroids—A Systematic Review and Network Meta-Analysis of Randomised Controlled Trials. *PLoS ONE* **2016**, *11*, e0149631. [CrossRef] [PubMed]
13. Gedeon Richter Pharma, G.m.b.H. Indikationseinschränkung, neue Kontraindikation sowie die Notwendigkeit zur Überwachung der Leberfunktion bei der Anwendung von Esmya®(Ulipristalacetat) 5 mg Tabletten. 2018. Available online: https://www.bfarm.de/SharedDocs/Risikoinformationen/Pharmakovigilanz/DE/RHB/2018/rhb-esmya-ec.pdf?__blob=publicationFile (accessed on 21 August 2023).
14. European Medicines Agency. *Ryeqo, INN: Relugolix/Estradiol/Norethisterone Acetate: An Overview of Ryeqo and Why It Is Authorised in the EU*; European Medicines Agency: Amsterdam, The Netherlands, 2021.
15. Parker, W.H.; Fu, Y.S.; Berek, J.S. Uterine sarcoma in patients operated on for presumed leiomyoma and rapidly growing leiomyoma. *Obstet. Gynecol.* **1994**, *83*, 414–418. [PubMed]
16. Ji, Y.; Hu, K.; Zhang, Y.; Gu, L.; Zhu, J.; Zhu, L.; Zhu, Y.; Zhao, H. High-intensity focused ultrasound (HIFU) treatment for uterine fibroids: A meta-analysis. *Arch. Gynecol. Obstet.* **2017**, *296*, 1181–1188. [CrossRef] [PubMed]
17. Hynynen, K. MRI-guided focused ultrasound treatments. *Ultrasonics* **2010**, *50*, 221–229. [CrossRef] [PubMed]

18. Yu, T.; Luo, J. Adverse events of extracorporeal ultrasound-guided high intensity focused ultrasound therapy. *PLoS ONE* **2011**, *6*, e26110. [CrossRef] [PubMed]
19. Izadifar, Z.; Izadifar, Z.; Chapman, D.; Babyn, P. An Introduction to High Intensity Focused Ultrasound: Systematic Review on Principles, Devices, and Clinical Applications. *J. Clin. Med.* **2020**, *9*, 460. [CrossRef] [PubMed]
20. Marinova, M.; Ghaei, S.; Recker, F.; Tonguc, T.; Kaverina, O.; Savchenko, O.; Kravchenko, D.; Thudium, M.; Pieper, C.C.; Egger, E.K.; et al. Efficacy of ultrasound-guided high-intensity focused ultrasound (USgHIFU) for uterine fibroids: An observational single-center study. *Int. J. Hyperth.* **2021**, *38*, 30–38. [CrossRef] [PubMed]
21. Tonguc, T.; Recker, F.; Ganslmeier, J.; Strunk, H.M.; Pieper, C.C.; Ramig, O.; Welz, S.; Egger, E.K.; Mutschler, N.; Warwas, L.; et al. Improvement of fibroid-associated symptoms and quality of life after US-guided high-intensity focused ultrasound (HIFU) of uterine fibroids. *Sci. Rep.* **2022**, *12*, 21155. [CrossRef] [PubMed]
22. Recker, F.; Thudium, M.; Strunk, H.; Tonguc, T.; Dohmen, S.; Luechters, G.; Bette, B.; Welz, S.; Salam, B.; Wilhelm, K.; et al. Multidisciplinary management to optimize outcome of ultrasound-guided high-intensity focused ultrasound (HIFU) in patients with uterine fibroids. *Sci. Rep.* **2021**, *11*, 22768. [CrossRef] [PubMed]

Disclaimer/Publisher's Note: The statements, opinions and data contained in all publications are solely those of the individual author(s) and contributor(s) and not of MDPI and/or the editor(s). MDPI and/or the editor(s) disclaim responsibility for any injury to people or property resulting from any ideas, methods, instructions or products referred to in the content.

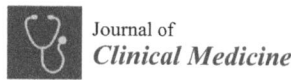 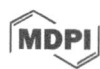

Case Report

Intraoperative Utilization of Indocyanine Green (ICG) Dye for the Assessment of Ovarian Perfusion—Case Report and Review of the Literature

Ruben Plöger [1,*], Mateja Condic [1], Damian J. Ralser [1], Hannah M. Plöger [2], Eva K. Egger [1], Lucia A. Otten [1] and Alexander Mustea [1]

1. Department of Gynecology and Gynecological Oncology, University Hospital Bonn, 53127 Bonn, Germany; mateja.condic@ukbonn.de (M.C.); damian.ralser@ukbonn.de (D.J.R.); eva-katharina.egger@ukbonn.de (E.K.E.); lucia.otten@ukbonn.de (L.A.O.); alexander.mustea@ukbonn.de (A.M.)
2. Department of Paediatrics, University Hospital Bonn, 53127 Bonn, Germany; hannah.ploeger@ukbonn.de
* Correspondence: ruben.ploeger@ukbonn.de; Tel.: +49-228-287-15444

Abstract: The assessment of ovarian perfusion after detorsion is crucial in the surgical management of patients with ovarian torsion. In current routine clinical practice, the surgical decision (preservation of the ovary versus oophorectomy) is based on the subjective impression of the surgeon. Intraoperative indocyanine green (ICG) angiography has been shown to sufficiently reflect tissue perfusion with a potential impact on the surgical procedure. Currently, there are only sparse data available on the utilization of ICG in the surgical treatment of ovarian torsion. Here, we describe the successful intraoperative use of ICG in a 17-year-old female patient with ovarian torsion who underwent ovary-preserving surgery. Further, a systematic literature review was performed. Based on the data available to date, the use of ICG in the surgical treatment of ovarian torsion is feasible and safe. The extent to which this might reduce the necessity for oophorectomy has to be evaluated in further investigations.

Keywords: ovarian torsion; oophorectomy; indocyanine green; fluorescence guides surgery; adnexal torsion

Citation: Plöger, R.; Condic, M.; Ralser, D.J.; Plöger, H.M.; Egger, E.K.; Otten, L.A.; Mustea, A. Intraoperative Utilization of Indocyanine Green (ICG) Dye for the Assessment of Ovarian Perfusion—Case Report and Review of the Literature. *J. Clin. Med.* **2023**, *12*, 5923. https://doi.org/10.3390/jcm12185923

Academic Editor: Yariv Yogev

Received: 31 July 2023
Revised: 3 September 2023
Accepted: 7 September 2023
Published: 12 September 2023

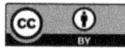

Copyright: © 2023 by the authors. Licensee MDPI, Basel, Switzerland. This article is an open access article distributed under the terms and conditions of the Creative Commons Attribution (CC BY) license (https://creativecommons.org/licenses/by/4.0/).

1. Introduction

Ovarian torsion is a rarely occurring gynecological emergency leading to an impairment of ovarian perfusion with consecutive hemorrhagic infarction and ovarian necrosis. This condition requires rapid surgical treatment by means of detorquing the twisted ovary to restore perfusion and thus to preserve ovarian function. The incidence is difficult to estimate, but the fact that ovarian torsion is sometimes defined as the fifth most common surgical emergency or that ovarian torsion accounts for 2.7% of all surgical emergencies [1] confirms that it is a highly relevant illness. Patient groups associated with ovarian torsion include women undergoing fertilization treatments [2]. Several case reports of ovarian torsion in pregnant patients and in the pediatric population [3–6] have been published. Furthermore, several studies reveal that right-sided torsions are more common [7,8]. Although some case reports describe conservative treatments [9], the most common treatment is surgical. Based on the location and time period of the published study, the main treatment methods differ between a laparoscopic approach and an approach with laparotomy [10,11]. In the developed world, the laparoscopic approach is currently the most common. The intraoperative assessment of restored ovarian perfusion is crucial for the surgical approach (ovarian preservation versus oophorectomy); however, the intraoperative decision is based on the subjective impression of the surgeon [12,13]. In this regard, a black or blue color and/or an enlargement of the ovary signify interrupted blood flow, whereas a regression of the ovarian size and—in the case of acute torsion—regained ovarian color represent signs of successful restoration of ovarian blood flow. These visual features of re-established ovarian perfusion might develop—especially after prolonged torsion—with delay, thereby leading to misjudgment and consequential oophorectomy. Therefore, alternative assessment methods are necessary to support decision making.

Laboratory findings proving the restoration of ovarian blood flow have not yet been discovered. Radiologic features indicating ovarian torsion have been described and could support diagnostic and therapeutic decision making, always in combination with clinical signs such as severe pain, nausea, vomiting, and adnexal tenderness. In B-mode during an ultrasound examination, ultrasound features of ovarian torsion [14] include evidence of an enlarged ovary, ovarian edema, minimal free fluid, shift in the ovarian position toward the midline, variable echogenicity as a sign of cystic or hemorrhagic degeneration in the case of a long-standing ovarian infarction, and a follicular ring sign [15]. These signs often coincide with the existence of risk factors, also determined using ultrasound in B-mode, which are large cystic ovaries, such as after hyperstimulation [16], or the presence of an ovarian mass between 5 and 10 cm [17]. However, these features take time to normalize after the restoration of ovarian blood flow. Doppler ultrasound enables the illustration of blood flow and thus provides an almost immediate proof after restored perfusion. The absence of arterial flow is a sign of poor prognosis [14], and the lack of ovarian venous flow shows a sensitivity of 100% and specificity of 97% for ovarian torsion [18]. In 13–88% of patients with ovarian torsion, the whirlpool sign appears to be caused by the swirling blood flow in the twisted ovarian pedicle [19–21]. This pathognomonic sign of ovarian torsion is also seen in one third of patients on CT or MRI [10,22]. Using CT and MRI, a subacute ovarian hematoma or an abnormal or absent ovarian enhancement are diagnosed more easily than by using ultrasound [23], while evidence of enlarged or shifted ovaries in CT and MRI, as signs of ovarian torsion, is seen with a similar precision as that achieved with ultrasound. Radiographic diagnostic tools such as ultrasound, MRI and CT provide the possibility of a conservative treatment of ovarian torsion, for example, when an ultrasound-guided aspiration of the ovarian cyst is performed, resulting in spontaneous detorsion of the ovary [9]. However, an intraoperative, real-time assessment tool to prove the successful restoration of ovarian blood flow is needed.

Indocyanine green (ICG) angiography is used across various medical fields for evaluation of tissue perfusion [24]. In gynecology [25], ICG is applied for visualization of the vascular perfusion of the vaginal cuff after total hysterectomy [26,27], of the ureteral course [28], and of endometriosis [29,30], as well as for detection of the sentinel lymph node [31–33]. The visualization of vascular perfusion of the vaginal cuff using ICG is feasible and complication-free but with unclear clinical profit, while a more objective analysis of its fluorescence has been established in colorectal surgery by applying the correlation between fluorescence and leakage of the colorectal anastomosis to determine further surgical steps [34]. This kind of correlation between vascular perfusion marked by ICG and the vaginal cuff dehiscence may allow a reduction in dehiscence rates in the future, which currently range between 0.64% and 1.35% [35]. The use of ICG to prevent iatrogenic ureteral injury via real-time delineation of the ureter has the advantage that only the tip of the ureteral catheter has to be inserted and a further intervention for the insertion for a ureteral stent is avoided. [36]. In the case of surgical management of endometriosis, ICG allows for a detection of the polymorphic-appearing endometriosis lesions based on their neovascularization, but its usefulness is inconsistent, as shown in a systematic review [37]. Furthermore, ICG is used for sentinel lymph node mapping after the preoperative lymphoscintigraphy in the diagnostics of breast cancer [38]. Therefore, the use of ICG for sentinel lymph node identification is superior to the established combined use of a radioactive tracer and a blue dye in regard to the logistical challenges between the operating room and radiology, its excellent safety profile without radiopharmaceutical material, with good tissue penetration, and with real-time intraoperative imaging capabilities [39,40]. Recently, a higher sentinel lymph node detection rate in breast surgery though the use of ICG compared to radio-guided surgery using radioisotope technetium, sometimes combined with blue dye, was shown [33]. Thus, ICG is a safe and effective alternative to technetium in breast surgery [33,41]. The use of ICG in sentinel diagnosis is documented in further gynecologic areas such as in the treatment of vulva cancer [32,42], in cervical cancer [32] and in endometrial cancer [43]. While various safe application possibilities of ICG dye have been demonstrated, its application in the treatment of ovarian torsion has not yet been established; however, it is promising to analyze ovarian perfusion after detorsion. Here, we describe the successful intraoperative use of ICG in a 17-year-old female patient with ovarian torsion who underwent ovary-preserving surgery. Further, a systematic literature review was performed.

2. Materials and Methods

The patient presented herself emergently during the night shift. She consented to the treatment and to the publication of the case. Her parents were informed and agreed as well. The literature search was performed using the PubMed database. Studies that were published until October 2022 were considered. The following terms were applied: 'Ovarian torsion' and 'ICG dye', 'adnexal torsion' and 'ICG dye' and 'gynecology' and 'ICG dye'. Duplications were removed. The title and abstract of the retrieved publications were read to assess their relevance. Publications with promising abstracts were full-text assessed for eligibility. Study design and language were not restricted (Figure 1).

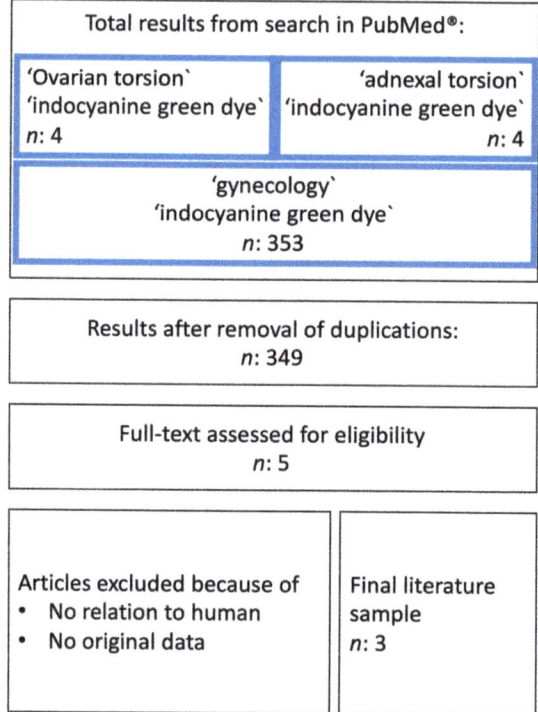

Figure 1. Flowchart of the PubMed search. *n*: number.

3. Results

3.1. Case Report

A 17-year-old female patient presented with severe, sudden onset of pain in the right lower abdomen. Furthermore, she suffered from pronounced nausea with repeated vomiting. The patient's history revealed the presence of a right ovarian cyst that was diagnosed several years ago. The rest of the patient's history was unremarkable. Blood tests showed no abnormalities except for mild leukocytosis (12.56 G/L, normal range: 4–10 G/L). Serum beta HCG and C-reactive protein were in normal range. The clinical examination revealed severe abdominal tenderness with localized tenderness in the right lower abdomen. Transvaginal ultrasound showed a cyst on the right ovary measuring 75 × 94 mm with the presence of ovarian stromal edema (Figure 2a,b) highly suspicious for right-sided ovarian torsion. Hence, laparoscopic surgery was conducted, which confirmed torsion of the right ovary (Figure 2c,d). Intraoperatively, the right ovary was livid and ischemic. The rest of the situs was normal. Detorsion and enucleation of the ovarian cyst were performed. Following detorsion, the ovary remained livid with no evidence of recovery. To assess the ovarian perfusion more sufficiently, ICG dye (Diagnostic Green®, Aschheim-Dornach, Germany) was applied intravenously (2 mL equivalent to 10 mg). ICG angiography using an endoscopic fluorescence imaging system (Stryker®, Duisburg, Germany) demonstrated restored ovarian perfusion (Figure 2e). Histopathological examination revealed a dermoid cyst. No signs of necrosis were reported. The postoperative course was unremarkable. The drainage could be removed on the first postoperative day and the patient was discharged on the second postoperative day. At 6 months of follow-up, there was no evidence of secondary ovarian necrosis or infection.

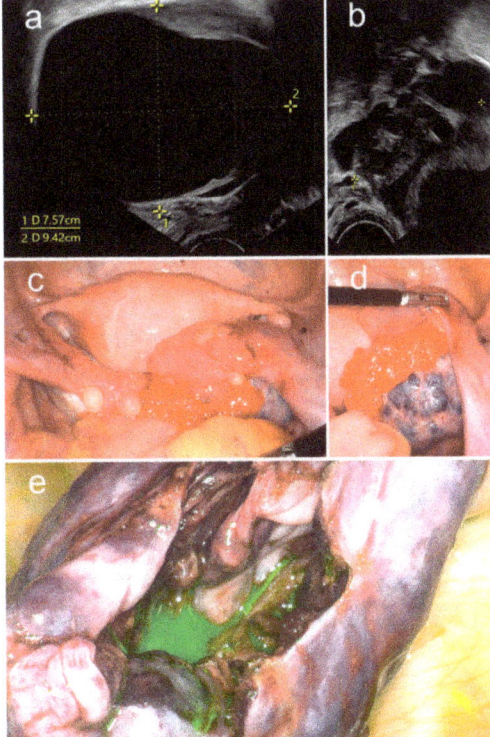

Figure 2. Ultrasonic (**a**,**b**) and intraoperative (**c**–**e**) presentation of the right ovary. The right ovary shows an ovarian cyst measuring 75.2 × 94.2 mm (**a**) with ovarian stromal edema and edema around the ovary (**b**). Intraoperatively, the right ovary appears lived and ischemic (**c**,**d**). Following detorsion and cystectomy, ICG angiography demonstrated restored ovarian perfusion (**e**). The photos were taken with the pinpoint endoscopic fluorescence imaging camera system (Stryker®, Duisburg, Germany).

3.2. Use of Indocyanine Green Dye

A systematic literature review (Figure 1 and Table 1) on ICG application for the evaluation of ovarian perfusion in the context of ovarian torsion was performed. There was no evidence for adverse events resulting from ICG application in $n = 34$ described cases [44–46]. Intraoperative ICG administration is reported to be feasible and its implementation in the treatment approach of ovarian torsion is unproblematic [44,46] given the already established use of ICG in other gynecological indications (s. above). Furthermore, Esposito et al. (2022) indicated that the use of the dye reduces surgery time. In five reported cases, a lack of ovarian perfusion on ICG angiography led to oophorectomy. In one case, necrosis was detected histopathologically [44]. The visualization of ICG perfusion was detected in a median time of 1 min [44]. The reported cases collectively demonstrate that the intraoperative utilization of ICG is beneficial in deciding whether to perform oophorectomy or to preserve the ovary [45,46]. In one study [46], ovary sparing based on the intraoperative use of ICG resulted in no long-term complications, as yearly follow-up ultrasound examinations showed normal ovaries with no evidence of pathologies. The high cost of the equipment needed in laparoscopy to use the ICG system is referred to as one of the main limitations [46].

Table 1. Results of the literature review.

	Cases (n)	Absent Perfusion (n)	Oophorectomy (n)	Histologic Confirmed Necrosis (n)	Surgery Time (min)	Amount of ICG Dye
Nicholson et al., 2022 [44]	12	2	2	1	74	n. r.
Klar et al., 2022 [45]	1	0	0	0	n. r.	5 mg
Esposito et al., 2022 [46]	20	n. r.	3	n. r.	39.2	n. r.
Present case	1	0	0	0	110	10 mg (2 mL)

n: number, n. r.: not reported.

4. Discussion

Ovarian torsion is commonly associated with younger age, as this case demonstrates [47]. This stresses that the indication for oophorectomy should be considered critically. The presented case displays the established risk factors for ovarian torsion such as an enlarged ovary (>5 cm) and presentation with typical clinical findings such as nausea, vomiting, and sudden onset of pain (s. above). Ultrasound findings were suggestive of ovarian torsion (ovarian stromal edema, presence of whirlpool sign) based on the known signs (see above, [21,48]). The right-sided bias of ovarian torsion [7,8] verified itself in this case. In the presented case, the application of ICG with consecutive visualization of restored ovarian perfusion prevented oophorectomy without signs of complications.

The application of ICG in the surgical treatment for ovarian torsion is documented in $n = 14$ cases of ovarian torsion in adult patients [44,45] and in $n = 20$ cases of ovarian torsion in children [46]. The low number of published case reports contrasts markedly with the prevalence of ovarian torsion [1] and thus demonstrates the low establishment rate of ICG in the treatment of ovarian torsion. In five cases, oophorectomy was performed because of the absence of ovarian perfusion in ICG angiography [44,46]. No complications were reported in the $n = 33$ cases with ovarian preservation. In only one case where oophorectomy was performed did the histopathological results report no evidence of ovarian necrosis [44]. However, due to the limited number of cases, a final evaluation of sensitivity and specificity cannot be carried out. Supportive data for the high sensitivity of ICG for ovarian necrosis are provided by a study based on a murine model. In this study, fluorescence intensity was shown to reliably predict ovarian necrosis [49]. Data on the future function of the ovary, such as the development of follicles or the level of anti-Müllerian hormone, are not reported and should be implemented in further investigations.

The amount of dye used differs in the reported cases (Table 1); however, 5 to 10 mg of ICG was applied in the majority of cases, which is in line with the recommendations by one ICG manufacturer [50]. The effect of ICG—in the case of re-perfusion—is reported to appear in a median time of 1 min [44] and suits the visualization of anatomic structures, such as in the testis though ICG application between 30 and 60 s [51]. Esposito et al. argue that ICG proves to be very useful for the assessment of the ovary's ischemic damage and of its re-perfusion, and thus for the decision making for or against an oophorectomy [46]. Further intraoperative decision aids may include the regression of ultrasound-detected absence of arterial flow, a lack of ovarian venous flow, and a whirlpool sign demonstrating the successful reperfusion of the ovary. However, intraoperative ultrasound lacks practicability based on the fact that the common laparoscopic approach requires the inflation of carbon dioxide gas, which limits ultrasound quality and visibility [52]. While CT and MRI are helpful diagnostic tools to evaluate perfusion in general, their intraoperative application to demonstrate the restoration of ovarian blood flow is irrelevant in most cases, as CT and MRI are rarely encountered in the surgery theater. Therefore, ICG may represent the only diagnostic tool to show reperfusion during surgery with the potential to reduce the rate of oophorectomy in patients with ovarian torsion. Postoperative histopathological evaluations of removed ovaries in patients with ovarian torsion confirm the presence of ischemia in only 43% [53,54] of cases, demonstrating the urgent need for a reliable diagnostic tool to support the sparing of the ovary. The resilience of ovaries argues for a general ovary-sparing technique in every case. There is increasing evidence for an ongoing hormonal ovarian function even in cases where ischemia is histologically confirmed [54]. On the contrary, the development of acute inflammation due to secondary ovarian necrosis may be a complication of ovarian sparing. Few case reports discuss the release of cytokines following ovarian necrosis as a reason for the death of infants after ovarian torsion [55,56]. Therefore, the sparing of every ovary after detorsion combined with the expectation of recovery may be harmful for the patient and lead to further surgical procedures. In order to differentiate these cases, the preoperative level of C-reactive protein may be useful, as it correlates with the necrosis of the ovary [57,58]. However, its use for the perfusion evaluation after detorsion is limited as it maintains a high level even after the successful restoration of ovarian blood flow and due to its long plasma half-life of about 19 h [59]. In conclusion, an intraoperative ICG-based evaluation of ovarian perfusion, in addition to a visual assessment carried out by the surgeon, represents a potential diagnostic tool to guide the intraoperative procedure (ovarian preservation versus no ovarian preservation). The extent to which secondary complications (re-operation, secondary inflammation, and limited fertility) could be diminished by the use of this technique, as opposed to general ovarian preservation, needs to be studied prospectively in larger collectives. The high cost can be shared either through the application of ICG in other fields of gynecological surgery [26,28–30] or in other disciplines [34,51]. These data and this case show an interesting new field of ICG's application in gynecology.

5. Conclusions

Based on the data available to date, the use of ICG in the surgical treatment of ovarian torsion is feasible and safe. The extent to which this might reduce the necessity for oophorectomy has to be evaluated in further investigations.

Author Contributions: All authors contributed to the study conception and design. Conceptualization, R.P., M.C., D.J.R. and A.M.; Methodology, R.P., H.M.P., D.J.R., L.A.O., E.K.E. and A.M.; Data Curation, R.P., D.J.R., H.M.P., L.A.O., E.K.E. and A.M.; Writing—Original Draft Preparation, R.P., D.J.R. and H.M.P.; Writing—Review and Editing, R.P., D.J.R., H.M.P., L.A.O., E.K.E. and A.M.; Visualization, R.P.; Supervision, A.M., Project Administration, A.M. All authors have read and agreed to the published version of the manuscript.

Funding: This research received no external funding.

Institutional Review Board Statement: The study was conducted in accordance with the Declaration of Helsinki. The patient provided written informed consent for publication. A distinct ethical approval was not required to the ethical committee of the University Hospital Bonn.

Informed Consent Statement: Written informed consent has been obtained from the patient to publish this paper.

Data Availability Statement: Data available upon request.

Conflicts of Interest: The authors declare that the research was conducted in the absence of any commercial or financial relationships that could be construed as potential conflicts of interest.

References

1. Bridwell, R.E.; Koyfman, A.; Long, B. High risk and low prevalence diseases: Ovarian torsion. *Am. J. Emerg. Med.* **2022**, *56*, 145–150. [CrossRef] [PubMed]
2. Gorkemli, H.; Camus, M.; Clasen, K. Adnexal torsion after gonadotrophin ovulation induction for IVF or ICSI and its conservative treatment. *Arch. Gynecol. Obstet.* **2002**, *267*, 4–6. [CrossRef] [PubMed]
3. Breech, L.L.; Hillard, P.J.A. Adnexal torsion in pediatric and adolescent girls. *Curr. Opin. Obstet. Gynecol.* **2005**, *17*, 483–489. [CrossRef] [PubMed]
4. Hasiakos, D.; Papakonstantinou, K.; Kontoravdis, A.; Gogas, L.; Aravantinos, L.; Vitoratos, N. Adnexal torsion during pregnancy: Report of four cases and review of the literature. *J. Obstet. Gynaecol. Res.* **2008**, *34*, 683–687. [CrossRef]
5. Erdemoğlu, M.; Kuyumcuoğlu, U.; Kale, A. Pregnancy and adnexal torsion: Analysis of 20 cases. *Clin. Exp. Obs. Gynecol.* **2010**, *37*, 224–225.
6. Corre, A.; Dandekar, S.; Lau, C.; Ranasinghe, L. A Case Report of Pediatric Ovarian Torsion: The Importance of Diagnostic Laparoscopy. *Clin. Pract. Cases Emerg. Med.* **2021**, *5*, 109. [CrossRef] [PubMed]
7. Chiou, S.-Y.; Lev-Toaff, A.S.; Masuda, E.; Feld, R.I.; Bergin, D. Adnexal Torsion: New Clinical and Imaging Observations by Sonography, Computed Tomography, and Magnetic Resonance Imaging. *J. Ultrasound Med.* **2007**, *26*, 1289–1301. [CrossRef]
8. Alkatout, I.; Mettler, L.; Anlauf, M.; Jonat, W.; Eckmann-Scholz, C.; Schollmeyer, T. Management of adnexal torsion by laparoscopic approach. *Gynecol. Surg.* **2012**, *9*, 405–409. [CrossRef]
9. Boswell, K.M.O.; Silverberg, K.M. Recurrence of ovarian torsion in a multiple pregnancy: Conservative management via transabdominal ultrasound–guided ovarian cyst aspiration. *Fertil. Steril.* **2010**, *94*, 1910.e1–1910.e3. [CrossRef]
10. Hiller, N.; Appelbaum, L.; Simanovsky, N.; Lev-Sagi, A.; Aharoni, D.; Sella, T. CT Features of Adnexal Torsion. *Am. J. Roentgenol.* **2007**, *189*, 124–129. [CrossRef]
11. Cohen, A.; Solomon, N.; Almog, B.; Cohen, Y.; Tsafrir, Z.; Rimon, E.; Levin, I. Adnexal Torsion in Postmenopausal Women: Clinical Presentation and Risk of Ovarian Malignancy. *J. Minim. Invasive Gynecol.* **2017**, *24*, 94–97. [CrossRef] [PubMed]
12. Huang, C.; Hong, M.-K.; Ding, D.-C. A review of ovary torsion. *Tzu-Chi Med. J.* **2017**, *29*, 143. [CrossRef]
13. Guile, S.L.; Mathai, J.K. Ovarian Torsion. In *StatPearls*; StatPearls Publishing: Treasure Island, FL, USA, 2022.
14. Moro, F.; Bolomini, G.; Sibal, M.; Vijayaraghavan, S.B.; Venkatesh, P.; Nardelli, F.; Pasciuto, T.; Mascilini, F.; Pozzati, F.; Leone, F.P.G.; et al. Imaging in gynecological disease (20): Clinical and ultrasound characteristics of adnexal torsion. *Ultrasound Obs. Gynecol.* **2020**, *56*, 934–943. [CrossRef] [PubMed]
15. Sibal, M. Follicular Ring Sign: A Simple Sonographic Sign for Early Diagnosis of Ovarian Torsion. *J. Ultrasound Med.* **2012**, *31*, 1803–1809. [CrossRef] [PubMed]
16. Mandelbaum, R.; Matsuo, K.; Awadalla, M.; Shoupe, D.; Chung, K. Risk of ovarian torsion in patients with ovarian hyperstimulation syndrome. *Fertil. Steril.* **2019**, *111*, e50–e51. [CrossRef]
17. Amirbekian, S.; Hooley, R.J. Ultrasound Evaluation of Pelvic Pain. *Radiol. Clin. N. Am.* **2014**, *52*, 1215–1235. [CrossRef] [PubMed]
18. Nizar, K.; Deutsch, M.; Filmer, S.; Weizman, B.; Beloosesky, R.; Weiner, Z. Doppler studies of the ovarian venous blood flow in the diagnosis of adnexal torsion. *J. Clin. Ultrasound* **2009**, *37*, 436–439. [CrossRef] [PubMed]
19. Lee, E.J.; Kwon, H.C.; Joo, H.J.; Suh, J.H.; Fleischer, A.C. Diagnosis of ovarian torsion with color Doppler sonography: Depiction of twisted vascular pedicle. *J. Ultrasound Med.* **1998**, *17*, 83–89. [CrossRef]
20. Albayram, F.; Hamper, U.M. Ovarian and adnexal torsion: Spectrum of sonographic findings with pathologic correlation. *J. Ultrasound Med.* **2001**, *20*, 1083–1089. [CrossRef]
21. Vijayaraghavan, S.B. Sonographic Whirlpool Sign in Ovarian Torsion. *J. Ultrasound Med.* **2004**, *23*, 1643–1649. [CrossRef]
22. Comerci, J.T., Jr.; Licciardi, F.; Bergh, P.A.; Gregori, C.; Breen, J.L. Mature cystic teratoma: A clinicopathologic evaluation of 517 cases and review of the literature. *Obstet. Gynecol.* **1994**, *84*, 22–28. [PubMed]
23. Duigenan, S.; Oliva, E.; Lee, S.I. Ovarian Torsion: Diagnostic Features on CT and MRI With Pathologic Correlation. *Am. J. Roentgenol.* **2012**, *198*, W122–W131. [CrossRef]
24. Reinhart, M.B.; Huntington, C.R.; Blair, L.J.; Heniford, B.T.; Augenstein, V.A. Indocyanine Green: Historical Context, Current Applications, and Future Considerations. *Surg. Innov.* **2016**, *23*, 166–175. [CrossRef] [PubMed]

25. Raffone, A.; Raimondo, D.; Oliviero, A.; Raspollini, A.; Travaglino, A.; Torella, M.; Riemma, G.; La Verde, M.; De Franciscis, P.; Casadio, P.; et al. The Use of near Infra-Red Radiation Imaging after Injection of Indocyanine Green (NIR–ICG) during Laparoscopic Treatment of Benign Gynecologic Conditions: Towards Minimalized Surgery. A Systematic Review of Literature. *Medicina* **2022**, *58*, 792. [CrossRef] [PubMed]
26. Beran, B.D.; Shockley, M.; Arnolds, K.; Escobar, P.; Zimberg, S.; Sprague, M.L. Laser Angiography with Indocyanine Green to Assess Vaginal Cuff Perfusion during Total Laparoscopic Hysterectomy: A Pilot Study. *J. Minim. Invasive Gynecol.* **2017**, *24*, 432–437. [CrossRef] [PubMed]
27. Beran, B.D.; Shockley, M.; Padilla, P.F.; Farag, S.; Escobar, P.; Zimberg, S.; Sprague, M.L. Laser Angiography to Assess the Vaginal Cuff During Robotic Hysterectomy. *JSLS* **2018**, *22*, e2018.00001. [CrossRef] [PubMed]
28. Park, H.; Farnam, R. Novel Use of Indocyanine Green for Intraoperative, Real-time Localization of Ureter During Robot-Assisted Excision of Endometriosis. *J. Minim. Invasive Gynecol.* **2015**, *22*, S69. [CrossRef]
29. De Neef, A.; Cadière, G.-B.; Bourgeois, P.; Barbieux, R.; Dapri, G.; Fastrez, M. Fluorescence of Deep Infiltrating Endometriosis During Laparoscopic Surgery: A Preliminary Report on 6 Cases. *Surg. Innov.* **2018**, *25*, 450–454. [CrossRef]
30. Vizzielli, G.; Cosentino, F.; Raimondo, D.; Turco, L.C.; Vargiu, V.; Iodice, R.; Mastronardi, M.; Mabrouk, M.; Scambia, G.; Seracchioli, R. Real three-dimensional approach vs two-dimensional camera with and without real-time near-infrared imaging with indocyanine green for detection of endometriosis: A case-control study. *Acta Obstet. Gynecol. Scand.* **2020**, *99*, 1330–1338. [CrossRef]
31. Soergel, P.; Hertel, H.; Nacke, A.K.; Klapdor, R.; Derlin, T.; Hillemanns, P. Sentinel Lymphadenectomy in Vulvar Cancer Using Near-Infrared Fluorescence from Indocyanine Green Compared with Technetium 99m Nanocolloid. *Int. J. Gynecol. Cancer* **2017**, *27*, 805–812. [CrossRef]
32. Soergel, P.; Kirschke, J.; Klapdor, R.; Derlin, T.; Hillemanns, P.; Hertel, H. Sentinel lymphadenectomy in cervical cancer using near infrared fluorescence from indocyanine green combined with technetium-99m-nanocolloid: Sentinel Lymphadenectomy in Cervical Cancer Using Icg. *Lasers Surg. Med.* **2018**, *50*, 994–1001. [CrossRef] [PubMed]
33. Bargon, C.A.; Huibers, A.; Young-Afat, D.A.; Jansen, B.A.M.; Borel-Rinkes, I.H.M.; Lavalaye, J.; Van Slooten, H.-J.; Verkooijen, H.M.; Van Swol, C.F.P.; Doeksen, A. Sentinel Lymph Node Mapping in Breast Cancer Patients Through Fluorescent Imaging Using Indocyanine Green: The INFLUENCE Trial. *Ann. Surg.* **2022**, *276*, 913–920. [CrossRef] [PubMed]
34. Son, G.M.; Kwon, M.S.; Kim, Y.; Kim, J.; Kim, S.H.; Lee, J.W. Quantitative analysis of colon perfusion pattern using indocyanine green (ICG) angiography in laparoscopic colorectal surgery. *Surg. Endosc.* **2019**, *33*, 1640–1649. [CrossRef] [PubMed]
35. Uccella, S.; Zorzato, P.C.; Kho, R.M. Incidence and Prevention of Vaginal Cuff Dehiscence after Laparoscopic and Robotic Hysterectomy: A Systematic Review and Meta-analysis. *J. Minim. Invasive Gynecol.* **2021**, *28*, 710–720. [CrossRef] [PubMed]
36. Siddighi, S.; Yune, J.J.; Hardesty, J. Indocyanine green for intraoperative localization of ureter. *Am. J. Obstet. Gynecol.* **2014**, *211*, 436.e1–436.e2. [CrossRef] [PubMed]
37. Ianieri, M.M.; Della Corte, L.; Campolo, F.; Cosentino, F.; Catena, U.; Bifulco, G.; Scambia, G. Indocyanine green in the surgical management of endometriosis: A systematic review. *Acta Obstet. Gynecol. Scand.* **2021**, *100*, 189–199. [CrossRef] [PubMed]
38. Abu-Rustum, N.R.; Khoury-Collado, F.; Pandit-Taskar, N.; Soslow, R.A.; Dao, F.; Sonoda, Y.; Levine, D.A.; Brown, C.L.; Chi, D.S.; Barakat, R.R.; et al. Sentinel lymph node mapping for grade 1 endometrial cancer: Is it the answer to the surgical staging dilemma? *Gynecol. Oncol.* **2009**, *113*, 163–169. [CrossRef] [PubMed]
39. Alander, J.T.; Kaartinen, I.; Laakso, A.; Pätilä, T.; Spillmann, T.; Tuchin, V.V.; Venermo, M.; Välisuo, P. A Review of Indocyanine Green Fluorescent Imaging in Surgery. *Int. J. Biomed. Imaging* **2012**, *2012*, 7. [CrossRef]
40. Ferri, F.; Montorfano, L.; Bordes, S.J.; Forleiter, C.; Newman, M.I. Near-Infrared Fluorescence Imaging for Sentinel Lymph Node Identification in Melanoma Surgery. *Cureus* **2021**, *13*, e14550. [CrossRef]
41. Kedrzycki, M.S.; Leiloglou, M.; Ashrafian, H.; Jiwa, N.; Thiruchelvam, P.T.R.; Elson, D.S.; Leff, D.R. Meta-analysis Comparing Fluorescence Imaging with Radioisotope and Blue Dye-Guided Sentinel Node Identification for Breast Cancer Surgery. *Ann. Surg. Oncol.* **2021**, *28*, 3738–3748. [CrossRef]
42. Di Donna, M.C.; Quartuccio, N.; Giallombardo, V.; Sturiale, L.; Arnone, A.; Ricapito, R.; Sozzi, G.; Arnone, G.; Chiantera, V. Detection of sentinel lymph node in vulvar cancer using 99mTc-labeled colloid lymphoscintigraphy, blue dye, and indocyanine-green fluorescence: A meta-analysis of studies published in 2010–2020. *Arch Gynecol Obstet.* **2022**, *307*, 1677–1686. [CrossRef] [PubMed]
43. Nagar, H.; Wietek, N.; Goodall, R.J.; Hughes, W.; Schmidt-Hansen, M.; Morrison, J. Sentinel node biopsy for diagnosis of lymph node involvement in endometrial cancer. *Cochrane Database Syst. Rev.* **2021**, *2021*, CD013021. [CrossRef]
44. Nicholson, K.; Urh, A.; Demertzis, K.; Holubyeva, A.; LaPier, Z.; Cisneros-Camacho, A.; Goldberg, G.L.; Schwartz, B. Intraoperative Indocyanine Green Dye Use in Ovarian Torsion: A Feasibility Study. *J. Minim. Invasive Gynecol.* **2022**, *29*, 738–742. [CrossRef] [PubMed]
45. Klar, M.; Matsuo, K.; Juhasz-Böss, I.; Hasanov, M.-F. Ovarian conservation in a patient with a large ovarian cyst and adnexal torsion—A confirmatory video with intravenous indocyanine green. *Fertil. Steril.* **2022**, *118*, 417–418. [CrossRef] [PubMed]
46. Esposito, C.; Fulvia, D.C.; Vincenzo, B.; Giorgia, E.; Roberto, C.; Lepore, B.; Castagnetti, M.; Califano, G.; Escolino, M. Review of a 25-Year Experience in the Management of Ovarian Masses in Neonates, Children and Adolescents: From Laparoscopy to Robotics and Indocyanine Green Fluorescence Technology. *Children* **2022**, *9*, 1219. [CrossRef]

47. Rabinovich, I.; Pekar-Zlotin, M.; Bliman-Tal, Y.; Melcer, Y.; Vaknin, Z.; Smorgick, N. Dermoid cysts causing adnexal torsion: What are the risk factors? *Eur. J. Obstet. Gynecol. Reprod. Biol.* **2020**, *251*, 20–22. [CrossRef] [PubMed]
48. Moro, K.; Kameyama, H.; Abe, K.; Tsuchida, J.; Tajima, Y.; Ichikawa, H.; Nakano, M.; Ikarashi, M.; Nagahashi, M.; Shimada, Y.; et al. Left colic artery aneurysm rupture after stent placement for abdominal aortic aneurysm associated with neurofibromatosis type 1. *Surg. Case Rep.* **2019**, *5*, 12. [CrossRef] [PubMed]
49. Oyama, K.; Nakamoto, K.; Omori, M.; Fukasawa, H.; Hirata, S. Prognostication of Ovarian Function after Ovarian Torsion Using Intraoperative Indocyanine Green Angiography. *J. Minim. Invasive Gynecol.* **2022**, *29*, 237–242. [CrossRef]
50. Diagnostic Green Verdye. Available online: https://diagnosticgreen.com/row/wp-content/uploads/sites/2/2020/08/Diagnostic-Green-ICG-Brochure-RoW-3.pdf (accessed on 29 January 2023).
51. Esposito, C.; Settimi, A.; Del Conte, F.; Cerulo, M.; Coppola, V.; Farina, A.; Crocetto, F.; Ricciardi, E.; Esposito, G.; Escolino, M. Image-Guided Pediatric Surgery Using Indocyanine Green (ICG) Fluorescence in Laparoscopic and Robotic Surgery. *Front. Pediatr.* **2020**, *8*, 314. [CrossRef]
52. Goudie, A. Detection of intraperitoneal free gas by ultrasound. *Australas. J. Ultrasound Med.* **2013**, *16*, 56–61. [CrossRef]
53. Bar-On, S.; Mashiach, R.; Stockheim, D.; Soriano, D.; Goldenberg, M.; Schiff, E.; Seidman, D.S. Emergency laparoscopy for suspected ovarian torsion: Are we too hasty to operate? *Fertil. Steril.* **2010**, *93*, 2012–2015. [CrossRef] [PubMed]
54. Soh, P.Q.; Cheng, C.; Reddington, C.; Dior, U.P.; Healey, M. Oophorectomy for ovarian torsion—Should this be abandoned? *Aust. N. Z. J. Obstet. Gynaecol.* **2022**, *62*, 548–552. [CrossRef] [PubMed]
55. Havlik, D.M.; Nolte, K.B. Sudden Death in an Infant Resulting from Torsion of the Uterine Adnexa. *Am. J. Forensic Med. Pathol.* **2002**, *23*, 289–291. [CrossRef] [PubMed]
56. Higa, G.; Pacanowski, J.P.; Jeck, D.T.; Goshima, K.R.; León, L.R. Vertebral Artery Aneurysms and Cervical Arteriovenous Fistulae in Patients with Neurofibromatosis 1. *Vascular* **2010**, *18*, 166–177. [CrossRef] [PubMed]
57. Tobiume, T.; Shiota, M.; Umemoto, M.; Kotani, Y.; Hoshiai, H. Predictive Factors for Ovarian Necrosis in Torsion of Ovarian Tumor. *Tohoku J. Exp. Med.* **2011**, *225*, 211–214. [CrossRef] [PubMed]
58. Shiota, M.; Kotani, Y.; Umemoto, M.; Tobiume, T.; Hoshiai, H. Clinical indices and histological changes over time in ovarian torsion related to ovarian tumors. *Gynecol. Surg.* **2012**, *9*, 347–350. [CrossRef]
59. Vigushin, D.M.; Pepys, M.B.; Hawkins, P.N. Metabolic and scintigraphic studies of radioiodinated human C-reactive protein in health and disease. *J. Clin. Investig.* **1993**, *91*, 1351–1357. [CrossRef]

Disclaimer/Publisher's Note: The statements, opinions and data contained in all publications are solely those of the individual author(s) and contributor(s) and not of MDPI and/or the editor(s). MDPI and/or the editor(s) disclaim responsibility for any injury to people or property resulting from any ideas, methods, instructions or products referred to in the content.

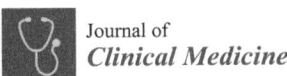

Systematic Review

Prenatal Diagnosis of an Intrathoracic Left Kidney Associated with Congenital Diaphragmatic Hernia: Case Report and Systematic Review

Giuliana Orlandi [1,2], Paolo Toscano [1,2], Olimpia Gabrielli [1,2], Enrica Di Lella [1,2], Antonia Lettieri [2], Luigi Manzo [1,2], Laura Letizia Mazzarelli [1,2], Carmine Sica [2], Letizia Di Meglio [3], Lavinia Di Meglio [4], Ferdinando Antonio Gulino [5,*], Giosuè Giordano Incognito [6], Attilio Tuscano [6], Stefano Cianci [7] and Aniello Di Meglio [2]

1. Department of Neuroscience, Reproductive Sciences and Dentistry, School of Medicine, University of Naples Federico II, 80131 Naples, Italy; giulianaorlandi@msn.com (G.O.); paol.toscano@gmail.com (P.T.); enrica_dilella@hotmail.it (E.D.L.); luigimanzo93@libero.it (L.M.); lauramazzarelli@gmail.com (L.L.M.)
2. Diagnostica Ecografica e Prenatale di A. Di Meglio, 80133 Naples, Italy; antonia_lettieri@libero.it (A.L.); sicacarmine111@gmail.com (C.S.); aniellodimeglio@gmail.com (A.D.M.)
3. Radiology Department, School of Medicine, University of Milan, 20133 Milan, Italy; letiziadimeglio@gmail.com
4. Pediatric Department, Bambino Gesù Children's Research Hospital IRCCS, 00165 Rome, Italy; laviniadimeglio@gmail.com
5. Department of Obstetrics and Gynaecology, Azienda di Rilievo Nazionale e di Alta Specializzazione (ARNAS) Garibaldi Nesima, 95124 Catania, Italy
6. Department of General Surgery and Medical Surgical Specialties, University of Catania, 95123 Catania, Italy; attiliotuscano@gmail.com (A.T.)
7. Department of Human Pathology of Adult and Childhood "G. Barresi", University of Messina, 98121 Messina, Italy; stefanoc85@hotmail.it
* Correspondence: docferdi@hotmail.it; Tel.: +39-3381111000

Abstract: Introduction: A congenital intrathoracic kidney (ITK) is a rare anomaly that is recognized to have four causes: renal ectopia with an intact diaphragm, diaphragmatic eventration, diaphragmatic hernia, and traumatic diaphragmatic rupture. We report a case of a prenatal-diagnosed ITK related to a congenital diaphragmatic hernia (CDH) and conducted a systematic review of all cases of the prenatal diagnosis of this association. Case presentation: A fetal ultrasound scan at 22 gestational weeks showed left CDH and ITK, hyperechoic left lung parenchyma, and mediastinal shift. The fetal echocardiography and karyotype were normal. Magnetic resonance imaging at 30 gestational weeks confirmed the ultrasound suspicion of left CDH in association with bowel and left kidney herniation. The fetal growth, amniotic fluid, and Doppler indices remained within the normal range over time. The woman delivered the newborn via an at-term spontaneous vaginal delivery. The newborn was stabilized and underwent non-urgent surgical correction; the postoperative course was uneventful. Conclusions: CDH is the rarest cause of ITK; we found only eleven cases describing this association. The mean gestational age at diagnosis was 29 ± 4 weeks and 4 days. There were seven cases of right and four cases of left CDH. There were associated anomalies in only three fetuses. All women delivered live babies, the herniated kidneys showed no functional damage after their surgical correction, and the prognosis was favorable after surgical repair. The prenatal diagnosis and counseling of this condition are important in planning adequate prenatal and postnatal management in order to improve neonatal outcomes.

Keywords: ectopic kidney; congenital diaphragmatic hernia; prenatal diagnosis; congenital malformation; case report

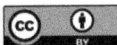

1. Introduction

Congenital intrathoracic kidney (ITK) is a rare malformation representing partial or complete protrusion of the kidney above the level of the diaphragm into the mediastinum. This pathological abnormality represents <5% of all renal ectopias. It is more common in the male sex than in the female sex (2:1), and it has a slight left-side predominance.

In most cases, a congenital intrathoracic kidney is asymptomatic and diagnosed incidentally, often after birth; however, it can be misdiagnosed as pneumonia because of its presentation on a chest X-ray as an opacity or lobar consolidation [1,2].

An ITK is recognized as having four main causes: "real" renal ectopia with an intact diaphragm, diaphragmatic eventration, congenital or acquired diaphragmatic hernia, and traumatic diaphragmatic rupture [3].

Congenital diaphragmatic hernia (CDH) is frequently associated with gastric, bowel, or hepatic herniation, whereas renal protrusion is extremely rare.

We report a case of a prenatal diagnosed ITK associated with CDH.

We also conducted a systematic review of all cases of this association diagnosed antenatally using MEDLINE, EMBASE, Scopus, ClinicalTrials.gov, OVID, and the Cochrane Library as electronic databases from January 1970 to December 2022. We used the medical subject heading (MeSH) term Kidney (MeSH Unique ID: D007668) in combination with Hernias, Diaphragmatic, and Congenital (MeSH Unique ID: D065630). No restrictions concerning language or geographic location were applied. The systematic review was performed in accordance with the Preferred Reporting Items for Systematic Reviews and Meta-Analyses (PRISMA) guidelines [4] (Figure 1). One author (F.A.G.) independently screened the titles and abstracts of each citation, after which they selected relevant ones for a full-text review. Each retrieved full-text article was independently evaluated for inclusion by another author (G.G.I.). Any potential disagreement was solved via a discussion with a third author (A.D.M.). After reading the abstracts and titles, 113 articles were excluded because they were not pertinent to the field; 33 articles were excluded after reading the text because the diagnosis of an intrathoracic left kidney was performed in the postnatal period.

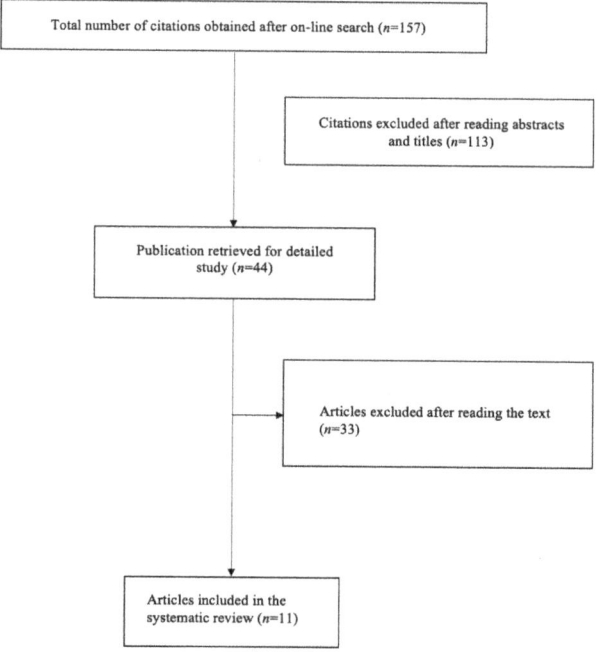

Figure 1. Selection process for the inclusion of suitable studies for the systematic review.

2. Case Presentation

A 37-year-old Caucasian woman, gravida 2 para 0, with a history of a previous miscarriage due to an unknown cause, was referred to our second-level center at 22 gestational weeks for a suspicious fetal intrathoracic mass and left CDH at a second-trimester ultrasound (US) screening. Her previous medical and family histories were unremarkable; she was a nonsmoker, had not consumed any alcohol during the pregnancy, and had never been exposed to drugs or toxins. The measurements of the dating examination in the first trimester were consistent with the dates of the last menstrual period, the nuchal translucency was normal, and toxoplasmosis, other agents, rubella, cytomegalovirus, and herpes simplex (TORCH) screening was negative. Our US examination was performed via the use of a Voluson E10 scanner (GE Healthcare Ultrasound, Milwaukee, WI, USA) equipped with a curved linear array transabdominal transducer (2–5 MHz). The fetal heart rate was within the normal range, fetal movements were visualized, the placenta was identified on the anterior portion of the uterus and showed a normal insertion, and the amniotic fluid, as well as the Doppler indices, were within normal limits. The fetal biometry was consistent with the gestational age (GA). An intrathoracic left hypoechoic mass with a maximum diameter of 26.8 mm was seen (Figure 2).

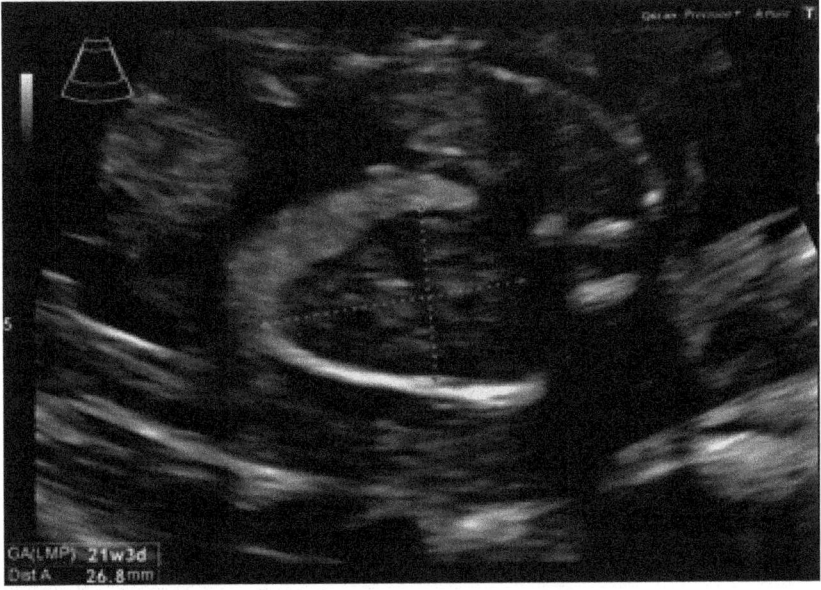

Figure 2. Ultrasound scan at 22 gestational weeks showing an intrathoracic left mass and hyperechoic left lung parenchyma.

The heart was displaced to the right (mediastinal shift), in normal levocardia. Furthermore, the left renal fossa was empty. In the left parasagittal view, the left kidney appeared lifted up toward the thorax (Figure 3).

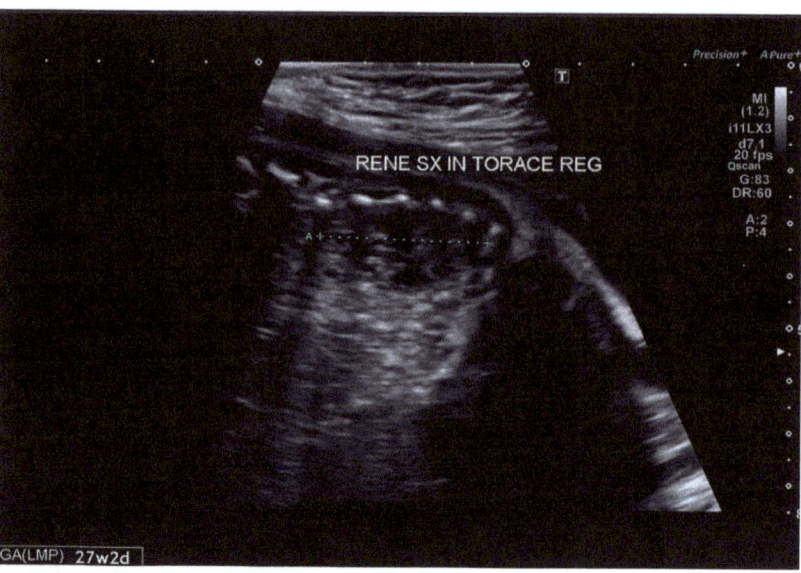

Figure 3. Sagittal view showed a left kidney in the thorax.

Power Doppler showed the abnormal course of the left renal artery, which started from the abdominal aorta and ended in the thoracic kidney (Figure 4).

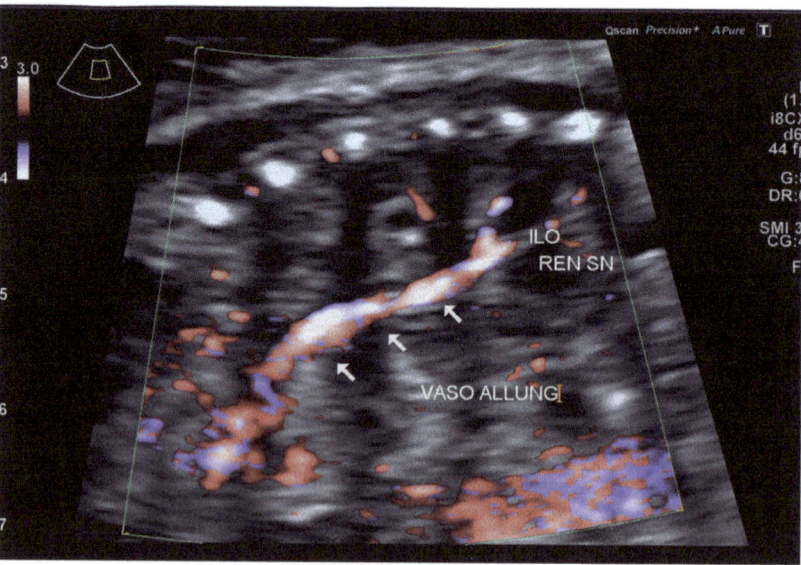

Figure 4. Power Doppler showed the course of the left renal artery, from the abdominal aorta toward the thorax and the renal hilum.

The scan did not show a clear herniation of the stomach, bowel, or liver. The lung-to-head circumference ratio (LHR) was greater than 1.4, and the observed-to-expected (o/e) LHR was 52.1%. The left lung parenchyma beside the mass was hyperechoic (Figure 2). The left renal biometry and echogenicity were normal, and no pyelectasia was found (Figure 3). The right kidney was normal, and no other anomalies were identified. Fetal echocardiography verified normal conotruncal anatomy, normal left and right ventricular cavity size as well as systolic function, and sinus rhythm with 1:1 atrioventricular conduction. Our clinical suspicion was of a left CDH and ITK. Furthermore, we suspected an association with a congenital cystic adenomatoid malformation. The patient underwent amniocentesis, and the traditional karyotype as well as comparative genomic hybridization (CGH) array showed a normal female karyotype (46, XX). Subsequently, prenatal management included serial US examinations, including biophysical profile scoring, to monitor fetal growth and assess the fetal heart. On subsequent scans, no changes in the US characteristics of the ectopic kidney were found, and the fetal growth, amniotic fluid, and Doppler indices remained within the normal range for GA. The fetus did not develop hydrothorax. The pregnant woman was referred for fetal magnetic resonance imaging (MRI) at 30 gestational weeks, which confirmed the US suspicion of left CDH in association with bowel and left kidney herniation. After 34 weeks of gestation, cardiotocography was performed weekly to monitor fetal wellbeing, which remained good. The patient was referred to a third-level center for delivery. A female infant weighing 3100 g was delivered via a spontaneous vaginal delivery at 37 weeks of gestation; her Apgar scores at 1 and 5 min were 8 and 9, respectively. The neonate cried immediately after birth, and she was pink and well-perfused. Nevertheless, she developed respiratory distress in the delivery room and required intubation. Chest radiography confirmed the prenatal suspicion of CDH, including bowel loops and the left kidney, with a mediastinal shift of the heart. Echocardiography showed normal heart function and morphology, with no pulmonary hypertension. Due to the hemodynamic stability, the newborn underwent non-urgent surgery on her second day of life through a transverse laparotomy. Surgical exploration confirmed the left kidney with the hernia sac. The organs herniated in the thoracic cavity included small bowel loops, the colon, and the left kidney. The intrathoracic ectopic right kidney was covered with retroperitoneum. After the hernia sac was excised, the small intestine, colon, and ITK were reduced with no difficulties into the abdominal cavity, in a near-to-normal site, without complication or hemodynamic changes. The defect of the diaphragm was primarily repaired using interrupted non-absorbable sutures. A chest tube was placed in the left hemithorax and removed on day four. The corrected kidney showed regular function, with a slight biometric reduction. The postoperative course was uneventful; the baby was extubated on day two and discharged from the hospital after about two months in good condition. She has remained asymptomatic at subsequent follow-ups 1 year after discharge, with normal physical as well as mental development and without any long-term complications, not requiring further monitoring.

3. Discussion

A congenital ectopic kidney is a rare malformation, caused by the malposition of the kidney during embryogenesis. Most ectopic kidneys are found in the pelvic and lumbar regions secondary to failure to ascend during fetal life. ITK is extremely rare, with a prevalence ranging from 0.5 to 5% and an incidence of 1 in every 10.000 cases of an ectopic kidney [1,2]. Males (63%) are affected more frequently than females (37%) [5]. It is found more frequently on the left than on the right side, and it is rarely bilateral [5]. It is considered a sporadic malformation and is not associated with an increased risk of recurrence. ITK may be differentiated from other intrathoracic and mediastinal masses using various diagnostic methods, including contrast-enhanced computed tomography scans and MRI. Differential diagnoses should include esophageal duplication cysts, bronchogenic cysts, microcystic adenomatoid malformation, bronchopulmonary sequestration, mediastinal teratoma, and aneurysm of the descending aorta [6]. ITK is recognized as having four main causes: "real" renal ectopia with an intact diaphragm, diaphragmatic eventration, congenital or acquired diaphragmatic hernia, and traumatic diaphragmatic rupture [3]. The "real" variant represents less than 5% of ectopic kidneys [7]. It possesses the following characteristics: rotation anomaly, elongated ureter, and vascularization from the thoracic aorta. Generally, it is asymptomatic, and, if not detected during the antenatal period, may remain silent for many years [8] and require no treatment [9]. Diaphragmatic eventration is a congenital anomaly related to a phrenic nerve injury that causes half or total diaphragm elevation, with an apparent ascent of abdominal viscera into the thorax and no diaphragm defect [10]. The incidence of diaphragmatic eventration is less than 0.05% [11].

CDH is a rare anomaly that affects 2.3–2.8 per 10,000 live births, with a male predominance [12]. The development of the musculotendinous diaphragm, which occurs from the 4th to 12th week of development, involves four embryologic structures: the septum trasversum, the pleuroperitoneal membranes, the mediastinum (dorsal mesentery of the esophagus), and body wall muscles. The gradual fusion of the pleuroperitoneal membranes and septum transversum starts during the fourth week of development [13]. At approximately the eighth week, the closure of the pleuroperitoneal canals occurs when the septum transversum fuses with the structures surrounding the esophagus, the esophageal mesentery, and connects to the pleuroperitoneal membranes [14]. The right and left pleuroperitoneal membranes close the communication between the pleural and peritoneal cavities. A delayed closure or the maldevelopment of the septum transversum and the two pleuroperitoneal folds leads to a diaphragmatic defect, with herniation of abdominal viscera into the thorax [9]. An alternative hypothesis is that lung hypoplasia may be the primary causal factor in the development of CDH [15,16]; it has also been reported in association with the maternal administration of medications such as thalidomide or antiepileptics [17]. The most frequent is a Bochdalek hernia, with a postero-lateral defect, described in 70–95% of CDH cases [10]. Right-sided CDHs are less common [18], due to either the presence of the liver on the right as a physical thoraco-abdominal barrier or the early fusion of the pleura-peritoneal channel on the right side [19]. CDH is usually diagnosed antenatally, the overall prenatal detection rate is 46–52% [20], and the average GA at diagnosis ranges from 24 to 25 weeks [21]. The prenatal diagnosis of CDH is quite straightforward, with echogenic contents seen in the thorax and a mediastinal shift; however, when the kidney is the only herniating organ it can be misdiagnosed as renal agenesis [14]. These signs are also typical of pulmonary sequestration [22]. Using the color Doppler to trace the aberrant renal artery arising from the aorta and coursing upward can help reach the correct diagnosis. In 10–30% of cases, there are associated chromosomal anomalies. The most common include trisomy 12, 18, and 21, Turner syndrome, partial trisomy 5, partial trisomy 20, tetraploidy 21, and tetrasomy 12p [23]. Fetal syndromes, such as Apert, Beckwith–Wiedemann, Coffin-Siris, and Pierre Robin, as well as many others, can be associated with CDH [24,25]. Structural defects are found in 25–57% of all cases [23], and cardiac defects worsen the prognosis most frequently among them (11–15%) [24]. Proof of this degraded prognosis was confirmed through research conducted by Graziano et al. [25], in which 2636 pediatric CDH patients from 82 centers were followed. The survival rate among CDH patients without any heart defect was 70%, whereas those patients with diagnosed heart defects had a significantly lower survival rate of 41.1%. These data were validated by Menon et al. [26], who found the survival rate of infants born with CDH and no heart defects to be 69%; for those with a heart defect, the survival rate was 36%.

Renal herniation related to CDH is rare, with eleven cases [27–37] described in the literature (Table 1).

Table 1. Studies included in the systematic review.

Study, Year	Country	Maternal Age (Years)	GA at Diagnosis (Weeks)	Side of CDH; Herniated Organs	Associated Anomalies	LHR o/e LHR	Karyotype	GA at Delivery (Weeks) and Mode of Delivery	Newborn Gender	Kidney Damage	Outcome
Singh et al., 2020 [27]	India	30	31	Left; small bowel, transverse colon, and left kidney	None	LHR 3.0; o/e 100%	NA	37 CS	F	None	Favorable after surgical repair
Masturzo et al., 2001 [28]	UK	30	33	Right; bowel, right lobe of the liver, and right kidney	None	NA	Normal	35 VD	M	None	Favorable after surgical repair
Juricic et al., 2015 [29]	France	35	33	Right; small bowel, transverse colon, and right kidney	None	NA	NA	39 VD	F	None	Favorable after surgical repair
Park, 2020 [30]	South Korea	31	28	Right; small intestine, colon, right lobe of the liver, and right kidney	Bronco-pulmonary sequestration	NA	NA	40 VD	F	None	Favorable after surgical repair
Thompson et al., 2019 [31]	USA	33	35	Right; small bowel, liver, and right kidney	None	NA	NA	39 CS	F	None	Favorable after surgical repair
Athanasiadis et al., 2011 [32]	Greece	25	22	Left; spleen, small intestine, and left kidney	None	NA	Normal	34 CS	M	None	Favorable after surgical repair
Hidaka et al., 2012 [33]	Japan	26	28	Left; stomach, small intestine, spleen, and left kidney	None	LHR 1.6	Normal	38 CS	M	None	Favorable after surgical repair

Table 1. *Cont.*

Study, Year	Country	Maternal Age (Years)	GA at Diagnosis (Weeks)	Side of CDH; Herniated Organs	Associated Anomalies	LHR o/e LHR	Karyotype	GA at Delivery (Weeks) and Mode of Delivery	Newborn Gender	Kidney Damage	Outcome
Panda et al., 2009 [34]	USA	23	28	Left; small intestine, spleen, and left kidney	Bicuspid aortic valve (postnatal)	LHR 1.6	NA	40 VD	M	None	Favorable after surgical repair
Takezoe et al., 2017 [35]	Japan	NA	33	Right; right lobe of the liver, right kidney	Hepatic-pulmonary fusion	NA	NA	39 NA	F	None	Favorable after surgical repair
Jeong et al., 2016 [36]	Korea	29	32	Right; right kidney	None	LHR 2.54	Normal	39 VD	F	None	Favorable after surgical repair
Cessans et al., 2015 [37]	France	35	22	Right; small bowel, colon, and right kidney	None	NA	NA	39 VD	F	None	Favorable after surgical repair

Abbreviations: CDH, congenital diaphragmatic hernia; CS, cesarean section; GA, gestational age; LHR, lung-to-head circumference ratio; o/e, observed to expected; NA, not applicable; and VD, vaginal delivery.

The mean maternal age was 30 ± 4 years. The mean GA at diagnosis was 29 ± 4 weeks and 4 days. The incidence of renal herniation in CDH was higher on the right side, with seven cases of right [28–31,35–37] and four cases of left CDH [27,32–34] reported. A karyotype with CGH array should be offered because of the association with chromosomal and genetic anomalies. None of the cases previously reported and the present one had any chromosomal abnormalities or associated genetic syndromes, although the fetal karyotype has only been determined in three previous cases [28,32,33]. Ultrasound is a fundamental diagnostic tool for the diagnosis of numerous obstetric and gynecological conditions [38–42], and in this case as well, an accurate fetal anatomy study must be offered to exclude associated anomalies. Fetal echocardiography is essential in assessing fetal heart function and structure, as well as in aiding in the detection of pulmonary hypertension and/or pulmonary hypoplasia, and it plays a vital role in prognosis prediction [18]. Associated anomalies have previously been described in three fetuses: one bronchopulmonary sequestration [30], one bicuspid aortic valve [34], and one hepatic pulmonary fusion [35]. Another feature of the present case is the presence of hyperechoic pulmonary parenchyma beside the herniated mass. These findings cannot exclude a concurrent congenital lung cystic adenomatoid malformation. The postnatal surgical evaluation confirmed a compressive effect. This suggests that, in the case of a huge CDH, pulmonary hyperechogenicity is more likely related to a compressive effect, rather than a congenital lung cystic adenomatoid malformation. A fetal MRI was never performed in any of the previous cases, despite its ability to provide further insights into numerous obstetric conditions [43]; this fact aside, it can be useful for the quantitative evaluation of fetal lungs and, in association with the US, can help to predict the neonatal outcomes of prenatally diagnosed CDH, such as total fetal lung volume (TFLV) estimation [44]. As with any case of antenatally diagnosed CDH, the o/e LHR offers the best positive predictive values for postnatal survival [45]. All women included in the systematic review delivered a live baby. The mean GA at delivery was 38 ± 2 weeks. Most cases of ITK reported in the literature have been incidental diagnoses in asymptomatic individuals who may not require any treatment [14]. When isolated, it is an innocuous condition that does not need further extensive investigation [46]; however, the presence of CDH and the associated herniation of abdominal viscera can cause respiratory distress, necessitating surgical repair [14]. According to the previous literature, the present case shows that the herniation of the kidney does not represent the worst prognosis factor for CDH. Indeed, the kidney is not usually damaged from the herniation, preserving its physiological functions, and the prognosis is favorable after surgical repair, as seen in our case.

Improvements in surgical techniques and perioperative care have led to better outcomes for patients with these conditions. For example, minimally invasive surgical approaches, such as laparoscopy and thoracoscopy, have reduced the morbidity associated with open surgery and improved patient recovery times. Similarly, advances in neonatal respiratory support, including extracorporeal membrane oxygenation (ECMO), have increased survival rates for infants with severe CDH. Overall, the implications of these advancements for clinical practice and patient outcomes are significant. Early and accurate diagnosis, as well as effective surgical and perioperative care, can greatly improve the prognosis for patients with an intrathoracic kidney and CDH. As such, continued research and innovation in this field are essential for further improving the outcomes and quality of life of affected individuals.

4. Conclusions

ITK associated with CDH is a rare malformation. An accurate study of fetal anatomy is necessary to exclude associated anomalies, and a fetal invasive karyotype must be offered. Fetal MRI can be complementary to the US for prognostic evaluation and differential diagnosis. Renal function is usually preserved, and the prognosis is favorable after surgical repair. In line with prior research, this case report underscores the favorable prognosis for fetuses with kidney herniation, offering guidance to obstetricians for the counseling of this uncommon anomaly. The differential diagnosis of the reported case is a highly involved undertaking that requires a broad spectrum of specialized healthcare professionals. Prenatal counseling should involve a multidisciplinary team involving maternal-fetal medicine, pediatric surgery, genetics, and neonatology. The long-term outlook varies considerably and is based on associated anomalies, preterm delivery, hernia position, and fetal lung volume.

Author Contributions: G.O.: Conceptualization and writing—original draft preparation; P.T.: data curation and resources; O.G. and E.D.L.: investigation; C.S., L.L.M., A.L. and L.M.: methodology; L.D.M. (Letizia Di Meglio), L.D.M. (Lavinia Di Meglio), F.A.G., G.G.I., A.T. and S.C.: writing—review and editing; A.D.M.: supervision. All authors have read and agreed to the published version of the manuscript.

Funding: This research received no external funding.

Institutional Review Board Statement: Not applicable.

Informed Consent Statement: Informed consent was obtained from the subject involved in the study. Written informed consent has been obtained from the patient to publish this paper.

Data Availability Statement: Not applicable.

Conflicts of Interest: The authors declare no conflict of interest.

References

1. Peñafiel-Freire, D.M.; Hernández-Martín, S.; Iceta-Lizarraga, A.; Urriza-Yeregui, L. Ectopia renal intratorácica (Intrathoracic ectopic kidney). *An. Pediatr. Engl. Ed.* **2020**, *92*, 113–114. (In Spanish) [CrossRef]
2. Al-Saqladi, A.W.; Akares, S.A. Intrathoracic kidney in a child with literature review. *Saudi J. Kidney Dis. Transpl.* **2015**, *26*, 349–354. [CrossRef] [PubMed]
3. Pfister-Goedeke, L.; Brunier, E. Intrathoracic kidney in childhood with special reference to secondary renal transport in Bochdalek's hernia. *Helv. Paediatr. Acta* **1979**, *34*, 345–357. [PubMed]
4. Moher, D.; Liberati, A.; Tetzlaff, J.; Altman, D.G.; PRISMA Group. Preferred reporting items for systematic reviews and meta-analyses: The PRISMA statement. *PLoS Med.* **2009**, *6*, e1000097. [CrossRef] [PubMed]
5. Donat, S.M.; Donat, P.E. Intrathoracic kidney: A case report with a review of the literature. *J. Urol.* **1988**, *140*, 131–132. [CrossRef]
6. Sarac, M.; Bakal, U.; Tartar, T.; Canpolat, S.; Kara, A.; Kazez, A. Bochdalek hernia and intrathoracic ectopic kidney: Presentation of two case reports and review of the literature. *Niger. J. Clin. Pract.* **2018**, *21*, 681–686. [CrossRef]
7. Sirikci, A.; Sarica, K.; Bayram, M. Thoracic kidney associated with superior ectopic spleen. *J. Urol.* **2000**, *163*, 1901. [CrossRef]
8. Gupta, R.; Gupta, A.; Ilyas, M.; Chauhan, K.S. Adult right-sided thoracic kidney: A very rare form of renal ectopia. *Lung India* **2017**, *34*, 400–402. [CrossRef] [PubMed]
9. Murphy, J.J.; Altit, G.; Zerhouni, S. The intrathoracic kidney: Should we fix it? *J. Pediatr. Surg.* **2012**, *47*, 970. [CrossRef]
10. Saroj, S.K.; Kumar, S.; Afaque, Y.; Bhartia, A.K.; Bhartia, V.K. Laparoscopic Repair of Congenital Diaphragmatic Hernia in Adults. *Minim. Invasive Surg.* **2016**, *2016*, 9032380. [CrossRef]
11. Groth, S.S.; Andrade, R.S. Diaphragm plication for eventration or paralysis: A review of the literature. *Ann. Thorac. Surg.* **2010**, *89*, S2146–S2150. [CrossRef]
12. Langham, M.R.; Kays, D.W.; Ledbetter, D.J.; Frentzen, B.; Sanford, L.L.; Richards, D.S. Congenital diaphragmatic hernia. Epidemiology and outcome. *Clin. Perinatol.* **1996**, *23*, 671–688. [CrossRef] [PubMed]
13. Schumpelick, V.; Steinau, G.; Schlüper, I.; Prescher, A. Surgical embryology and anatomy of the diaphragm with surgical applications. *Surg. Clin. N. Am.* **2020**, *80*, 213–239. [CrossRef]
14. Keijzer, R.; Puri, P. Congenital diaphragmatic hernia. *Semin. Pediatr. Surg.* **2010**, *19*, 180–185. [CrossRef]
15. Koo, C.W.; Johnson, T.F.; Gierada, D.S.; White, D.B.; Blackmon, S.; Matsumoto, J.M.; Choe, J.; Allen, M.S.; Levin, D.L.; Kuzo, R.S. The breadth of the diaphragm: Updates in embryogenesis and role of imaging. *Br. J. Radiol.* **2018**, *91*, 20170600. [CrossRef]
16. Iritani, I. Experimental study on embryogenesis of congenital diaphragmatic hernia. *Anat. Embryol.* **1984**, *169*, 133–139. [CrossRef]
17. Detti, L.; Mari, G.; Ferguson, J.E. Color Doppler ultrasonography of the superior mesenteric artery for prenatal ultrasonographic diagnosis of a left-sided congenital diaphragmatic hernia. *J. Ultrasound Med.* **2001**, *20*, 689–692. [CrossRef] [PubMed]
18. Kirby, E.; Keijzer, R. Congenital diaphragmatic hernia: Current management strategies from antenatal diagnosis to long-term follow-up. *Pediatr. Surg. Int.* **2020**, *36*, 415–429. [CrossRef]
19. Moore, K.L.; Persaud, T.V.N.; Torchia, M.G. *The Developing Human: Clinically Oriented Embryology*, 8th ed.; Saunders: London, UK; Elsevier: Amsterdam, The Netherlands, 2008.

20. Dingeldein, M. Congenital Diaphragmatic Hernia: Management & Outcomes. *Adv. Pediatr.* **2018**, *65*, 241–247.
21. Gallot, D.; Coste, K.; Francannet, C.; Laurichesse, H.; Boda, C.; Ughetto, S.; Vanlieferinghen, P.; Scheye, T.; Vendittelli, F.; Labbe, A.; et al. Antenatal detection and impact on outcome of congenital diaphragmatic hernia: A 12-year experience in Auvergne, France. *Eur. J. Obstet. Gynecol. Reprod. Biol.* **2006**, *125*, 202–205. [CrossRef] [PubMed]
22. Smulian, J.C.; Guzman, E.R.; Ranzini, A.C.; Benito, C.W.; Vintzileos, A.M. Color and duplex Doppler sonographic investigation of in utero spontaneous regression of pulmonary sequestration. *J. Ultrasound Med.* **1996**, *15*, 789–792. [CrossRef] [PubMed]
23. Graham, G.; Devine, P.C. Antenatal diagnosis of congenital diaphragmatic hernia. *Semin. Perinatol.* **2005**, *29*, 69–76. [CrossRef]
24. Lin, A.E.; Pober, B.R.; Adatia, I. Congenital diaphragmatic hernia and associated cardiovascular malformations: Type, frequency, and impact on management. *Am. J. Med. Genet. C Semin. Med. Genet.* **2007**, *145C*, 201–216. [CrossRef] [PubMed]
25. Graziano, J.N. Cardiac anomalies in patients with congenital diaphragmatic hernia and their prognosis: A report from the Congenital Diaphragmatic Hernia Study Group. *J. Pediatr. Surg.* **2005**, *40*, 1045–1050. [CrossRef] [PubMed]
26. Menon, S.C.; Tani, L.Y.; Weng, H.Y.; Lally, P.A.; Lally, K.P.; Yoder, B.A.; Congenital Diaphragmatic Hernia Study Group. Congenital Diaphragmatic Hernia Study Group: Clinical characteristics and outcomes of patients with cardiac defects and congeni-al diaphragmatic hernia. *J. Pediatr.* **2013**, *162*, 114–119. [CrossRef] [PubMed]
27. Singh, C.; Shahnaz, G.; Handa, R.; Gupta, N.P.; Sundar, J. A missing kidney and a hidden congenital diaphragmatic hernia. *J. Clin. Ultrasound.* **2021**, *49*, 401–404. [CrossRef]
28. Masturzo, B.; Kalache, K.D.; Cockell, A.; Pierro, A.; Rodeck, C.H. Prenatal diagnosis of an ectopic intrathoracic kidney in right-sided congenital diaphragmatic hernia using color Doppler ultrasonography. *Ultrasound Obstet. Gynecol.* **2001**, *18*, 173–174. [CrossRef]
29. Juricic, M.; Cambon, Z.; Baunin, C.; Abbo, O.; Puget, C.; Crouzet, K.; Galinier, P.; Bouali, O. Prenatal diagnosis of right-sided diaphragmatic hernia and ipsilateral intrathoracic kidney in a female fetus: A rare observation. *Surg. Radiol. Anat.* **2016**, *38*, 419–423. [CrossRef]
30. Park, J. Right intrathoracic ectopic kidney and pulmonary sequestration associated with right sided congenital diaphragmatic hernia. *J. Pediatr. Surg. Case Rep.* **2020**, *61*, 101600. [CrossRef]
31. Thompson, E.; Simmons, L.Q.; Baker, A.L. A Rare Finding: Right-Sided Congenital Diaphragmatic Hernia With an Intrathoracic Kidney. *J. Diagn. Med. Sonogr.* **2019**, *35*, 241–246. [CrossRef]
32. Athanasiadis, A.P.; Zafrakas, M.; Arnaoutoglou, C.; Karavida, A.; Papasozomenou, P.; Tarlatzis, B.C. Prenatal diagnosis of thoracic kidney in the 2nd trimester with delayed manifestation of associated diaphragmatic hernia. *J. Clin. Ultrasound* **2011**, *39*, 221–224. [CrossRef]
33. Hidaka, N.; Fujita, Y.; Satoh, Y.; Fukushima, K.; Wake, N. Sonographic appearance of intrathoracic kidney in a fetus with left diaphragmatic hernia. *J. Clin. Ultrasound* **2012**, *40*, 600–602. [CrossRef]
34. Panda, B.; Rosenberg, V.; Cornfeld, D.; Stiller, R. Prenatal diagnosis of ectopic intrathoracic kidney in a fetus with a left diaphragmatic hernia. *J. Clin. Ultrasound* **2009**, *37*, 47–49. [CrossRef] [PubMed]
35. Takezoe, T.; Nomura, M.; Ogawa, K.; Tomonaga, K.; Ohno, M.; Tahara, K.; Watanabe, T.; Hishiki, T.; Fujino, A.; Miyasaka, M.; et al. Prenatally diagnosed, right- sided congenital diaphragmatic hernia complicated by hepatic pulmonary fusion and intrathoracic kidney. *Birth Defect* **2017**, *1*, 1–3. [CrossRef]
36. Jeong, B.D.; Ahn, S.H.; Song, J.W.; Shim, J.Y.; Lee, M.Y.; Won, H.S.; Lee, P.R.; Kim, A. Impaction of an intrathoracic kidney acted as a shield against herniation of the abdominal viscera in a case of right congenital diaphragmatic hernia. *Obstet. Gynecol. Sci.* **2016**, *59*, 58–61. [CrossRef]
37. Cessans, C.; Pharamin, J.; Crouzet, K.; Kessler, S.; Puget, C.; Bouali, O.; Galinier, P.; Marcoux, M.O. Prenatal diagnosis of a right thoracic congenital ectopic kidney with a diaphragmatic hernia: A combination with a good prognosis. *Arch. Pediatr.* **2015**, *22*, 1176–1179. [CrossRef] [PubMed]
38. Leanza, V.; Incognito, G.G.; Gulino, F.A.; Tuscano, A.; Cimino, M.; Palumbo, M. Cesarean Scar Pregnancy and Successful Ultrasound-Guided Removal after Uterine Artery Ligation. *Case Rep Obstet Gynecol.* **2023**, *2023*, 6026206. [CrossRef] [PubMed]
39. Leanza, V.; D'Urso, V.; Gulisano, M.; Incognito, G.G.; Palumbo, M. Bulging of both membranes and fetal lower limbs: Conservative management. *Minerva Obstet Gynecol.* **2021**, *73*, 654–658. [CrossRef]
40. Pappalardo, E.; Gulino, F.A.; Ettore, C.; Cannone, F.; Ettore, G. Body Stalk Anomaly Complicated by Ectopia Cordis: First-Trimester Diagnosis of Two Cases Using 2- and 3-Dimensional Sonography. *J. Clin. Med.* **2023**, *12*, 1896. [CrossRef]
41. Incognito, G.G.; D'Urso, G.; Incognito, D.; Lello, C.; Miceli, A.; Palumbo, M. Management of a giant uterine smooth muscle tumor of uncertain malignant potential in a 32-year-old woman: Case report and review of the literature. *Minerva Obstet. Gynecol.* **2022**, *74*, 466–470. [CrossRef] [PubMed]
42. Di Guardo, F.; Incognito, G.G.; Lello, C.; D'Urso, G.; Genovese, F.; Palumbo, M. Efficacy of sonohysterography and hysteroscopy for evaluation of endometrial lesions in tamoxifen treated patients: A systematic review. *Eur. J. Gynaecol. Oncol.* **2022**, *43*, 78–86.
43. Leanza, V.; Incognito, G.G.; Gulisano, M.; Incognito, D.; Correnti, S.G.; Palumbo, M. Herlyn-Werner-Wunderlich syndrome and central placenta previa in a COVID-19 positive pregnant woman: A case report. *Ital J. Gynaecol. Obstet.* **2023**, 35. [CrossRef]
44. Wataganara, T.; Ebrashy, A.; Aliyu, L.D.; Moreira de Sa, R.A.; Pooh, R.; Kurjak, A.; Sen, C.; Adra, A.; Stanojevic, M. Fetal magnetic resonance imaging and ultrasound. *J. Perinat. Med.* **2016**, *44*, 533–542. [CrossRef]

45. Jani, J.; Keller, R.L.; Benachi, A.; Nicolaides, K.H.; Favre, R.; Gratacos, E.; Laudy, J.; Eisenberg, V.; Eggink, A.; Vaast, P.; et al. Prenatal prediction of survival in isolated left-sided diaphragmatic hernia. *Ultrasound Obstet. Gynecol.* **2006**, *27*, 18–22. [CrossRef]
46. Kirshenbaum, A.S.; Puri, H.C.; Rama Rao, B. Congenital intrathoracic kidney. *J. Urol.* **1981**, *125*, 412–413. [CrossRef] [PubMed]

Disclaimer/Publisher's Note: The statements, opinions and data contained in all publications are solely those of the individual author(s) and contributor(s) and not of MDPI and/or the editor(s). MDPI and/or the editor(s) disclaim responsibility for any injury to people or property resulting from any ideas, methods, instructions or products referred to in the content.

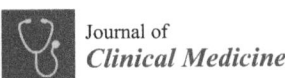

Systematic Review

Umbilical Vein Blood Flow in Uncomplicated Pregnancies: Systematic Review of Available Reference Charts and Comparison with a New Cohort

Moira Barbieri [1], Giulia Zamagni [2], Ilaria Fantasia [1], Lorenzo Monasta [2], Leila Lo Bello [1], Mariachiara Quadrifoglio [1], Giuseppe Ricci [1,3], Gianpaolo Maso [1], Monica Piccoli [1], Daniela Denis Di Martino [4], Enrico Mario Ferrazzi [4,5] and Tamara Stampalija [1,3,*]

1. Department of Mother and Neonate, Institute for Maternal and Child Health IRCCS "Burlo Garofolo", 34100 Trieste, Italy; moira.barbieri@unimi.it (M.B.)
2. Clinical Epidemiology and Public Health Research Unit, Institute for Maternal and Child Health IRCCS "Burlo Garofolo", 34100 Trieste, Italy
3. Department of Medicine, Surgery and Health Sciences, University of Trieste, 34100 Trieste, Italy
4. Department of Mother, Child and Neonate, Fondazione IRCCS Ca' Granda Ospedale Policlinico di Milano, 20100 Milan, Italy
5. Department of Clinical and Community Sciences, University of Milan, 20100 Milan, Italy
* Correspondence: tamara.stampalija@burlo.trieste.it; Tel.: +39-0403-785-237

Abstract: The objectives of the study were (1) to perform a systematic review of the available umbilical vein blood flow volume (UV-Q) reference ranges in uncomplicated pregnancies; and (2) to compare the findings of the systematic review with UV-Q values obtained from a local cohort. Available literature in the English language on this topic was identified following the PRISMA guidelines. Selected original articles were further grouped based on the UV sampling sites and the formulae used to compute UV-Q. The 50th percentiles, the means, or the best-fitting curves were derived from the formulae or the reported tables presented by authors. A prospective observational study of uncomplicated singleton pregnancies from 20^{+0} to 40^{+6} weeks of gestation was conducted to compare UV-Q with the results of this systematic review. Fifteen sets of data (fourteen sets belonging to manuscripts identified by the research strategy and one obtained from our cohort) were compared. Overall, there was a substantial heterogeneity among the reported UV-Q central values, although when using the same sampling methodology and formulae, the values overlap. Our data suggest that when adhering to the same methodology, the UV-Q assessment is accurate and reproducible, thus encouraging further investigation on the possible clinical applications of this measurement in clinical practice.

Keywords: umbilical vein blood flow volume; reproducibility; Doppler ultrasound; reference ranges; umbilical cord; fetus; nutrition; oxygenation

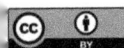

1. Introduction

The umbilical vein blood flow volume (UV-Q) reflects the amount of metabolites and oxygen delivered to the fetus [1]. An adequate UV-Q is essential to guarantee fetal needs for oxidative metabolism and growth [2]. The UV-Q increases progressively and exponentially throughout pregnancy, from 63 mL/min at 20 weeks to 373 mL/min at 38 weeks [3]. However, UV-Q normalized for estimated fetal weight (UV-Q/EFW) shows a progressive reduction in relation to the increasing fetal mass [4]. This suggests a progressive mismatch between fetal demands and placental availability, suggesting a possible role for UV-Q in clinical settings [5]. In fact, studies have shown a reduced UV-Q and UV-Q/EFW in fetal growth restriction (FGR) [6,7]. Lower UV-Q values have also been found in normally grown fetuses that experienced intrapartum distress [8,9], suggesting a potential role for UV-Q as an admission test [10]. The first reports regarding UV-Q measurement in human fetuses go back to the early 1980s [11,12]. Despite a great interest over the past four decades in the possibility of assessing the blood flow delivery to the fetus, this biophysical assessment has not gained ground, and it is still used only in research settings [13,14]. One of the main reasons is related to the questions raised regarding the accuracy, reproducibility, and technical aspects of the UV-Q measurement [15,16]. Over time, doubts about quantitative inaccuracies have been challenged [17,18], thanks to the improvement of ultrasound machines and the introduction of high-resolution ultrasound probes. Although UV-Q calculation has shown moderate to good intra- and inter-observer reproducibility [19], arguments against the accuracy and reproducibility of UV-Q measurement are still limiting its possible clinical use. On this ground, we performed a systematic review of the available reference ranges of UV-Q in the human fetus. We also prospectively recruited a cohort of uncomplicated singleton pregnancies between 20^{+0} and 40^{+6} weeks of gestation and performed UV-Q measurements with the aim to compare the obtained values with the results of this systematic review.

2. Materials and Methods

2.1. Systematic Review of the Available UV-Q Reference Ranges

A comprehensive systematic review was performed to identify studies that evaluated UV-Q in low-risk pregnancies. The study was registered with the International Prospective Register of Systematic Reviews database (PROSPERO registration number: CRD42021276868) [20]. The Preferred Reporting Items for Systematic Reviews and Meta-analysis (PRISMA) guidelines [21] were followed in the review report.

2.1.1. Study Identification and Selection

A systematic literature search in the English language was conducted from inception until December 2021 in PubMed (Medline) and Scopus. The search strategy consisted of relevant Medical Subject Headings (MeSH) terms and keywords, including "umbilical vein blood flow"/"umbilical venous blood flow" and "volume". Inclusion criteria were studies focusing on UV-Q values in singleton pregnancies without congenital abnormalities that were conducted in hospital settings. Study protocols, case reports, animal experimental studies, in vitro studies, review articles, editorials, letters to the editor, and conference proceedings/posters that did not appear as full-text papers were excluded. We aimed to identify studies that reported the algorithm for the calculation of the central values for UV-Q and/or UV-Q/EFW. Methods to plot the 50th percentile or the best-fitting curves were derived from the formulae presented in the manuscripts or from the reported tables of percentiles, when available. An absence of a central value for each week of gestation disqualified a study from further assessment. The following data were extracted: authors, year of publication, study type, number of participants, gestational age, type of population, sampling site of the UV, equation, and percentiles and mean values of UV-Q and UV-Q/EFW. Relevant articles were searched manually to identify manuscripts not obtained from the research strategy. The assessment of study eligibility, methodological quality, and data extraction of the included studies were completed by two independent investigators. Data from each eligible study were extracted without modification of the original information onto custom-made data collection forms. Disagreements were resolved by consensus with a third reviewer.

A distinction between uncomplicated pregnancies and unselected or mixed high- and low-risk populations was performed. To improve the synthesis and understanding of the different issues on this topic, selected original articles were further grouped based on:

- The sampling site: (a) studies investigating UV-Q on the intra-abdominal (IA) portion of the UV; and (b) studies investigating UV-Q at the free-floating (FF) portion of the UV;
- The formula used to compute the UV-Q.

2.1.2. Quality Assessment

The quality assessment of each included study was performed using the Quality Assessment of Diagnostic Accuracy Studies (QUADAS-2) criteria [22] in four domains related to the risk of bias: patient selection; index test; reference standard; and flow and timing. Each domain was categorized as "low risk", "high risk", or "some concerns" of bias if the data regarding the domain were "reported and adequate", "reported but inadequate", or "not reported", respectively. The first three domains were assessed in respect to applicability. The overall judgement was then established based on the rating of individual domains. The robvis tool web app [23] was then used to visualize the risk-of-bias after applying the separate quality criteria.

2.2. Prospective Cohort Study on UV-Q, UV-Q/AC, and UV-Q/EFW

A prospective cross-sectional monocentric observational study of singleton low-risk uncomplicated pregnancies from 20^{+0} to 40^{+6} weeks of gestation was conducted to obtain reference ranges for UV-Q, UV-Q/AC, and UV-Q/EFW. The study protocol was approved by the local Ethics Committee (CEUR-2019-EM-225). Criteria for inclusion were first-trimester dating based on crown-rump length measurement, low-risk singleton uncomplicated pregnancy, and compliance with the study protocol. Exclusion criteria were twin pregnancies, premature rupture of membranes, signs of pathological obstetric condition, pregnancies complicated by the fetal structure, chromosomal abnormalities, or intrauterine infections. Eligible women were consecutively allocated to an additional ultrasound examination > 20 weeks of gestation for UV-Q, UV-Q/AC, and UV-Q/EFW measurements, together with fetal biometry and Doppler velocimetry. UV-Q, UV-Q/EFW, and UV-Q/AC were calculated as already reported [24]. We planned to recruit at least 20 women for each gestational age group. Each woman was considered once and allocated to a biweekly gestational age group (20–21; 22–23; etc.). Fetal biometry and Doppler velocimetry were performed following the International Society of Ultrasound in Obstetrics and Gynecology guidelines [25,26]. The EFW was calculated by using the Hadlock formula [27]. UV-Q, UV-Q/AC, and UV-Q/EFW were calculated, blinded to the physician, and plotted and compared to the UV-Q and UV-Q/EFW values from other manuscripts considered eligible for this systematic review.

Statistical Analysis

For each variable of interest and for each gestational week, data points > Q3 + 3 × IQR (Interquartile Range) were identified as outliers and removed from the analysis. Centile curves were constructed using Generalized Additive Models for Location, Scale and Shape (GAMLSS) with the Box–Cox power exponential distribution (BCPE) or the Box–Cox Cole and Green distribution (BCCG) specified for the considered variables. Cubic or penalized splines with different degrees of freedom were used to model the scale and shape parameters. Different models were estimated for each variable using a combination of distributions and splines and the best model was selected, i.e., the model with the lowest value of the Akaike's Information Criterion (AIC). UV-Q was modelled using penalized splines with 1 d.f. for σ, 1 d.f. for τ, and 2 d.f. for η. For UV-Q/EFW, cubic splines were used to model the scale and shape parameters, with 2 d.f. for σ, 1 d.f. for τ, and 2 d.f. for η. Cubic splines were also used in the model for UV-Q/AC, with 1 d.f. for σ, 1 d.f. for τ, and 1 d.f. for η. The distances between the estimated central curves were calculated in terms of z-scores, as proposed by DeVore et al. [28], where:

$$z = \frac{value\ from\ published\ study - predicted\ value\ from\ current\ study}{predicted\ SD\ from\ current\ study}$$

Z-score values between −1 and 1 were considered not significantly different [29]. The statistical analyses were conducted using the software R Core Team (2020) [30].

A calculator that allows UV-Q and UV-Q/EFW computation as well as the respective z-score and percentile for a specific gestational week age, by using our data as the reference point, is provided at the following webpage https://giuliazamagni.shinyapps.io/UV_Calculator/ (accessed on 7 August 2022).

3. Results

3.1. Systematic Review of the Available UV-Q Reference Ranges

The research identified 587 publications (Table S1). After the removal of duplicates, a total of 397 studies were obtained. Figure 1 shows the PRISMA flow diagram of the study selection.

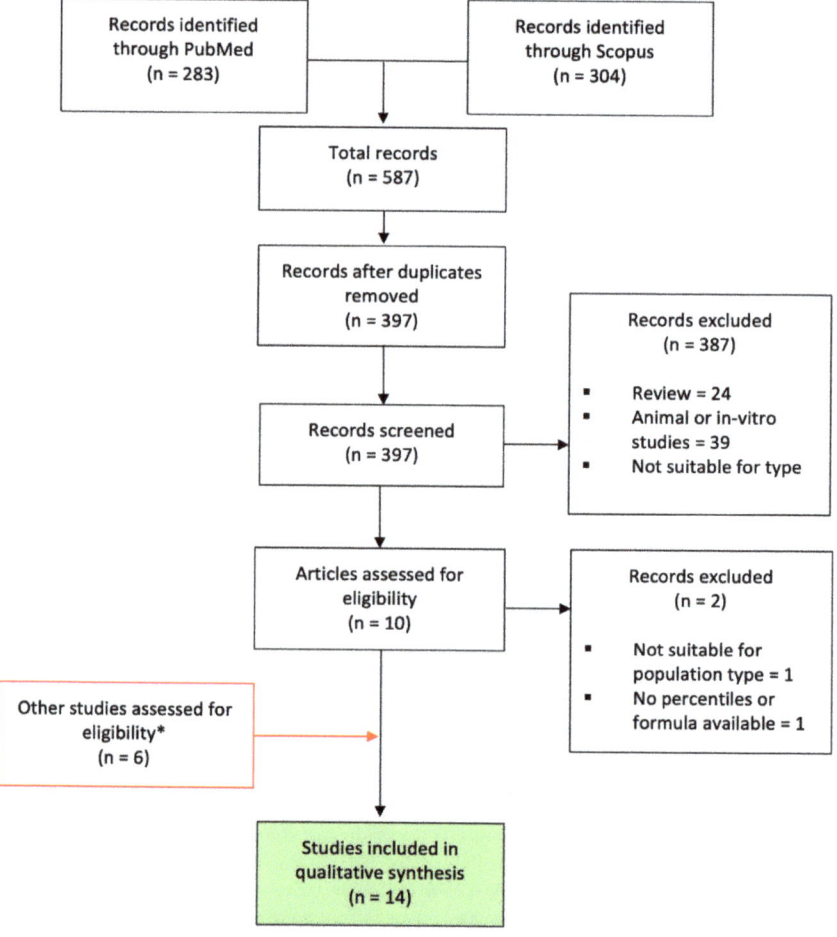

Figure 1. PRISMA flow diagram of the study selection. * Not identified through Pubmed or Scopus search strategy but cited in other articles similar to this systematic review or found by evaluating the bibliography of studies obtained from the research strategy. In red, the articles not found through the search strategy; in green, the articles selected for this systematic review.

Reviews, animal studies, and in vitro studies were excluded, as well as all articles that were not suitable for study type (i.e., conference proceedings, book chapters) or not suitable for the topic (not related to the research). This left 10 articles that were assessed to be eligible. A full-text review of the 10 articles excluded two additional manuscripts that were considered not suitable for the population type (Widnes et al. [31] investigated gestational age-specific serial changes in UV-Q, establishing sex-specific reference ranges) or because percentiles and/or equations were not provided by the authors (Lees et al. [32]). The evaluation of the bibliographies of the included studies further added six articles that were considered suitable for evaluation. Thus, fourteen manuscripts were included in the systematic review: eight articles [18,33–39] found with the research strategy and six articles [3,28,40–43] found by evaluating the bibliographies of studies obtained from the research strategy.

3.1.1. Risk of Bias within Studies According to QUADAS Criteria

Figure S1 shows the assessment of the included studies by QUADAS-2 criteria. In the "patient selection" domain, two studies [37,38] were classified as having a high risk of bias because fetuses with growth impairments or women with high-risk pregnancies were also included. The remaining 12 studies were considered to have a low risk of bias. In the "index domain", five studies [34,39,41–43] were classified as having 'some concerns' because it was not explicit if any action had been taken to test the inter- and intra-observer variability. The remaining nine studies were considered as low-risk. In the "reference range" domain, one study [3] was classified as having a high risk of bias because the exponential curve formula of the UV-Q reported by the authors did not correspond to the reported values. The remaining 13 studies were considered as low-risk. In the "flow and timing" domain, one study [36] was classified as having a high risk of bias because of its small sample size (32 low-risk pregnant women). The remaining 13 studies were considered as having a low risk of bias.

3.1.2. Description of the Included Studies

The main characteristics and results of the 14 studies are summarized in Table 1. One study [38] recruited women retrospectively, while all others were prospective. Eleven studies [3,18,34,36–43] published reference algorithms for the central values of UV-Q. For the remaining three articles [28,33,35], UV-Q values were derived from the percentile data. Six studies [3,18,28,33,36,37] investigated UV-Q at the FF portion of the umbilical vein, six studies [34,35,38,40,41,43] at the IA portion, and two studies [39,42] both at the FF and IA portions of the UV. For one study [3], the formula for the UV-Q exponential curve reported by authors did not correspond to the exponential values. For this reason, we decided to exclude the study from the comparison. On the contrary, the UV-Q/EFW values were considered plausible and therefore were included in the analysis. UV-Q and UV-Q/EFW central values were not reported homogeneously. In three studies [34,36,38], the central values of UV-Q and UV-Q/EFW of the entire observational period were reported. In six studies [28,39–43], the central UV-Q and UV-Q/EFW values were not reported, while Sutton et al. [18] reported only UV-Q/EFW values. The remaining studies [3,33,35,37] provided UV-Q and UV-Q/EFW values, considering the gestational period at the enrolment and at the end of observation separately. Gestational time intervals and the mean values are reported in Table 1.

3.2. Prospective Cohort Study on UV-Q

We recruited 277 women, and of those, 12 were excluded due to an onset of pregnancy complications. This left a total of 255 low-risk women from 20^{+0} to 40^{+6} gestational weeks for UV-Q, UV-Q/EFW, and UV-Q/AC calculation. Demographic, obstetric, and neonatal characteristics of the cohort are shown in Table 2.

Table 1. Main characteristics and results of the included studies, divided according to the sampling site (i.e., intra-abdominal [IA], free floating [FF]) and the formula used to compute umbilical vein blood flow volume (UV-Q).

First Author, Year of Publication	Study Type	Popula-tion (N)	Gestational Age	Description of Population	Available Percentiles	Formula for Q-UV Measurement	Mean Values of Q UV (mL/min)	Mean Values of Q-UV Normalized to EFW (mL/min/kg)
				Free-floating portion				
1 DeVore et al., 2021 [28]	Prospective cross-sectional study	240	20 to 40 weeks	Singleton low-risk pregnancies	Yes	$0.5 \times \text{TaMXV} \times \pi(D/2)^2 \times 60$		
2 Flo et al., 2010 [33]	Prospective longitudinal study	53	22 to 39^{+6} weeks	Singleton low-risk pregnancies	Yes	Two formulae used separately: (1) $0.5 \times \text{TaMXV} \times \pi(D/2)^2 \times 60$ (2) $\text{Vwmean} \times \pi(D/2)^2 \times 60$	1st formula: from 53 to 250 (22–39^{+6} weeks) 2nd formula: from 66 to 313 (22–39^{+6} weeks)	1st formula: from 110 to 68 (22–39^{+6} weeks)
3 Boito et al., 2003 [36]	Cross-sectional matched control study	64	18 to 36 weeks	32 low-risk $^{£}$ and 32 diabetic women	No	$0.06 \times \text{TaMXV} \times \pi \times (D/2)^2$	100.5 (in diabetic women) versus 106.2 (in controls)	94.2 (in diabetic women) versus 109.4 (in controls)
4 Boito et al., 2002 [37]	Prospective cross-sectional study	133	20 to 36 weeks	100 low-risk $^{£}$ and 33 SGA	No	$\text{TaMXV} \times \pi \times (D/2)^2$	33.2 (at 20 weeks) 221.0 (at 36 weeks)	117.5 (at 20 weeks) 78.3 (at 36 weeks)
5 Barbera et al., 1999 [3]	Prospective cross-sectional study	70	20 to 38 weeks	Singleton low-risk pregnancies	No	$0.5 \times \text{TaMXV} \times \pi \times (D/2)^2 \times 60$	54 (at 23 weeks) 320 (at 38 weeks)	125 (at 23 weeks) 104 (at 38 weeks)
6 Sutton et al., 1990 [18]	Prospective cross-sectional study	74	19 to 42 weeks	Singleton low-risk pregnancies	No	$\text{FVI}_{UV}/s \times \pi \times (D/2)^2 \times 60$		105–130
				Intra-abdominal portion				
7 Rizzo et al., 2016 [40]	Prospective cross-sectional study	852	14 to 40 weeks	Singleton low-risk pregnancies	No	$0.5 \times \text{TaMXV} \times \pi(D/2)^2 \times 60$		
8 Tchirikov et al., 2009 [34]	Prospective cross-sectional study	181	17 to 41 weeks	148 low-risk and 33 with poor fetal outcome	No	$\text{TaMXV} \times \pi \times (D/2)^2$	160.2 (in compromised fetuses) versus 253.3 (in controls)	115.1 (in compromised fetuses) versus 200.3 (in controls)
9 Acharya et al., 2005 [35]	Prospective longitudinal study	130	19 to 42 weeks	Singleton low-risk pregnancies	Yes	Two formulae used separately: (1) $0.5 \times \text{Vmax} \times \pi(D/2)^2 \times 60$ (2) $\text{Vwmean} \times \pi(D/2)^2 \times 60$	1st formula: from 27.6 to 271.1 (19–41 weeks) 2nd formula: from 27.13 to 273.4 (19–41 weeks)	1st formula: from 74.7 to 63.2 (19–41 weeks) 2nd formula: from 73.5 to 63.3 (19–41 weeks)

Table 1. *Cont.*

	First Author, Year of Publication	Study Type	Popula-tion (N)	Gestational Age	Description of Population	Available Percentiles	Formula for Q-UV Measurement	Mean Values of UV Q (mL/min)	Mean Values of Q-UV Normalized to EFW (mL/min/kg)
10	Tchirikov et al., 2002 [38]	Retrospective, cross-sectional clinical study	85	17 to 41 weeks	of whom 15 had poor fetal outcomes	No	iVmean × π(D/2)²	17 *	−2.2 **
11	Kiserud et al., 2000 [41]	Prospective cross-sectional study	197	18 to 41 weeks	Singleton low-risk pregnancies	No	Vwmean × π × (D/2)²		
12	Tchirikov et al., 1998 [43]	Prospective cross-sectional study	−75 (singleton) −10 (twin pregnancies)	100 to 300 days	Singleton: −55 low-risk £ −20 FGR	No			
	Both at free-floating and intra-abdominal portions								
13	Wang et al., 2021 [39]	Prospective cross-sectional study	907	20 to 39 weeks	Singleton low-risk pregnancies	No	iVmean × 60 × π(D/2)²	FL: from 32.6 to 381.9 (20–39 weeks) IA: from 31.5 to 360.1 (20–39 weeks)	
14	Bellotti et al., 2000 [42]	Prospective cross-sectional study	137	20 to 38 weeks	Singleton low-risk pregnancies	No	0.5 × TaMXV × π × (D/2)²		

Blank cells correspond to data not provided by the authors. Green lines correspond to authors using our same methodology in the computing of UV-Q, both in terms of sampling site and formula used. D, diameter; FF, free floating; FVI, flow velocity integral; IA, intra-abdominal; iVmean, intensity-weighted mean velocity; Q-UV, umbilical vein blood flow volume; SD, standard deviation; SGA, small for gestational age; TaMXV, time averaged mean velocity; Vmax, maximum velocity; Vmean, mean velocity; Vwmean, weighted mean velocity. * mL/min/week. ** mL/min/kg/week;sexpressed as the mean of three successive measurements of the inner diameter of the vessel, £ UV-Q curve returned by the authors is based only on low-risk pregnant women.

Table 2. Demographic, obstetric, and neonatal characteristics of the cohort. Data are represented as number and percentage, mean ± standard deviation, or median with interquartile range, as appropriate.

	Population (n = 255)
Maternal age (years)	33 (29–36)
Non-Caucasian ethnicity	3 (1.2%)
Maternal pre-pregnancy BMI (kg/m^2)	22 (20–24)
Nulliparous	122 (47.7%)
EFW percentile	50 (36–63)
GA at delivery	40^{+3} (39^{+1}–40^{+5})
Birthweight (g)	3420 (3175–3645)
Male fetuses	133 (52.2%)

BMI, body mass index; EFW, estimated fetal weight; GA, gestational age.

Based on this cohort, we established the 5th, 10th, 50th, 90th, and 95th percentiles for UV-Q, UV-Q/EFW, and UV-Q/AC for each gestational week, both combined (Table 3) and sex-specific (Table S2).

Table 3. The 5th, 10th, 50th, 90th, and 95th percentiles for UV-Q, UV-Q/EFW, and UV-Q/CA at each gestational week are represented. Sex-combined percentiles are represented.

GA (Weeks)	UV-Q					UV-Q/EFW					UV-Q/AC				
	5th	10th	50th	90th	95th	5th	10th	50th	90th	95th	5th	10th	50th	90th	95th
20	28	31	45	60	64	92	101	137	174	51	0.19	0.21	0.30	0.41	0.44
21	36	40	57	75	80	95	103	139	178	66	0.21	0.24	0.35	0.47	0.51
22	45	50	69	92	98	97	105	140	181	95	0.24	0.27	0.39	0.53	0.57
23	55	60	83	109	117	99	106	141	183	112	0.27	0.30	0.43	0.59	0.63
24	65	71	97	128	136	99	106	141	184	132	0.29	0.33	0.48	0.64	0.70
25	76	82	112	147	156	98	105	139	182	154	0.32	0.36	0.52	0.70	0.75
26	85	93	129	165	175	96	103	136	177	176	0.34	0.38	0.55	0.75	0.81
27	95	103	140	182	194	93	99	131	171	198	0.36	0.41	0.59	0.80	0.86
28	104	113	154	200	212	89	95	126	163	220	0.38	0.43	0.62	0.84	0.91
29	112	122	167	217	230	84	91	121	154	241	0.40	0.45	0.65	0.88	0.96
30	120	131	181	234	248	80	87	116	147	261	0.42	0.47	0.68	0.92	1.00
31	127	140	194	252	267	76	83	111	140	281	0.44	0.49	0.71	0.96	1.04
32	135	149	208	270	286	73	80	108	135	300	0.45	0.51	0.73	0.99	1.07
33	142	158	222	289	307	70	77	104	131	319	0.47	0.53	0.76	1.03	1.11
34	148	166	235	307	328	67	74	101	127	337	0.48	0.54	0.78	1.05	1.14
35	153	173	247	326	349	64	71	98	124	355	0.49	0.55	0.80	1.08	1.17
36	157	178	258	344	369	60	67	94	121	371	0.50	0.57	0.81	1.1	1.19
37	159	182	267	360	389	55	62	91	119	385	0.51	0.58	0.83	1.12	1.21
38	158	184	274	376	409	50	57	87	117	397	0.52	0.59	0.84	1.14	1.23
39	156	183	279	389	428	45	53	83	115	406	0.53	0.60	0.86	1.16	1.25
40	150	181	282	402	446	39	48	80	113	415	0.54	0.60	0.87	1.17	1.27
41	143	176	283	412	464	34	43	76	111	422	0.54	0.61	0.88	1.19	1.29

Overall, there was an increase in UV-Q and UV-Q/AC, while UV-Q/EFW showed a decreasing trend (Figure 2).

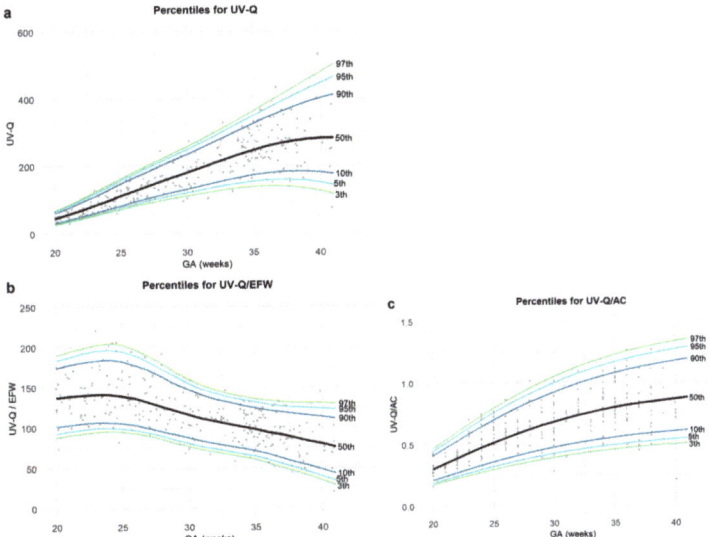

Figure 2. The figure represents the percentiles for (**a**) umbilical vein blood flow volume (UV-Q); (**b**) UV-Q normalized for estimated fetal weight (UV-Q/EFW); and (**c**) UV-Q normalized for abdominal circumference (UV-Q/AC).

Comparison between Reference Range Values for UV-Q and UV-Q/EFW

A comparison was performed for the 14 manuscripts included in the systematic review (Table 1) and the 15th set of data represented by our local cohort. Because the examined gestational age interval was heterogeneous among the studies (Table 1), we decided to consider a gestational age interval common to all studies (i.e., from 22^{+0} to 39^{+0} gestational weeks). Since neither crude data nor confidence intervals were available to perform a statistical comparison, all estimated curves were superimposed on a single plot in order to detect graphical differences in relation to the gestational age (Figure 3).

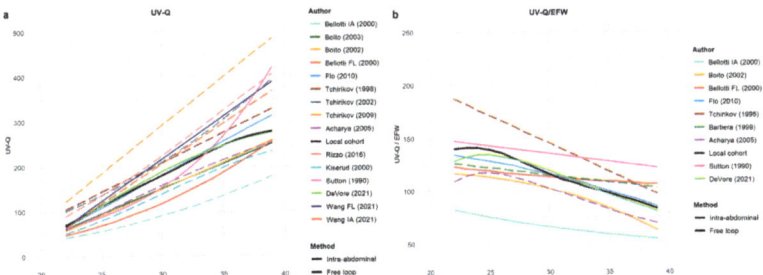

Figure 3. The figure represents (**a**) absolute and (**b**) normalized-for-estimated-fetal-weight (EFW) umbilical vein blood flow central values (UV-Q) from studies included in systematic review and our set of data. Straight lines (—): studies investigating UV-Q at the intra-abdominal portion of the umbilical cord; dashed lines (- -): studies investigating UV-Q at the free-floating portion of the umbilical cord. Different colors represent the first author's name and the year of publication [18,28,33–43].

The comparison among UV-Q and UV-Q/EFW central curves, including low-risk and unselected populations both on IA and FF, is represented in Figures S2 and S3, while each author's UV-Q and UV-Q/EFW central values are reported in relation to the gestational age in Tables S3 and S4, respectively.

Figures 4 and 5 represent UV-Q and UV-Q/EFW central values only in low-risk populations according to the UV sample site.

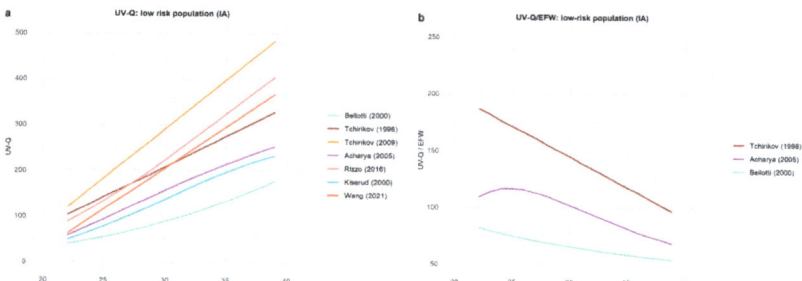

Figure 4. This figure represents umbilical vein blood flow volume (UV-Q) central values in low-risk populations in studies that investigated UV-Q in the intra-abdominal (IA) portion of the umbilical vein: (**a**) UV-Q absolute value; and (**b**) normalized for estimated fetal weight (UV-Q/EFW). Different colors represent the first author's name and the year of publication [34,35,39–43].

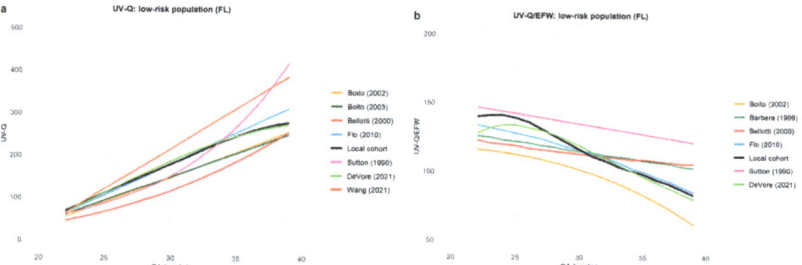

Figure 5. This figure represents umbilical vein blood flow volume (UV-Q) central values in low-risk populations in studies that investigated UV-Q on the free-floating (FF) portion of the umbilical cord: (**a**) UV-Q absolute value; and (**b**) normalized for estimated fetal weight (UV-Q/EFW). Different colors represent the first author's name and the year of publication [18,28,33,36,37,39,42].

In order to detect the deviations among available curves, we used our cohort as the reference, and we computed z-scores for all UV-Q and UV-Q/EFW computed with the same methodology (i.e., sampled at an FF portion of the UV and computed with the same formulae) (Table 4). Figure 6 represents UV-Q and UV-Q/EFW central values in low-risk populations sampled on an FF umbilical vein and computed with our same formula for UV-Q [3,28,33].

Table 4. Standardized scores for umbilical vein blood flow volume (UV-Q) and UV-Q normalized for estimated fetal weight (UV-Q/EFW) on free-floating umbilical vein calculated using our cohort as the reference. Values in bold italics represent z-scores in the interval [−1, 1].

	UV-Q						UV-Q/EFW				
GA (Weeks)	Sutton 1990	Bellotti 2000	Boito 2003	Flo 2010	DeVore 2021	Wang 2021	GA (Weeks)	Sutton 1990	Barbera 1999	Bellotti 2000	Flo 2010	DeVore 2021
22	−0.56	−1.92	−0.67	−0.25	−0.33	−0.34	22	*0.32*	−0.65	−0.79	−0.28	−0.56
23	−0.60	−1.36	−0.50	−0.18	*−0.09*	*0.04*	23	*0.13*	−0.45	−0.56	−0.25	−0.25
24	−0.68	−1.32	−0.50	*−0.14*	*−0.04*	*0.21*	24	*0.07*	−0.45	−0.52	−0.27	*−0.17*
25	−1.18	−2.10	−0.83	−0.24	*0.00*	*0.48*	25	*0.13*	−0.63	−0.74	−0.41	*−0.18*

Table 4. Cont.

	UV-Q							UV-Q/EFW				
GA (Weeks)	Sutton 1990	Bellotti 2000	Boito 2003	Flo 2010	DeVore 2021	Wang 2021	GA (Weeks)	Sutton 1990	Barbera 1999	Bellotti 2000	Flo 2010	DeVore 2021
26	−1.05	−1.85	−0.75	−0.19	0.07	0.56	26	0.21	−0.63	−0.79	−0.42	−0.17
27	−1.02	−1.80	−0.76	−0.13	0.13	0.67	27	0.39	−0.55	−0.69	−0.32	−0.05
28	−0.86	−1.57	−0.70	−0.08	0.14	0.68	28	0.40	−0.27	−0.37	−0.17	0.03
29	−0.69	−1.39	−0.63	−0.02	0.16	0.70	29	0.64	−0.21	−0.29	−0.12	0.08
30	−0.61	−1.39	−0.66	0.00	0.17	0.78	30	0.76	−0.04	−0.12	0.00	0.12
31	−0.53	−1.49	−0.75	0.05	0.19	0.98	31	1.07	0.14	0.05	0.10	0.14
32	−0.39	−1.55	−0.83	0.07	0.17	1.12	32	1.67	0.28	0.21	0.14	0.14
33	−0.14	−1.18	−0.68	0.07	0.07	0.95	33	1.09	0.29	0.25	0.12	0.04
34	0.10	−1.36	−0.84	0.13	0.04	1.23	34	1.55	0.50	0.44	0.11	0.00
35	0.43	−1.20	−0.80	0.18	0.00	1.30	35	1.72	0.58	0.64	0.12	−0.12
36	0.53	−0.69	−0.50	0.15	−0.03	0.91	36	1.33	0.54	0.58	0.08	−0.08
37	1.00	−0.68	−0.55	0.26	−0.04	1.20	37	1.42	0.64	0.68	0.08	−0.13
38	1.79	−0.63	−0.59	0.44	−0.07	1.67	38	1.89	0.89	1.00	0.11	−0.16
39	1.75	−0.27	−0.34	0.42	−0.04	1.35	39	1.67	0.87	1.00	0.09	−0.13

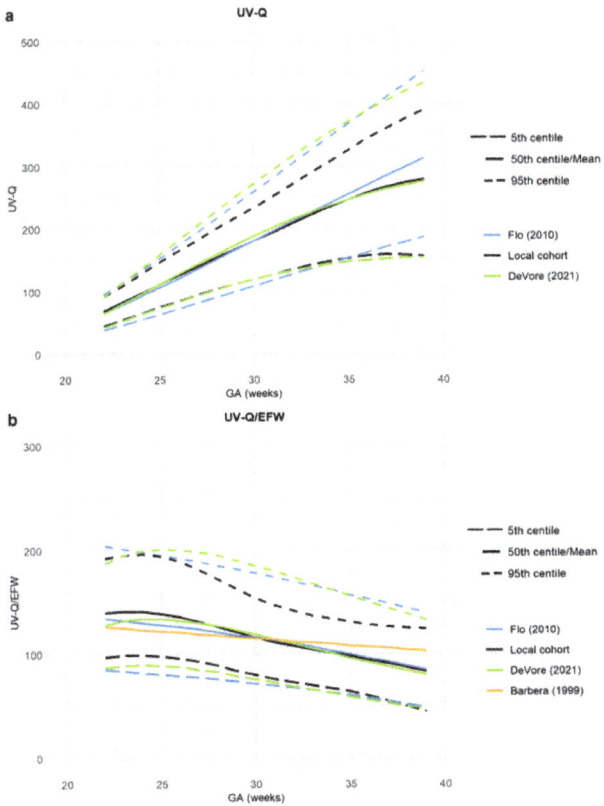

Figure 6. (**a**,**b**) Umbilical vein blood flow (UV-Q) 5th, 50th, and 95th percentiles, both (**a**) absolute and (**b**) normalized for estimated fetal weight (UV-Q/EFW) computed with the same methodology (i.e., on a free-floating loop of umbilical vein, in low-risk population, and with the same formula). Different colors represent the first author's name and the year of publication [3,28,33].

4. Discussion

4.1. The Main Findings of the Study

We found a substantial heterogeneity among UV-Q and UV-Q/EFW central values reported from 1990 to the present, selected by the robust standard procedures required for systematic reviews. We report our reference ranges for UV-Q, UV-Q/EFW, and UV-Q/AC, combined and sex-specific sampled at an FF UV portion. Part of the heterogeneity seems to be attributable to the sampling site used to compute UV-Q. In fact, the reported central values for the UV-Q sampled at FF UV portions were overall lower than those sampled on IA portions. When UV-Q central values computed with the same methodology as ours [28,33] were compared, there was an impressive overlap. Particularly, when comparing exclusively studies in which UV-Q calculations were performed using the same methodology [3,28,33] both in terms of population, sampling site, and formulae, we found an impressive overlap in central values. At 22 and 39 weeks, UV-Q corresponded to 66.6 ± 2.1 and 289.3 ± 20.5 mL/min, while UV-Q/EFW corresponded to 132.0 ± 6.2 to 87.7 ± 10.3 mL/min/kg, with an overall %err of 7%. These findings suggest that the assessment of UV-Q, assessed with the same methodology, may be reproducible and accurate, which opens a window of possible clinical applications.

4.2. Comment

Heterogeneity among reference ranges used in perinatology is not a novelty [44], and it has been reported for fetal biometry, Doppler velocimetry, and birthweight [44–46]. Reasons behind this heterogeneity are numerous and are beyond the scope of this manuscript. Despite the reported heterogeneity, most of these are used for clinical management in everyday practice.

Our systematic review highlights substantial differences among available reference charts for UV-Q and UV-Q/EFW that might be referred to various technological and methodological discrepancies. Some of the heterogeneity may be also related to the study design; most studies are cross-sectional [3,18,28,34,36–43], while relatively fewer are longitudinal studies [33,35]. Moreover, part of the heterogeneity seems to be related to the sampling site. UV-Q sampled at the IA portion of the UV showed greater values than those sampled at the FF portion and a greater dispersion among the reported values. The values reported in the low-risk population for UV-Q and UV-Q/EFW sampled at the IA portion are 80 ± 31 mL/min and 330 ± 112 mL/min at 22 weeks of gestation, and 125 ± 55 mL/min/kg and 73 ± 22 mL/min/kg at 39 weeks of gestation (%err of 36%), respectively [34,35,39–43]. These values sampled at the FF portion, at 22 and 39 weeks of gestation, are 62 ± 8 mL/min and 304 ± 63 mL/min for UV-Q and 130 ± 10 mL/min/kg and 93 ± 18 mL/min/kg for UV-Q/EFW (%err of 15%), respectively [18,28,33,36,37,39,42]. Part of the heterogeneity might also be attributed to the different sample sizes of the studies and different statistical procedures used to assess the central values and their percentiles.

4.2.1. Methodology

Theoretically, the blood flow measured through the UV should be parabolic, regardless of the measurement site. However, in practice, this concept does not apply, while it has been shown that the velocity distribution coefficient changes according to the sampling site [47], affecting the evaluation of UV-Q. Thus, the choice of the sampling site is important and should be made a priori in order to make the results comparable. The preference of IA over the FF sampling site, and vice versa, has some argumentations. The main advantage of using the IA portion is its fixed location, thus making the reproducibility of the sampling site apparently easier. The angle of insonation is of crucial importance for the accurate measurement of UV-Q, and it should be maintained close to 0° for precise flow velocity evaluation. Fixed fetal position, bone shadowing, and other technical aspects, especially toward term, might represent an important obstacle of IA evaluation. In addition, flow velocity at the umbilical inlet is affected by possible turbulences caused by the umbilical ring and the change of diameter along the amniotic portion to the intra-hepatic portion of the vein. These are easily overcome by UV-Q assessment at the FF portion. On the other side, due to its length and mobility, doubts have been raised regarding the reliability of repeated measurements from the FF portion [48].

Despite the difficulties in standardizing the sampling site, measurements obtained at the FF portion proved to be reproducible, especially when performed far from the placental insertion [2,3]. The use of the FF portion of the umbilical cord for UV-Q measurement has been validated by Galan et al. [49] in an animal model and more recently by Figueras et al. [19], thus being a candidate for methodological recommendation. Sampling at the UV FF portion has another advantage. UV-Q is a measure based on the formula: $UV\text{-}Q = CSA \times$ mean velocity $\times\ 60$, where flow is expressed in mL/min, the CSA is the cross-sectional area expressed in mm^2, and the mean velocity is computed as mm/s. When UV-Q is evaluated at the FF portion, it is also possible to evaluate the CSA directly [32,37] or indirectly from the measurement of the diameters [3,6] through the formula: $CSA = \pi \times (diameter/2)^2$. The radius-squared itself represents a source of inaccuracy, as any error in its measurement is squared and amplified. To minimize this error, it is recommended to use an average of 3 to 5 successive measurements on a straight segment of the UV [50].

Moreover, ultrasound software extracts the mean velocity from the instantaneous Doppler shift analysis as an intensity-weighted mean velocity (IVmean). This creates a second source of inaccuracy, especially when peak velocities are relatively slow (14–18 cm/s from 20 to 38 weeks of gestation). The ideal flow model is a perfect parabolic flow uniformly distributed in the lumen of vessel. The mean velocity can be calculated by adding a correction coefficient which considers the ideal flow shape in the CSA, thus using the following formula:

$$mean\ velocity = TAMXV \times 0.5$$

Consequently, it is not only the sampling site that is relevant but the whole methodology that allows the calculation of the blood flow volume, which also depends on the ultrasound equipment.

4.2.2. Experimental Research

In vivo models have been used for assessing the accuracy of umbilical vein blood flow. Doppler measurements of umbilical venous blood flow have been found to be accurate when compared with several gold standards for in vivo flow calculation. The simple "diameter-peak velocity $\times\ 0.5$" methodology was applied to two veins of fetal lambs versus historical measurements of flow obtained with invasive techniques [3]. Gestational ages and fetal weights were not different between the animals studied (129.6 ± 2.8 days, 2.75 ± 0.26 kg, respectively) and the steady-state data (131.6 ± 4.1 days, 2.94 ± 0.68, respectively). A study by Galan et al. [48] was then performed in an ovine model [48]. Their results showed that umbilical venous blood flow volume determined by triplex-mode ultrasonography differed by less than 1% from the true flow measurement obtained by the steady-state diffusion technique (207 ± 9 vs. 208 ± 7 mL/min/kg).

4.3. Strengths and Limitations of the Study

We used the best available methodology and predefined protocol to perform this systematic review, allowing for an objective quality evaluation of the studies. We aimed to perform an objective comparison and to quantify the differences among the reported reference ranges, but the lack of some crucial statistical data made this evaluation not feasible. This is the rationale behind the decision to use our data as a reference point and to express the distance between the curves in terms of z-scores instead of performing only a visive, subjective evaluation. It has to be acknowledged that the calculation involved values derived from different estimation methods for the construction of the curves (i.e., best fits, median, or mean). For these reasons, these z-scores should be carefully evaluated.

The fact that we used our cohort as the reference point made the comparison with UV reference ranges obtained on the IA portion impossible. Thus, our conclusions are mainly related to the UV-Q assessment on the UV FF portion.

Similarly to other authors [3,28,33], we provided an automatic UV-Q and UV-Q/EFW calculator as well as respective z-scores and percentiles for specific gestational weeks.

5. Conclusions

The measurement of UV-Q defines the blood flow volume delivered from the placenta to the fetus. The clinical value of UV-Q in understanding fetal adaptation to poor oxygenation and hypo-nutrition seems intuitive. However, its application, both in research and clinical settings, is still underestimated, mainly due to the concerns and criticisms regarding the measurement accuracy and reproducibility [16]. Our data suggest that when the same methodology is used for the UV-Q calculation, reproducible values may be obtained in line with other studies [19,32,37]. These findings should encourage further investigation on the potential role of UV-Q.

Supplementary Materials: The following supporting information can be downloaded at: https://www.mdpi.com/article/10.3390/jcm12093132/s1. Figure S1. Risk of bias author's judgement review based on Quality Assessment of Diagnostic Accuracy Studies Tool (QUADAS). (a) Risk of bias in each domain are presented as percentages across included studies. Green, low risk of bias; red, high risk of bias; yellow, some concerns of bias; blue, unclear risk of bias. (b) Concerns regarding applicability. Figure S2: The Figure represents umbilical vein blood flow volume (UV-Q) central values in low-risk and general population in studies that investigated UV-Q in an intra-abdominal (IA) portion of the umbilical vein: (a) UV-Q absolute value; and (b) normalized for estimated fetal weight (UV-Q/EFW). Different colors represent the first author's name and the year of publication [34,35,38–43]. Figure S3: The Figure represents umbilical vein blood flow volume (UV-Q) central values in low-risk and general population in studies that investigated UV-Q on a free-floating (FF) portion of the umbilical cord: (a) UV-Q absolute value; and (b) normalized for estimated fetal weight (UV-Q/EFW). Different colors represent the first author's name and the year of publication [3,18,28,33,36,37,39,42]. Table S1. Literature search strategy in Pubmed and Scopus. Table S2. The Table represents the 5th, 10th, 50th, 90th and 95th sex-specific percentiles for umbilical vein blood flow volume (UV-Q), UV-Q normalized for estimated fetal weight (UV-Q/EFW) and UV-Q normalized for the abdominal circumference (UV-Q/AC) from our local cohort. Table S3. The Table represents the central values for umbilical vein blood flow volume (UV-Q) of each manuscript included in this systematic review. Table S4. The Table represents the central values for umbilical vein blood flow volume normalized for estimated fetal weight (UV-Q/EFW) of each manuscript included in this systematic review.

Author Contributions: M.B., I.F. and T.S. developed the study; M.B., I.F., L.L.B., M.Q. and T.S. collected the data; G.Z. and L.M. analyzed the data; M.B. wrote the manuscript; G.R., G.M., M.P., D.D.D.M. and E.M.F. contributed to the scientific contents; T.S. revised the manuscript. All authors have read and agreed to the published version of the manuscript.

Funding: This research received no external funding.

Institutional Review Board Statement: The study protocol was approved by the Ethics Committee (CEUR-2019-EM-225).

Informed Consent Statement: Informed consent was obtained from all subjects involved in the study.

Data Availability Statement: The data presented in this study are available on request from the corresponding author.

Acknowledgments: This work was supported by the Italian Ministry of Health, through the contribution given to the Institute for Maternal and Child Health IRCCS Burlo Garofolo—Trieste, Italy.

Conflicts of Interest: The authors declare no conflict of interest.

References

1. Tchirikov, M.; Strohner, M.; Scholz, A. Cardiac output and blood flow volume redistribution during acute maternal hypoxia in fetal sheep. *J. Perinat. Med.* **2010**, *38*, 387–392. [CrossRef]
2. Flo, K.; Wilsgaard, T.; Acharya, G. Agreement between umbilical vein volume blood flow measurements obtained at the intra-abdominal portion and free loop of the umbilical cord. *Ultrasound Obstet. Gynecol.* **2009**, *34*, 171–176. [CrossRef]
3. Barbera, A.; Galan, H.L.; Ferrazzi, E.; Rigano, S.; Józwik, M.; Battaglia, F.C.; Pardi, G. Relationship of umbilical vein blood flow to growth parameters in the human fetus. *Am. J. Obstet. Gynecol.* **1999**, *181*, 174–179. [CrossRef]
4. Flo, K.; Wilsgaard, T.; Vartun, A.; Acharya, G. A longitudinal study of the relationship between maternal cardiac output measured by impedance cardiography and uterine artery blood flow in the second half of pregnancy. *BJOG* **2010**, *117*, 837–844. [CrossRef]
5. Najafzadeh, A.; Dickinson, J.E. Umbilical venous blood flow and its measurement in the human fetus. *J. Clin. Ultrasound* **2012**, *40*, 502–511. [CrossRef]
6. Ferrazzi, E.; Rigano, S.; Bozzo, M.; Bellotti, M.; Giovannini, N.; Galan, H.; Battaglia, F.C. Umbilical vein blood flow in growth-restricted fetuses. *Ultrasound Obstet. Gynecol.* **2000**, *16*, 432–438. [CrossRef]
7. Rizzo, G.; Mappa, I.; Bitsadze, V.; Słodki, M.; Khizroeva, J.; Makatsariya, A.; D'antonio, F. Role of Doppler ultrasound at time of diagnosis of late-onset fetal growth restriction in predicting adverse perinatal outcome: Prospective cohort study. *Ultrasound Obstet. Gynecol.* **2020**, *55*, 793–798. [CrossRef]
8. Prior, T.; Mullins, E.; Bennett, P.; Kumar, S. Umbilical venous flow rate in term fetuses: Can variations in flow predict intrapartum compromise? *Am. J. Obstet. Gynecol.* **2014**, *210*, 61.e1–61.e8. [CrossRef]
9. Prior, T.; Mullins, E.; Bennett, P.; Kumar, S. Prediction of fetal compromise in labor. *Obstet. Gynecol.* **2014**, *123*, 1263–1271. [CrossRef]
10. Parra-Saavedra, M.; Crovetto, F.; Triunfo, S.; Savchev, S.; Parra, G.; Sanz, M.; Gratacos, E.; Figueras, F. Added value of umbilical vein flow as a predictor of perinatal outcome in term small-for-gestational-age fetuses. *Ultrasound Obstet. Gynecol.* **2013**, *42*, 189–195. [CrossRef]
11. Jouppila, P.; Kirkinen, P. Umbilical vein blood flow as an indicator of fetal hypoxia. *Br. J. Obstet. Gynaecol.* **1984**, *91*, 107–110.
12. Gill, R.W.; Kossoff, G.; Warren, P.S.; Garrett, W.J. Umbilical venous flow in normal and complicated pregnancy. *Ultrasound Med. Biol.* **1984**, *10*, 349–363. [CrossRef]
13. Ferrazzi, E.; Di Martino, D.; Stampalija, T. Doppler interrogation of the umbilical venous flow. In *Maulik and Lees book on Doppler Ultrasound*; Springer: Cham, Switzerland, 2023.
14. Ferrazzi, E.; Di Martino, D.; Stampalija, T. Blood flow volume in umbilical vein in fetal growth restriction. In *Placental-Fetal Growth Restriction*; University of Cambridge: Cambridge, UK, 2018; pp. 155–163.
15. Giles, W.B.; Lingman, G.; Marsal, K.; Trudinger, B.J. Fetal volume blood flow and umbilical artery flow velocity waveform analysis: A comparison. *Br. J. Obstet. Gynaecol.* **1986**, *93*, 461–465. [CrossRef]
16. Van Splunder, I.P.; Huisman, T.W.; Stijnen, T.; Wladimiroff, J.W. Presence of pulsations and reproducibility of waveform recording in the umbilical and left portal vein in normal pregnancies. *Ultrasound Obstet. Gynecol.* **1994**, *4*, 49–53. [CrossRef]
17. Reed, K.L.; Meijboom, E.J.; Sahn, D.J.; Scagnelli, S.A.; Valdes-Cruz, L.M.; Shenker, L. Cardiac Doppler flow velocities in human fetuses. *Circulation* **1986**, *73*, 41–46. [CrossRef]
18. Sutton, M.S.J.; Theard, M.A.; Bhatia, S.J.; Plappert, T.; Saltzman, D.H.; Doubilet, P. Changes in placental blood flow in the normal human fetus with gestational age. *Pediatr. Res.* **1990**, *28*, 383–387. [CrossRef]
19. Figueras, F.; Fernandez, S.; Hernandez-Andrade, E.; Gratacos, E. Umbilical venous blood flow measurement: Accuracy and reproducibility. *Ultrasound Obstet. Gynecol.* **2008**, *32*, 587–591. [CrossRef]
20. PROSPERO. International Prospective Register of Systematic Reviews [Homepage on the Internet]. Available online: https://www.crd.york.ac.uk/prospero/ (accessed on 15 December 2021).
21. Shamseer, L.; Moher, D.; Clarke, M.; Ghersi, D.; Liberati, A.; Petticrew, M.; Shekelle, P.; Stewart, L.A. Preferred reporting items for systematic review and meta-analysis protocols (PRISMA-P) 2015: Elaboration and explanation. *BMJ* **2015**, *350*, g7647. [CrossRef]
22. Whiting, P.F.; Rutjes, A.W.; Westwood, M.E.; Mallett, S.; Deeks, J.J.; Reitsma, J.B.; Leeflang, M.M.; Sterne, J.A.; Bossuyt, P.M. QUADAS-2: A revised tool for the quality assessment of diagnostic accuracy studies. *Ann. Intern. Med.* **2011**, *155*, 529–536. [CrossRef]
23. McGuinness, L.A.; Higgins, J.P.T. Risk-of-bias VISualization (robvis): An R package and Shiny web app for visualizing risk-of-bias assessments. *Res. Synth. Methods* **2021**, *12*, 55–61. [CrossRef]
24. Stampalija, T.; Monasta, L.; Barbieri, M.; Chiodo, A.; Quadrifoglio, M.; Fantasia, I.; Bello, L.L.; Barresi, V.; Ottaviani, C.; Di Martino, D.D.; et al. Late-term fetuses with reduced umbilical vein blood flow volume: An under-recognized population at increased risk of growth restriction. *Eur. J. Obstet. Gynecol. Reprod. Biol.* **2022**, *272*, 182–187. [CrossRef]
25. Salomon, L.J.; Alfirevic, Z.; Da Silva Costa, F.; Deter, R.L.; Figueras, F.; Ghi, T.A.; Glanc, P.; Khalil, A.; Lee, W.; Napolitano, R.; et al. ISUOG Practice Guidelines: Ultrasound assessment of fetal biometry and growth. *Ultrasound Obstet. Gynecol.* **2019**, *53*, 715–723. [CrossRef]
26. Bhide, A.; Acharya, G.; Bilardo, C.M.; Brezinka, C.; Cafici, D.; Hernandez-Andrade, E.; Kalache, K.; Kingdom, J.; Kiserud, T.; Lee, W.; et al. ISUOG practice guidelines: Use of Doppler ultrasonography in obstetrics. *Ultrasound Obstet. Gynecol.* **2013**, *41*, 233–239.

27. Hadlock, F.P.; Harrist, R.B.; Sharman, R.S.; Deter, R.L.; Park, S.K. Estimation of fetal weight with the use of head, body, and femur measurements–a prospective study. *Am. J. Obstet. Gynecol.* **1985**, *151*, 333–337. [CrossRef]
28. DeVore, G.R.; Epstein, A. Computing Z-Score Equations for Clinical Use to Measure Fetal Umbilical Vein Size and Flow Using Six Independent Variables of Age and Size. *J. Ultrasound Med.* **2021**. [CrossRef]
29. Salomon, L.J.; Duyme, M.; Crequat, J.; Brodaty, G.; Talmant, C.; Fries, N.; Althuser, M. French fetal biometry: Reference equations and comparison with other charts. *Ultrasound Obstet. Gynecol.* **2006**, *28*, 193–198. [CrossRef]
30. A Language and Environment for Statistical Computing. Foundation for Statistical Computing, Vienna, Austria. Available online: https://www.R-project.org/ (accessed on 15 December 2021).
31. Widnes, C.; Flo, K.; Wilsgaard, T.; Odibo, A.O.; Acharya, G. Sexual Dimorphism in Umbilical Vein Blood Flow During the Second Half of Pregnancy: A Longitudinal Study. *J. Ultrasound Med.* **2017**, *36*, 2447–2458. [CrossRef]
32. Lees, C.; Albaiges, G.; Deane, C.; Parra, M.; Nicolaides, K.H. Assessment of umbilical arterial and venous flow using color Doppler. *Ultrasound Obstet. Gynecol.* **1999**, *14*, 250–255. [CrossRef]
33. Flo, K.; Wilsgaard, T.; Acharya, G. Longitudinal reference ranges for umbilical vein blood flow at a free loop of the umbilical cord. *Ultrasound Obstet. Gynecol.* **2010**, *36*, 567–572. [CrossRef]
34. Tchirikov, M.; Strohner, M.; Forster, D.; Huneke, B. A combination of umbilical artery PI and normalized blood flow volume in the umbilical vein: Venous-arterial index for the prediction of fetal outcome. *Eur. J. Obstet. Gynecol. Reprod. Biol.* **2009**, *142*, 129–133. [CrossRef]
35. Acharya, G.; Wilsgaard, T.; Rosvold Berntsen, G.K.; Maltau, J.M.; Kiserud, T. Reference ranges for umbilical vein blood flow in the second half of pregnancy based on longitudinal data. *Prenat. Diagn.* **2005**, *25*, 99–111. [CrossRef]
36. Boito, S.M.; Struijk, P.C.; Ursem, N.T.; Stijnen, T.; Wladimiroff, J.W. Assessment of fetal liver volume and umbilical venous volume flow in pregnancies complicated by insulin-dependent diabetes mellitus. *BJOG* **2003**, *110*, 1007–1013. [CrossRef]
37. Boito, S.; Struijk, P.C.; Ursem, N.T.; Stijnen, T.; Wladimiroff, J.W. Umbilical venous volume flow in the normally developing and growth-restricted human fetus. *Ultrasound Obstet. Gynecol.* **2002**, *19*, 344–349. [CrossRef]
38. Tchirikov, M.; Rybakowski, C.; Huneke, B.; Schoder, V.; Schroder, H.J. Umbilical vein blood volume flow rate and umbilical artery pulsatility as 'venous-arterial index' in the prediction of neonatal compromise. *Ultrasound Obstet. Gynecol.* **2002**, *20*, 580–585. [CrossRef]
39. Wang, L.; Zhou, Q.; Zhou, C.; Wang, J.; Shi, C.; Long, B.; Hu, L.; Peng, Y.; Liu, Y.; Xu, G. Response to Comment on "Z-Score Reference Ranges for Umbilical Vein Diameter and Blood Flow Volume in Normal Fetuses". *J. Ultrasound Med.* **2022**, *41*, 2383–2385. [CrossRef]
40. Rizzo, G.; Rizzo, L.; Aiello, E.; Allegra, E.; Arduini, D. Modelling umbilical vein blood flow normograms at 14-40 weeks of gestation by quantile regression analysis. *J. Matern. Fetal Neonatal Med.* **2016**, *29*, 701–706. [CrossRef]
41. Kiserud, T.; Rasmussen, S.; Skulstad, S. Blood flow and the degree of shunting through the ductus venosus in the human fetus. *Am. J. Obstet. Gynecol.* **2000**, *182*, 147–153. [CrossRef]
42. Bellotti, M.; Pennati, G.; De Gasperi, C.; Battaglia, F.C.; Ferrazzi, E. Role of ductus venosus in distribution of umbilical blood flow in human fetuses during second half of pregnancy. *Am. J. Physiol. Heart Circ. Physiol.* **2000**, *279*, H1256–H1263. [CrossRef]
43. Tchirikov, M.; Rybakowski, C.; Huneke, B.; Schroder, H.J. Blood flow through the ductus venosus in singleton and multifetal pregnancies and in fetuses with intrauterine growth retardation. *Am. J. Obstet. Gynecol.* **1998**, *178*, 943–949. [CrossRef]
44. Stampalija, T.; Ghi, T.; Rosolen, V.; Rizzo, G.; Ferrazzi, E.M.; Prefumo, F.; Dall'Asta, A.; Quadrifoglio, M.; Todros, T.; Frusca, T. Current use and performance of the different fetal growth charts in the Italian population. *Eur. J. Obstet. Gynecol. Reprod. Biol.* **2020**, *252*, 323–329. [CrossRef]
45. Wolf, H.; Stampalija, T.; Lees, C.C.; Group, T.S. Fetal cerebral blood-flow redistribution: Analysis of Doppler reference charts and association of different thresholds with adverse perinatal outcome. *Ultrasound Obstet. Gynecol.* **2021**, *58*, 705–715. [CrossRef]
46. Giuliani, F.; Ohuma, E.; Spada, E.; Bertino, E.; Al Dhaheri, A.S.; Altman, D.G.; Conde-Agudelo, A.; Kennedy, S.H.; Villar, J.; Cheikh Ismail, L. Systematic review of the methodological quality of studies designed to create neonatal anthropometric charts. *Acta Paediatr.* **2015**, *104*, 987–996. [CrossRef]
47. Pennati, G.; Bellotti, M.; De Gasperi, C.; Rognoni, G. Spatial velocity profile changes along the cord in normal human fetuses: Can these affect Doppler measurements of venous umbilical blood flow? *Ultrasound Obstet. Gynecol.* **2004**, *23*, 131–137. [CrossRef]
48. Galan, H.L.; Jozwik, M.; Rigano, S.; Regnault, T.R.; Hobbins, J.C.; Battaglia, F.C.; Ferrazzi, E. Umbilical vein blood flow determination in the ovine fetus: Comparison of Doppler ultrasonographic and steady-state diffusion techniques. *Am. J. Obstet. Gynecol.* **1999**, *181*, 1149–1153. [CrossRef]
49. Galan, H.L.; Anthony, R.V.; Rigano, S.; Parker, T.A.; de Vrijer, B.; Ferrazzi, E.; Wilkening, R.B.; Regnault, T.R. Fetal hypertension and abnormal Doppler velocimetry in an ovine model of intrauterine growth restriction. *Am. J. Obstet. Gynecol.* **2005**, *192*, 272–279. [CrossRef]
50. Kiserud, T.; Saito, T.; Ozaki, T.; Rasmussen, S.; Hanson, M.A. Validation of diameter measurements by ultrasound: Intraobserver and interobserver variations assessed in vitro and in fetal sheep. *Ultrasound Obstet. Gynecol.* **1999**, *13*, 52–57. [CrossRef]

Disclaimer/Publisher's Note: The statements, opinions and data contained in all publications are solely those of the individual author(s) and contributor(s) and not of MDPI and/or the editor(s). MDPI and/or the editor(s) disclaim responsibility for any injury to people or property resulting from any ideas, methods, instructions or products referred to in the content.

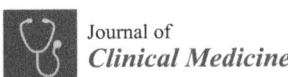

Case Report

Body Stalk Anomaly Complicated by Ectopia Cordis: First-Trimester Diagnosis of Two Cases Using 2- and 3-Dimensional Sonography

Elisa Pappalardo, Ferdinando Antonio Gulino *, Carla Ettore, Francesco Cannone and Giuseppe Ettore

Department of Obstetrics and Gynaecology, Azienda di Rilievo Nazionale e di Alta Specializzazione (ARNAS) Garibaldi Nesima, 95124 Catania, Italy
* Correspondence: docferdi@hotmail.it; Tel.: +39-33-8111-1000

Abstract: Introduction: Body stalk anomaly is a severe defect of the abdominal wall, characterized by the evisceration of abdominal organs and, in more severe cases, thoracic organs as well. The most serious condition in a body stalk anomaly may be complicated by ectopia cordis, an abnormal location of the heart outside the thorax. The aim of this scientific work is to describe our experience with the prenatal diagnosis of ectopia cordis as part of the first-trimester sonographic screening for aneuploidy. Methods: We report two cases of body stalk anomalies complicated by ectopia cordis. The first case was identified during a first ultrasound examination at 9 weeks of gestation. The second was identified during an ultrasound examination at 13 weeks of gestation. Both of these cases were diagnosed using high-quality 2- and 3-dimensional ultrasonographic images obtained by the Realistic Vue and Crystal Vue techniques. The chorionic villus sampling showed that the fetal karyotype and CGH-array were both normal. Results: In our clinical case reports, the patients, immediately after the diagnosis of a body stalk anomaly complicated by ectopia cordis, opted for the termination of pregnancies. Conclusion: Performing an early diagnosis of a body stalk anomaly that is complicated by ectopia cordis is desirable, considering their poor prognoses. Most of the reported cases in the literature suggest that an early diagnosis can be made between 10 and 14 weeks of gestation. A combination of 2- and 3-dimensional sonography could allow an early diagnosis of body stalk anomalies complicated by ectopia cordis, particularly using new ultrasonographic techniques, the Realistic Vue and the Crystal Vue.

Keywords: body stalk anomaly; malformation; ultrasound; ectopia cordis

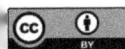

1. Introduction

Body stalk anomaly is a congenital abnormality of the abdominal wall, depending on the evisceration of abdominal organs and, in more complicated clinical cases, thoracic organs. This anomaly is usually characterized also by kyphoscoliosis and by a defect of the umbilical cord, which is usually short or not present [1]. This pathological condition could also be related to neural tube anomalies, genital and urinary abnormalities, chest wall defects, bowel atresia, and craniofacial defects. The most serious condition in a body stalk anomaly may be complicated by ectopia cordis, an abnormal location of the heart outside the thorax. The wide number of phenotypes reported in the scientific literature has allowed the use of different medical terms to define this congenital pathology, such as "amniotic band syndrome" or "short umbilical cord syndrome" [2].

The possible causes of a body stalk anomaly include early amnion rupture with direct mechanical pressure and amniotic bands, vascular disruption of the early embryo, or an abnormality in the germinal disk.

Body stalk anomaly is a rare congenital defect with an incidence rate of 1 in 14,000 to 1 in 31,000 pregnancies, according to large epidemiologic data. In a scientific work published in the last few years, based on the evaluation of 106,727 fetuses between 10 and 14 weeks of gestational age, the rate is approximately 1/7500 pregnancies, considering the elevated incidence of miscarriages related to this condition [3,4].

Although in the scientific literature there are many works on body stalk anomalies with a diagnosis performed in an advanced stage of pregnancy, studies about diagnosis between 10 and 14 weeks of gestational age are still few [5,6]. This study was based on the evaluation of the sonographic characteristics of this infrequent abnormality in the first three months of pregnancy using 2-dimensional (2D) and 3-dimensional (3D) sonography. We present the prenatal diagnosis and management of two cases of body stalk anomaly complicated by ectopia cordis, large abdominal wall defects, limb deformities, kyphoscoliosis, spina bifida, and acrania in the first trimester: the first case at 10 weeks of gestation and the second at 13 weeks of gestation.

The purpose of this scientific work is to describe our clinical experience with the prenatal diagnosis of ectopia cordis in routine sonographic screening performed in the first three months of pregnancy for the risk of chromosomal abnormalities. The description of the case reports was performed following the CARE criteria (https://www.care-statement.org/checklist (accessed on 30 December 2022). The study protocol was approved by the Ethics Committee of the ARNAS Garibaldi Hospital and conformed to the ethical guidelines of the Helsinki Declaration. The women signed informed consent before entering the study, and their anonymity was preserved.

The ultrasonographic images and video were obtained by a Samsung Hera W10 ultrasound, and the high-quality 2D and 3D images were obtained by Realistic Vue and Crystal Vue techniques.

REALISTIC VUE allows a high-resolution 3D visualization of anatomical details with extremely realistic depth perception. The direction of the light source can be selected by the operator, creating graduated shadows that allow better definition of the different anatomical structures.

CRYSTAL VUE is a 3D rendering software that helps locate fetal morphological anomalies through intuitive visualization of internal and external structures. Its diffusion is due to the progress made in terms of the quality of images, technologies, and ease of use. Crystal Vue is one of the most modern volumetric rendering technologies that retains the context and surface information of 3D ultrasound. This new method facilitates differentiation between soft tissue contours and anatomical structures with automatic settings in order to obtain optimal images in complex situations. Crystal Vue also displays the internal and external structures and provides additional information to enable detailed anatomical evaluation and the diagnosis of anomalies. It can also be activated in combination with the color doppler mode.

2. Cases Description

2.1. Case Report 1

A 25-year-old woman was referred for an ultrasound scan at 9 weeks of gestation.

There was no relevant medical history, and she was taking no medication. There were no teratogenic risk factors in the clinical history of the woman. It was her second pregnancy, and her first pregnancy was uneventful. The ultrasound scan showed a normal fetal crown-rump length and a not-normal site of the inferior part of the embryo in the coelomic cavity, and there were multiple fetal abnormalities. The abnormal findings were an anterior thoracoabdominal wall defect containing liver and bowel, ectopia cordis, severe kyphoscoliosis, deformed lower limbs, a spina bifida, and an acrania with exencephaly. All these findings were compatible with the diagnosis of a body stalk anomaly complicated by ectopia cordis. The umbilical cord was also located extra-amniotically but had a normal length.

Realistic Vue and Crystal Vue ultrasonographic techniques allow an early diagnosis of this pathological condition at 9 weeks of gestation, but to confirm this diagnosis, the woman was scheduled for a second ultrasound scan at 11 weeks of gestation (Figure 1). Unfortunately, we do not have any images of the first ultrasound scan, performed at

9 weeks of gestation, but only images of the second ultrasound scan. The ultrasound findings at 11 weeks of gestation confirmed the abnormal aspects evaluated at 9 weeks. The Realistic Vue and Crystal Vue ultrasonographic techniques were extremely useful to achieve this diagnostic objective because they allowed an accurate visualization of internal and external structures of the thoracoabdominal wall.

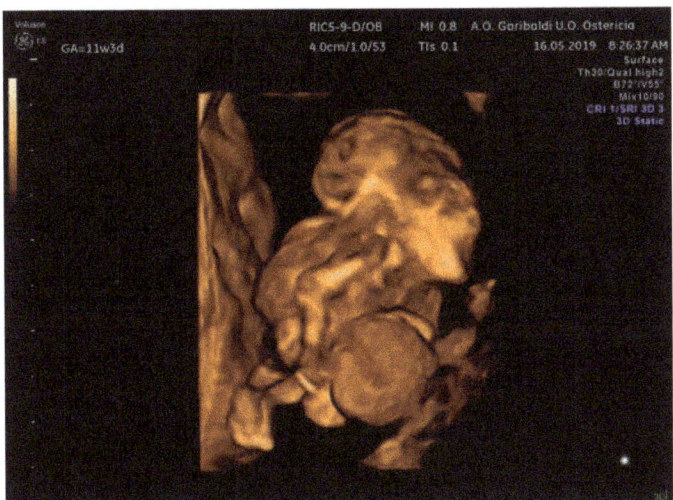

Figure 1. 3D Image of case report 1 at 11 weeks.

Chorionic villus sampling showed that the fetal karyotype and CGH-array were both normal. Considering that this malformation was not compatible with life, the patient decided to plan the termination of her pregnancy.

After the procedure, the embryo and the placenta were sent to the department of pathology, which showed these morphologic characteristics: a non-normal cephalic extremity with acrania and rachischisis, regular upper limbs, no presence of the right leg, the left leg bent toward the chest, and an abnormal omphalocele in which there was the presence of the bowels and liver. The placenta measured 5 × 4 cm. The umbilical cord was positioned anteriorly, characterized by a central insertion and a short length of 2 cm and 0.3 cm diameter, wrapped by amniotic membranes that trapped the fetus. The fetus was affected by a severe malformation and showed the presence of ectopia cordis, with a heart outside the thorax. There was an important anomaly of the anterior and lower thoracic walls and the abdominal wall, with an external presence of the bowel, spleen, and liver (Figure 2).

2.2. Case Report 2

A 43-year-old woman was referred for routine sonographic screening for chromosomic abnormalities at 13 weeks of gestational age. It was her third pregnancy, and her previous pregnancies were uneventful. There was no relevant medical history, and she was taking no other medication.

The ultrasonographic findings by Realistic Vue image (Figures 3 and 4) and Crystal Vue image (Figure 5) at 13 weeks (Supplementary File: Video S1) showed a regular crown-rump length (CRL) of 4 cm and multiple fetal abnormalities. The combination of defects was represented by a large skull and brain defect, an anterior thoracoabdominal wall defect, a heart pulsating outside the thorax, severe kyphoscoliosis and deformed lower limbs, a liver directly attached to the placenta without an interposed umbilical cord, increased distortion of the spine, a separation between the celomatic and amniotic cavities, and a short umbilical cord. All these abnormalities were compatible with the diagnosis of a body stalk anomaly.

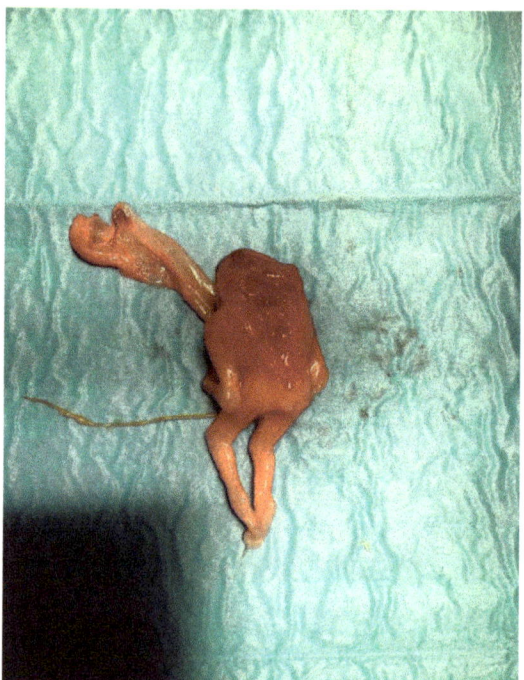

Figure 2. Macroscopic pathological examination of case report 1 at 11 weeks.

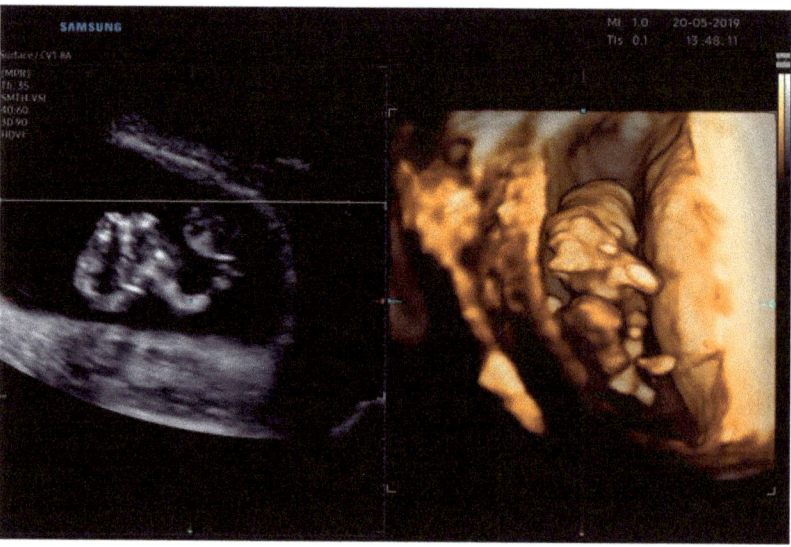

Figure 3. Realistic Vue image of case report 2 at 13 weeks.

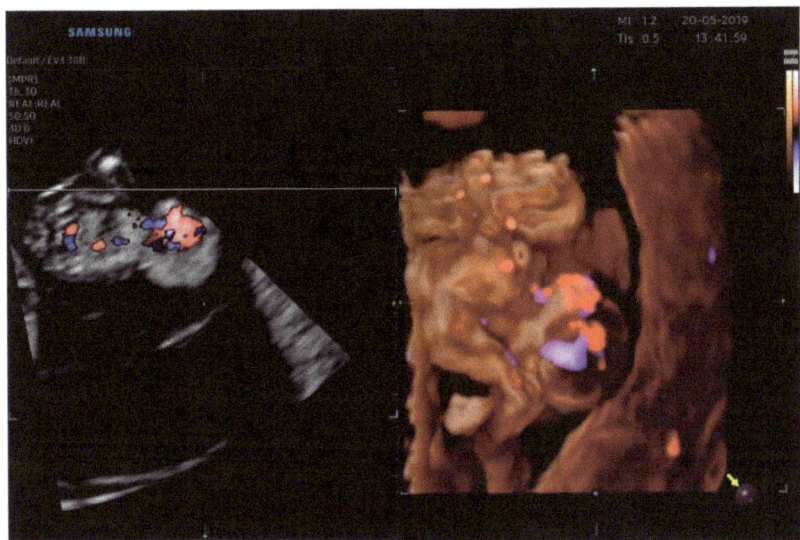

Figure 4. Realistic Vue image of case report 2 at 13 weeks.

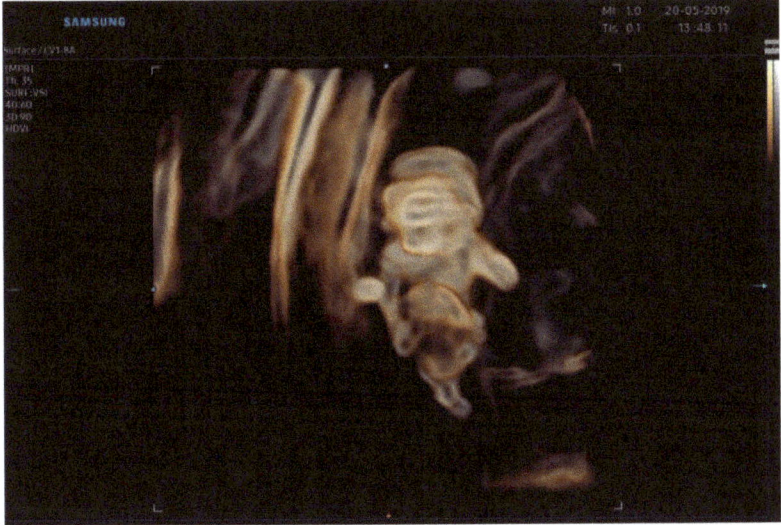

Figure 5. Crystal Vue image of case report 2 at 13 weeks.

The chorionic villus sampling showed that the fetal karyotype and CGH-array were both normal.

Considering that this diagnosis was considered to be incompatible with life, the patient decided to proceed with a termination of pregnancy.

The embryo and the placenta were sent to pathology; the embryo showed exencephaly, severe kyphoscoliosis, increased distortion of the spine, defects of the neural tube, ectopia cordis, and deformed lower and upper limbs (Figure 6).

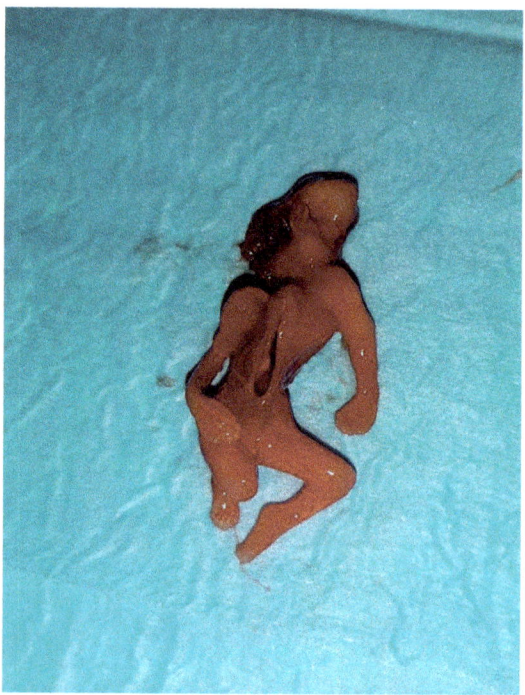

Figure 6. Macroscopic pathological examination of case report 2 at 13 weeks.

3. Discussion

In our scientific work, we described our experience with two cases of prenatal diagnosis of a body stalk anomaly complicated by ectopia cordis during a routine sonographic screening for chromosomic abnormalities in the first trimester. A body stalk anomaly is defined as a pathological congenital condition of multiple abnormalities, which are, in most of the reported scientific cases, not compatible with life. As described above, this condition should be suspected when a large abdominal defect is observed and is associated with other abnormalities in the axial skeleton, such as kyphosis or scoliosis, or a short or absent umbilical cord. Body stalk defects could be detected by ultrasound at the end of the first trimester of pregnancy.

This congenital syndrome has an incidence rate of 1/14,000 to 1/31,000 pregnancies. In a recent multicenter scientific study performed by Daskalakis et al. [3] there was a rate of 1/7500 pregnancies. This big difference in the incidence rates could be related to the high rate of miscarriages associated with body stalk anomalies, which could not allow a diagnosis during the first trimester of pregnancy; therefore, the exact incidence rate might be underestimated [6–12].

Van Allen et al. described this syndrome for the first time in 1987 [1], and they mentioned three essential features:

- Exencephaly, or facial clefts, or encephalocele;
- Thoraco or abdominoschisis;
- Limb defects.

In the study of Van Allen et al. "body stalk anomaly" is defined as a defect of embryonic blood flow in the first phases of embryonic development, between 4 and 6 gestational weeks. This condition determines a defect in the ventral wall's closure and maintains the coelomic cavity's persistence. The clinical evaluation that found cocaine abuse could raise the risk of a body stalk anomaly confirms this etiopathogenetic theory of vascular impairment [13]. Furthermore, another study proposed as an etiopathogenetic defect an early failure of fetal folding along the cephalic, lateral, and caudal axes [4]. In the scientific literature, body stalk anomaly is represented as two distinct phenotypes: the "placenta-cranial" phenotype, where cranial abnormalities and cranio-placental attachment are the main signs, and the "placenta-abdominal" phenotype, where the lower part of the fetus is sited within the not-obliterated extraembryonic cavity [14]. Our case reports describe placenta-abdominal phenotypes.

The actual mechanism, however, remains unclear. In most of the described cases, the karyotypes of the affected fetuses have been completely normal, and only in two cases have there been chromosomal abnormalities associated with uniparental disomy of chromosome 16 and with a trisomy of chromosome 2 [15]. This is probably due to confined placental mosaicism. Hence, what is known about the defects of the body stalk is that environmental and genetic factors play an important role in the pathophysiology of this complex and poorly understood condition.

In a review of 11 cases of body stalk anomaly by Smrcek et al. [4], four cases (36%) were complicated by ectopia cordis. On the other hand, two (50%) of four cases of ectopia cordis were associated with a body stalk anomaly, as was seen in a review by Sepulveda et al. [5]. Ectopia cordis is another pathological congenital condition with a complete or partial shift of the heart outside the thorax. The etiopathology of ectopia cordis is represented by a stop in the heart's infolding, which normally occurs after four weeks of pregnancy [14]. Ectopia cordis is subdivided into four types following the site of the heart [14]:

- Cervical (3% of cases);
- Thoracic (60% of cases);
- Thoracoabdominal (7% of cases);
- Abdominal (30% of cases).

The outcome of this condition is unfavorable due to intracardiac and extracardiac structural anomalies. Although usually the diagnosis is easy and clear and could be made at 10 weeks of gestational age, cases of thoraco-abdominal ectopia cordis could be difficult to diagnose if only the apex of the heart is extra-thoracic, and visualization is hindered by extruded abdominal organs [16–20].

Considering the increasing quality of first trimester ultrasonographic evaluation as a screening tool for aneuploidy in current clinical practice, it is reasonable to expect that most cases of ectopia cordis will be diagnosed at an early gestational age. For this reason, several cases describing the diagnosis before 14 weeks of gestational age have been reported in the scientific literature, but most of them are only isolated case reports [21–25].

An appropriate ultrasound scan of the first trimester with the right measurement of the crown-rump length should make a diagnosis of all cases of body stalk anomaly between 11 and 13 weeks of pregnancy [22]. A final diagnosis should exclude the following differential congenital pathological conditions: omphalocele, gastroschisis, vesical exstrophy, Cantrell pentalogy, amniotic band syndrome, Beckwith-Wiedemann syndrome, and the OEIS complex.

In our scientific work, we did not find any signs that could be related to environmental exposure to teratogens. However, in some case series described in scientific literature, it has been demonstrated that 50% of pregnant women with a fetal diagnosis of a body stalk anomaly smoke cigarettes or drink alcohol, and 30% of them smoke marijuana [24]. In our clinical cases, we also found that the fetal karyotype and CGH-18 array were both normal; these findings confirmed that the pathogenetic basis of these syndromes is not genetically based but rather a disruption.

The advantages of 3D ultrasound are its multiplanar and surface-rendering modalities. The multiplanar view helps the sonographer better correlate the anomaly in the three orthogonal planes simultaneously, providing more details. Then, the surface mode could provide a "sculpture-like" picture that could be rotated in all directions, allowing inspection from different angles. In this study, 2D ultrasound combined with 3D ultrasound showed more detailed features than 2D ultrasound alone.

The strength of our work is the description of two rare cases of body stalk anomaly complicated by ectopia cordis using new ultrasonographic techniques, the REALISTIC VUE and the CRYSTAL VUE, which could allow diagnosis of these malformations in an early stage of pregnancy with high accuracy. The knowledge of body stalk anomaly aetiology may guide the sonographer to carry out a diagnosis at an early stage and to eventually prevent a recurrence.

The main limitation of our work is related to the descriptions of only two case reports; in the scientific literature, the main limitation of this pathological condition is represented by the heterogeneity of the description of its features, based mainly on the report of single case reports. Further research on this topic is needed.

4. Conclusions

Body stalk anomaly is a congenital pathological condition with uncertain etiopathogenesis, uncertain pathophysiology, and an uncertain incidence rate. In the scientific literature, most of the reported clinical cases described an early diagnosis performed between 10 and 14 weeks of gestation; in our first case report, the diagnosis of a body stalk anomaly complicated by ectopia cordis was suspected earlier, at nine weeks of pregnancy, thanks to the use of 2- and 3-dimensional Sonography, particularly by new ultrasonographic techniques, the Realistic Vue and the Crystal Vue. This could represent an important turning point in the diagnosis of this pathological congenital syndrome because it could allow knowing the fetus's condition early and giving appropriate counseling to the parents and prompt management to the physicians.

Supplementary Materials: The following supporting information can be downloaded at: https://www.mdpi.com/article/10.3390/jcm12051896/s1, Video S1. (Body stalk anomaly by Crystal Vue sonographic imaging).

Author Contributions: E.P.: project development; C.E.: data collection; F.A.G.: manuscript writing/editing; F.C.: data analysis; G.E.: coordinator of the study. All authors have read and agreed to the published version of the manuscript.

Funding: This research received no external funding.

Institutional Review Board Statement: The study was conducted in accordance with the Declaration of Helsinki, and approved by the Institutional Review Board (or Ethics Committee) of Azienda di Rilievo Nazionale e di Alta Specializzazione (ARNAS) Garibaldi, Catania (N° Prot. 263/C.E approved on 21 December 2021) (Report n° 68/2021/CECT2).

Informed Consent Statement: Informed consent was obtained from all subjects involved in the study.

Data Availability Statement: Data is contained within the article.

Acknowledgments: The authors acknowledge the mentorship provided by Giuseppe Ettore, Department of Obstetrics and Gynecology, Azienda di Rilievo Nazionale e di Alta Specializzazione (ARNAS) Garibaldi, Catania, Italy, throughout the preparation of this manuscript.

Conflicts of Interest: The authors declare that they have no conflict of interest.

References

1. Van Allen, M.I.; Curry, C.; Gallagher, L. Limb-body wall complex, I: Pathogenesis. *Am. J. Med. Genet.* **1987**, *28*, 529–548. [CrossRef] [PubMed]
2. Van Allen, M.I.; Curry, C.; Walden, C.E.; Gallagher, L.; Patten, R.M. Limb-body wall complex, II: Limb and spine defects. *Am. J. Med. Genet.* **1987**, *28*, 549–565. [CrossRef] [PubMed]
3. Daskalakis, G.; Sebire, N.J.; Jurkovic, D.; Snijders, R.J.M.; Nicolaides, K.H. Body stalk anomaly at 10–14 weeks' gestation. *Ultrasound Obstet. Gynecol.* **1997**, *10*, 416–418. [CrossRef]
4. Smrcek, J.M.; Germer, U.; Krokowski, M.; Berg, C.; Krapp, M.; Geipel, A.; Gembruch, U. Prenatal ultrasound diagnosis and management of body stalk anomaly: Analysis of nine singleton and two multiple pregnancies. *Ultrasound Obstet. Gynecol.* **2003**, *21*, 322–328. [CrossRef]
5. Sepulveda, W.; Wong, A.E.; Simonetti, L.; Gomez, E.; Dezerega, V.; Gutierrez, J. Ectopia cordis in a first-trimester sonographic screening program for aneuploidy. *J. Ultrasound Med.* **2013**, *32*, 865–871. [CrossRef]

6. Murphy, A.; Platt, L.D. First-trimester diagnosis of body stalk anomaly using 2- and 3-dimensional sonography. *J. Ultrasound Med.* **2011**, *30*, 1739–1743. [CrossRef] [PubMed]
7. Singh, A.; Singh, J.; Gupta, K. Body stalk anomaly: Antenatal sonographic diagnosis of this rare entity with review of literature. *J. Ultrason.* **2017**, *17*, 133–135. [CrossRef]
8. Shibata, Y.; Terada, K.; Igarashi, M.; Suzuki, S. Body stalk anomaly complicated by ectopia cordis in the first trimester. *J. Clin. Diagn. Res.* **2014**, *8*, OD06–OD07.
9. Tsirka, A.; Korkontzelos, I.; Diamantopoulos, P.; Tsirkas, P.; Stefos, T. Prenatal diagnosis of body stalk anomaly in the first trimester of pregnancy. *J. Matern. Fetal Neonatal Med.* **2007**, *20*, 183–184. [CrossRef]
10. Takeuchi, K.; Fujita, I.; Nakajima, K.; Kitagaki, S.; Koketsu, I. Body stalk anomaly: Prenatal diagnosis. *Int. J. Gynaecol. Obstet.* **1995**, *51*, 49–52. [CrossRef] [PubMed]
11. Morrow, R.J.; Whittle, M.J.; McNay, M.B.; Raine, P.A.; Gibson, A.A.; Crossley, J. Prenatal diagnosis and management of anterior abdominal wall defects in the west of Scotland. *Prenat. Diagn.* **1993**, *13*, 111–115. [CrossRef] [PubMed]
12. Routhu, M.; Thakkallapelli, S.; Mohan, P.; Ahmed, N. Role of Ultrasound in Body Stalk Anomaly and Amniotic Band Syndrome. *Int. J. Reprod. Med.* **2016**, *2016*, 3974139. [CrossRef]
13. Viscarello, R.R.; Ferguson, D.D.; Nores, J.; Hobbins, J.C. Limb-body wall complex associated with cocaine abuse: Further evidence of cocaine's teratogenicity. *Obstet. Gynecol.* **1992**, *80*, 523–526. [PubMed]
14. Bianchi, D.; Crombleholme, T.; D'Alton, M. Body stalk anomaly. In *Fetology: Diagnosis and Management of the Fetal Patient*; McGraw-Hill: New York, NY, USA, 2000; pp. 453–456.
15. Chan, Y.; Silverman, N.; Jackson, L.; Wapner, R.; Wallerstein, R. Maternal uniparental disomy of chromosome 16 and body stalk anomaly. *Am. J. Med. Genet.* **2000**, *94*, 284–286. [CrossRef] [PubMed]
16. Quijano, F.E.; Rey, M.M.; Echeverry, M.; Axt-Fliedner, R. Body stalk anomaly in a 9-week pregnancy. *Case Rep. Obstet. Gynecol.* **2014**, *2014*, 357285. [CrossRef]
17. Costa, M.L.; Couto, E.; Furlan, E.; Zaccaria, R.; Andrade, K.; Barini, R.; Nomura, M.L. Body stalk anomaly: Adverse maternal outcomes in a series of 21 cases. *Prenat. Diagn.* **2012**, *32*, 264–267. [CrossRef]
18. Bianchi, D.W.; Crombleholme, T.M.; D'Alton, M.E.; Malone, F.D. (Eds.) Ectopia cordis. In *Fetology: Diagnosis and Management of the Fetal Patient*; McGraw-Hill: New York, NY, USA, 2010; pp. 411–415.
19. Amato, J.J.; Douglas, W.I.; Desai, U.; Burke, S. Ectopia cordis. *Chest Surg. Clin. N. Am.* **2000**, *10*, 297–316.
20. Liang, R.I.; Huang, S.E.; Chang, F.M. Prenatal diagnosis of ectopia cordis at 10 weeks of gestation using two-dimensional and three-dimensional ultra-sonography. *Ultrasound Obstet. Gynecol.* **1997**, *10*, 137–139. [CrossRef]
21. Sadler, T.W. The embryologic origin of ventral body wall defects. *Semin. Pediatr. Surg.* **2010**, *19*, 209–214. [CrossRef]
22. Syngelaki, A.; Chelemen, T.; Dagklis, T.; Allan, L.; Nicolaides, K.H. Challenges in the diagnosis of fetal non-chromosomal abnormalities at 11-13 weeks. *Prenat. Diagn.* **2011**, *31*, 90–102. [CrossRef]
23. Kähler, C.; Humbsch, K.; Schneider, U.; Seewald, H.J. A case report of body stalk anomaly complicating a twin pregnancy. *Arch. Gynecol. Obstet.* **2003**, *268*, 245–247. [CrossRef] [PubMed]
24. Luehr, B.; Lipsett, J.; Quinlivan, J.A. Limb-body wall complex: A case series. *J. Matern. Fetal Neonatal Med.* **2002**, *12*, 132–137. [PubMed]
25. Daskalakis, G.J.; Nicolaides, K.H. Monozygotic twins discordant for body stalk anomaly. *Ultrasound Obstet. Gynecol.* **2002**, *20*, 79–81. [CrossRef] [PubMed]

Disclaimer/Publisher's Note: The statements, opinions and data contained in all publications are solely those of the individual author(s) and contributor(s) and not of MDPI and/or the editor(s). MDPI and/or the editor(s) disclaim responsibility for any injury to people or property resulting from any ideas, methods, instructions or products referred to in the content.

MDPI
St. Alban-Anlage 66
4052 Basel
Switzerland
www.mdpi.com

Journal of Clinical Medicine Editorial Office
E-mail: jcm@mdpi.com
www.mdpi.com/journal/jcm

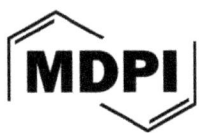

Disclaimer/Publisher's Note: The statements, opinions and data contained in all publications are solely those of the individual author(s) and contributor(s) and not of MDPI and/or the editor(s). MDPI and/or the editor(s) disclaim responsibility for any injury to people or property resulting from any ideas, methods, instructions or products referred to in the content.

www.ingramcontent.com/pod-product-compliance
Lightning Source LLC
LaVergne TN
LVHW070711100526
838202LV00013B/1068